Current Review of Chinese MEDICINE

Quality Control of Herbs and Herbal Material

Annals of Traditional Chinese Medicine – Vol. 2

Current Review of Chinese Medicine

Quality Control of Herbs and Herbal Material

Chief Editor

Ping-Chung Leung

The Chinese University of Hong Kong

Editors

Harry Fong

University of Illinois at Chicago, USA

Charlie Changli Xue

RMIT University, Australia

World Scientific

NEW JERSEY • LONDON • SINGAPORE • BEIJING • SHANGHAI • HONG KONG • TAIPEI • CHENNAI

Published by

World Scientific Publishing Co. Pte. Ltd.
5 Toh Tuck Link, Singapore 596224
USA office: 27 Warren Street, Suite 401-402, Hackensack, NJ 07601
UK office: 57 Shelton Street, Covent Garden, London WC2H 9HE

British Library Cataloguing-in-Publication Data
A catalogue record for this book is available from the British Library.

Annals of Traditional Chinese Medicine — Vol. 2
CURRENT REVIEW OF CHINESE MEDICINE
Quality Control of Herbs and Herbal Material

ISBN 981-256-707-0

Printed in Singapore by World Scientific Printers (S) Pte Ltd

Contents

Contributors

Jue Bai
Anatomy Department
Shanghai University of Traditional Chinese Medicine
Shanghai, China

Suzanne Banuvar
UIC/NIH Center for Botanical Dietary Supplements Research
Northwestern University Feinberg School of Medicine
Chicago, USA

Judy L. Bolton
Program for Collaborative Research in the Pharmaceutical Sciences
UIC/NIH Center for Botanical Dietary Supplements Research
Department of Medicinal Chemistry and Pharmacognosy
College of Pharmacy, University of Illinois at Chicago
Chicago, USA

Barrie R. Cassileth
Integrative Medicine Service
Memorial Sloan-Kettering Cancer Center
New York, USA

King-Fai Cheng
Institute of Chinese Medicine
The Chinese University of Hong Kong
Hong Kong, China

Gary Deng
Integrative Medicine Service
Memorial Sloan-Kettering Cancer Center
New York, USA

Norman R. Farnsworth
Program for Collaborative Research in the Pharmaceutical Sciences
UIC/NIH Center for Botanical Dietary Supplements Research
Department of Medicinal Chemistry and Pharmacognosy
WHO Collaborating Center for Traditional Medicine
College of Pharmacy, University of Illinois at Chicago
Chicago, USA

Harry H.-S. Fong
Program for Collaborative Research in the Pharmaceutical Sciences
UIC/NIH Center for Botanical Dietary Supplements Research
Department of Medicinal Chemistry and Pharmacognosy
WHO Collaborating Center for Traditional Medicine
College of Pharmacy, University of Illinois at Chicago
Chicago, USA

Kwok-Pui Fung
Institute of Chinese Medicine
The Chinese University of Hong Kong
Hong Kong, China

Stacie E. Geller
UIC/NIH Center for Botanical Dietary Supplements Research
Department of Obstetrics and Gynecology
College of Medicine, University of Illinois at Chicago
Chicago, USA

Baolin Guo
Institute of Medicinal Plant Development
Chinese Academy of Medical Sciences and Peking Union Medical College
Beijing, China

Guozhu Han
Department of Pharmacology
Dalian Medical University
Dalian, China

Yan Hong
Temasek Life Sciences Laboratory
National University of Singapore

Osamu Iida
Research Center for Medicinal Plant Resources
National Institute of Biomedical Innovation
Ibaraki, Japan

Hwee-Ling Koh
Department of Pharmacy, Faculty of Science
National University of Singapore

Aik-Jiang Lau
Department of Pharmacy, Faculty of Science
National University of Singapore

Mavis Y.-H. Lee
Institute of Chinese Medicine
The Chinese University of Hong Kong
Hong Kong, China

Ping-Chung Leung
Institute of Chinese Medicine
The Chinese University of Hong Kong
Hong Kong, China

Chun-Guang Li
The RMIT Chinese Medicine Research Group
Division of Chinese Medicine, School of Health Sciences
World Health Organization Collaborating Center for Traditional Medicine
RMIT University
Victoria, Australia

Lan Ling
Department of Endocrinology
Quang An Men Hospital
Traditional Chinese Medicine Research Institute of China
Beijing, China

Changxiao Liu
Tianjin State Key Laboratory of Pharmacokinetics and Pharmacodynamics
Tianjin Institute of Pharmaceutical Research
Tianjin, China

Shen-Biao Luo
Zhijiang Academy of Traditional Chinese Medicine
Hangzhou, China

Qing Ni
Department of Endocrinology
Quang An Men Hospital
Traditional Chinese Medicine Research Institute of China
Beijing, China

E. Pang
The RMIT Chinese Medicine Research Group
Division of Chinese Medicine, School of Health Sciences
World Health Organization Collaborating Center for Traditional Medicine
RMIT University
Victoria, Australia

Guido F. Pauli
Program for Collaborative Research in the Pharmaceutical Sciences
UIC/NIH Center for Botanical Dietary Supplements Research
Department of Medicinal Chemistry and Pharmacognosy
College of Pharmacy, University of Illinois at Chicago
Chicago, USA

Lee Schulman
UIC/NIH Center for Botanical Dietary Supplements Research
Northwestern University Feinberg School of Medicine
Chicago, USA

Baishui Shao
Anatomy Department
Shanghai University of Traditional Chinese Medicine
Shanghai, China

Han-Chen Shen
Zhijiang Academy of Traditional Chinese Medicine
Hangzhou, China

S.-J. Sheng
The RMIT Chinese Medicine Research Group
Division of Chinese Medicine, School of Health Sciences
World Health Organization Collaborating Center for Traditional Medicine
RMIT University
Victoria, Australia

David F. Story
The RMIT Chinese Medicine Research Group
Division of Chinese Medicine, School of Health Sciences
World Health Organization Collaborating Center for Traditional Medicine
RMIT University
Victoria, Australia

Suqin Sun
Department of Chemistry
Tsinghua University
Beijing, China

Richard B. van Breemen
Program for Collaborative Research in the Pharmaceutical Sciences
UIC/NIH Center for Botanical Dietary Supplements Research
Department of Medicinal Chemistry and Pharmacognosy
College of Pharmacy, University of Illinois at Chicago
Chicago, USA

Andrew Vickers
Integrative Medicine Service
Memorial Sloan-Kettering Cancer Center
New York, USA

Peishan Xie
Guangzhou Institute for Drug Control
Guangdong, China

Charlie Chang-Li Xue
The RMIT Chinese Medicine Research Group
Division of Chinese Medicine, School of Health Sciences
World Health Organization Collaborating Center for Traditional Medicine
RMIT University
Victoria, Australia

Zhengguo Yan
Anatomy Department
Shanghai University of Traditional Chinese Medicine
Shanghai, China

Zhijun Yang
School of Chinese Medicine
Hong Kong Baptist University
Hong Kong, China

K. Simon Yeung
Integrative Medicine Service
Memorial Sloan-Kettering Cancer Center
New York, USA

Jianhua Zhang
Anatomy Department
Shanghai University of Traditional Chinese Medicine
Shanghai, China

Zhongzhen Zhao
School of Chinese Medicine
Hong Kong Baptist University
Hong Kong, China

Xian-Ru Zhu
Zhijiang Academy of Traditional Chinese Medicine
Hangzhou, China

Preface to Series

Does Traditional Chinese Medicine Work?

History should be acknowledged and respected. Despite this, the historical value of Chinese medicine in China and some parts of Asia should not be used as the only important evidence of efficacy.

While clinical science has followed closely the principles of deductive research in science and developed its methodology of wide acceptance, there is a natural demand from both users and service providers that the same methodology be applied to the traditional art of healing. There should be only one scale for the measurement of efficacy. Thus, evidence-based medicine, which apparently is the only acceptable form of treatment, would also claim its sovereignty in Chinese medicine.

In spite of influential proponents and diligent practitioners, efforts relating to the application of evidence-based medicine methodology to Chinese medicine research have been slow and unimpressive. This should not come as a surprise. Evidence-based medicine requires the knowledge of the exact chemistry of the drug used, the exact physical or chemical activities involved and above all, the biological responses in the recipient. All these are not known. Working back from the black box of old historical records of efficacy requires huge resources and time, if at all possible. Insistence on this approach would result in either unending frustrations or utter desperation.

Parallel with the modern attempts, respectable Chinese medicine practitioners have unendingly and relentlessly cried out their objection to the evidence-based approach. They insisted that all the evidences were already there from the Classical Records. Forcing the classical applications through a rigid modern framework of scrutiny is artificially coating Chinese medicine with a scientific clothing that does not fit.

Thus, the modern proponents are facing an impasse when they rely totally on modern scientific concepts. The traditional converts are persisting to push their pilgrims of defense. Where do we stand so as to achieve the best results of harmonisation?

There must be a compromise somewhere. Classic evidences can be transformed into a universal language to be fairly evaluated and to be decided whether suitable for further research, using the deductive methodology or an innovative one after intelligent modifications.

There is a need for a platform on which a direction can be developed in the attempt to modernise the traditional art and science of healing, while remaining free and objective to utilise the decaying wisdom without prejudice.

With the growing demand for complementary/alternative medicine from the global public and a parallel interest from the service providers, there is an urgent need for the provision of valuable information in this area.

The Annals of Chinese Medicine is a timely serial publication responding to this need. It will be providing authoritative and current information about Chinese medicine in the areas of clinical trials, biological activities of herbs, education, research and quality control requirements. Contributors are invited to send in their reports and reviews to ensure quality and value. Clinicians and scientists who are willing to submit their valuable observations, resulting from their painstaking researches are welcome to send in their manuscripts. *The Annals of Chinese Medicine* has the objective of providing a lasting platform for all who concentrate their efforts on the modernization of Chinese medicine.

Professor Ping-chung Leung
Institute of Chinese Medicine
The Chinese University of Hong Kong

Chapter 1

The Basic Requirement for Modernisation of Chinese Herbal Medicine

Peishan Xie

Abstract

Authentication and consistent quality are the basic requirements for TCHM and its commercial products, regardless of the kind of research conducted to modernise the TCM. The complexities of TCHM challenge the current official quality control mode, for which only a few markers were selected for identification and quantitative assay. Referring to too many unknown factors existed in TCHM, it is impossible and unnecessary to pinpoint qualitatively and quantitatively every single component contained in the herbal drug. Chromatographic fingerprinting is a rational option to meet the need for more effective and powerful quality assessment to TCHM. The optimised chromatographic fingerprint is not only an alternative analytical tool for identification, but also an approach to express the various pattern of chemical ingredients distribution in the herbal drugs and preserve such "database" for further multi-faceted sustainable studies. Some examples demonstrated the role of fingerprinting in quality control and assessment.

Keywords: Chromatographic Fingerprint; Sustainable Quality Assessment Mode.

The paradigms of traditional Chinese herbal medicine (TCHM) are featured as holistic system; the common clinical use of Chinese medicines requires the complex recipes and formulae derived from historical and anecdotal evidence of Chinese medicinal practitioners. Based on ancient Chinese philosophy, a typical therapeutic formula is symbolised as an active "cabinet" consisted of "Monarch" drug, "ministers" drug, "assistants" drug and "messengers" or "servants" drug, which work together harmoniously and serve various functions respectively to adjust, balance, and restore the body's function guided by Chinese ancient philosophy and culture. Consequently, no single active constituent is responsible for the overall efficacy of the whole formula, even single herbal drugs, which usually contain numerous chemical compounds with holistic efficacy rather than a single active compound. It is definitely different from the Western single chemical drug, and is also distinguished from Western herbal/botanical medicine because TCHM is the carriers loading the information of the philosophy and culture of traditional Chinese medicine. Hence, we should keep in mind it will be nothing different from Western herbal drugs once the TCM information is unloaded from TCHM matrices. On the new wave of modernisation of TCM under the economic globalisation environment, there is a trend towards the seeking of TCHM as a source for discovery of new chemical drugs without considering the synergic effect of all of the ingredients in the herbal drugs. That means such an approach is mostly concerned with only the interested single target and ignores the total quality of the herbal drug itself. The consequence would lead to a loss of ancestors' wisdom (the culture and philosophy of TCM and exclusive clinical experiences) accumulated through generations. Referring to the complexity and difficulty in merging ancient Chinese culture and modern Western science, the first step in the process of TCM modernisation, we should preserve the total information loaded in the TCHM as much as possible in order to avoid any rash affirmation on the pros and cons of TCM without discreet study. From the viewpoint of chemistry and biology, the total chemical ingredients pattern in every entity of TCHM should be preferably expressed in the appropriate chromatograms — chromatographic fingerprint consisted of detectable ingredients. The optimised fingerprints can serve as "chemical signatures" of the TCHM for consecutive multi-faceted research. The following examples illustrate the role of chromatographic fingerprints in TCHM.

1.1 Authentication of the Species Prone to Confusion

Ginseng (root of *Panax ginseng*) and American ginseng (root of *Panax quinqueefolium*) are two close species containing very similar chemical

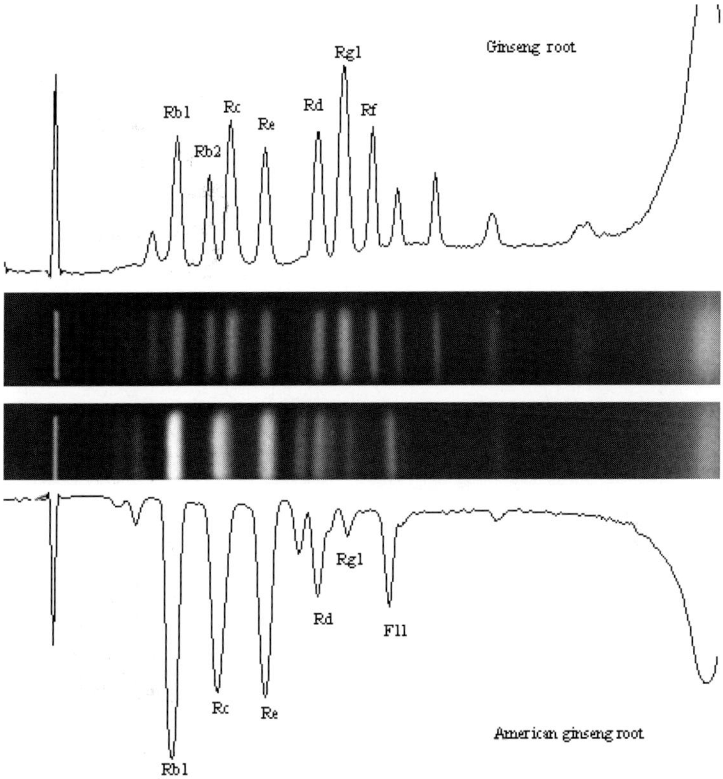

Fig. 1.1. HPTLC fingerprints of Ginseng and American ginseng.

ingredients. The functions of the two species are different according to TCM in clinical use. It is difficult to distinguish them by only selecting single ginsenosides, but the HPTLC images with digital scanning profiles as a whole can easily differentiate between them (Xie, 2005a) (Fig. 1.1).

1.2 Quality Evaluation of the Crude Drugs

There are two species of *Ge Gen* (Kudzu root) in Chinese Pharmacopoeia — *Ye Ge* (*Radix Pueraria lobatae*) and *Gan Ge* (*Radix P. thomsonii*), which were used as the same herbal drug for a long time (Xiao, 2002). But the content determination of main isoflavonoid, Puerarin and HPTLC fingerprint analysis showed the great disparity of the content of puerarin, and the total chemical pattern expressed by the fingerprint revealed that the puerarin content and the chemical components concentration distribution in the *Gan Ge* fingerprint was eight to 15 times lower than that of *Ye Ge* (Figs. 1.2 and 1.3), thus, it is impossible that both species are bio-equivalent. Hence, *Ye Ge* should be the appropriate candidate for *Ge Gen* (Kudzu root) in the prescription by TCM practitioners.

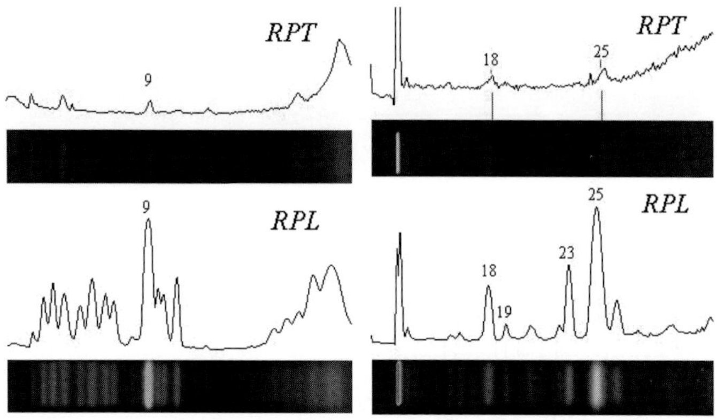

Fig. 1.2. HPTLC fingerprints of *Ye Ge* (root of *Puerariae lobatae*) and *Gan Ge* (root of *Puerarae thomsonii*). Left: Isoflavonoides, Right: Aglycones, PRL: Root of *Pueraria lobata*, PRT: Root of *Pueraria thomsonii*.

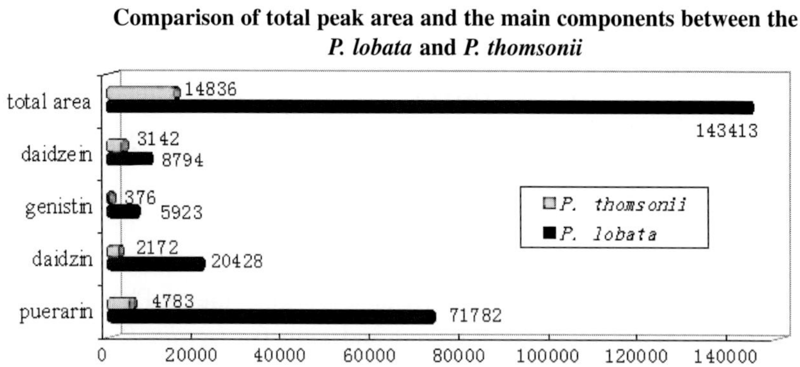

Fig. 1.3. Comparison of the discrepancy of total peak area and the main components between *Ye Ge* (black bar) and *Gan Ge* (grey bar).

1.3 Distinguishing the Adulterant from the Authentic Sample

The general practice of quality assessment of extracts of *Ginkgo biloba* leaves (EGb) is the determination of 24% of the total flavonoides and 6% of total terpene lactones without the provision of other detailed quality information. The HPLC fingerprint of total flavonoides disclosed the

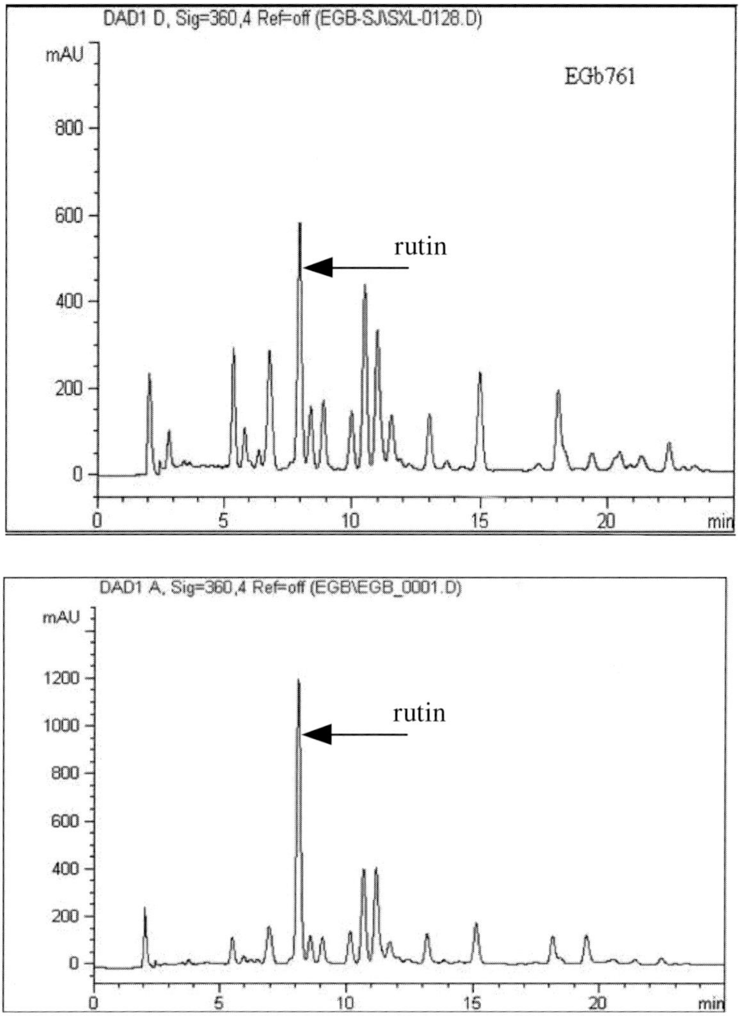

Fig. 1.4. HPLC fingerprint of the extracts of Ginkgo leaves (EGb). Upper: Standardised EGb fingerprint, Lower: A commercial EGb product fingerprint.

distribution pattern with the detectable peaks intensities and peak-to-peak ratio, which expresses the inherent quality. Any significant change in the pattern appearance will hint at the quality fluctuation of the products. For example, in a quality survey of commercial products in the market by means of comparative study of the HPLC fingerprinting, three batches of commercial extracts of *Ginkgo biloba* leaves (EGb) revealed that the rutin peak, which unexpectedly predominated in the fingerprints of those commercial products in comparison to that of standardised EGb (Fig. 1.4), is likely to be adulterated with the inexpensive flavonoid rutin to artificially increase the total flavonoids content (Qian and Xie, 2005). It would however not be evident if the adulterated ginkgo extracts had only been analysed by quantitation of total flavonoides by conventional HPLC assay.

1.4 Monitoring Rationality of Dosage Forms During R&D Period

Renewal of dosage forms of TCHM industrial products from an aged one to the modernised form, from conventional pill to tablets for example, is a trend in current modernisation of TCM industries. But it does not assure that the renewed dosage forms with modified extraction process will be successful without any analytical evidence. A typical example of fingerprint disclosed the outcome of a compound formula TCHM product BJW. It was clearly demonstrated that the chemical components of the said formula in the fingerprint were diminished more and more from pill to concentrated pill, to tablets, and finally to oral liquid (Fig. 1.5). We can say that such "innovation" of dosage forms with claimed renewed process techniques was obviously a failure in comparison to the HPLC fingerprint of the original dosage form, the pills (Fig. 1.5, top). It is noteworthy that although only part of chemical structures were elucidated currently in the chromatogram, the quality information was also able to be provided specifically with the total chemical pattern (peaks concentration distribution and peak-to-peak ratio) for comparative study between the different dosage forms. This example also demonstrated that chromatographic fingerprint is a sustainable quality assessment approach; it can be started from "black box" of fingerprint as a wholeness without reference substance being available at the beginning gradually to "grey box" and finally to a "clear box", where step-by-step detailed phytochemical studies are exploited.

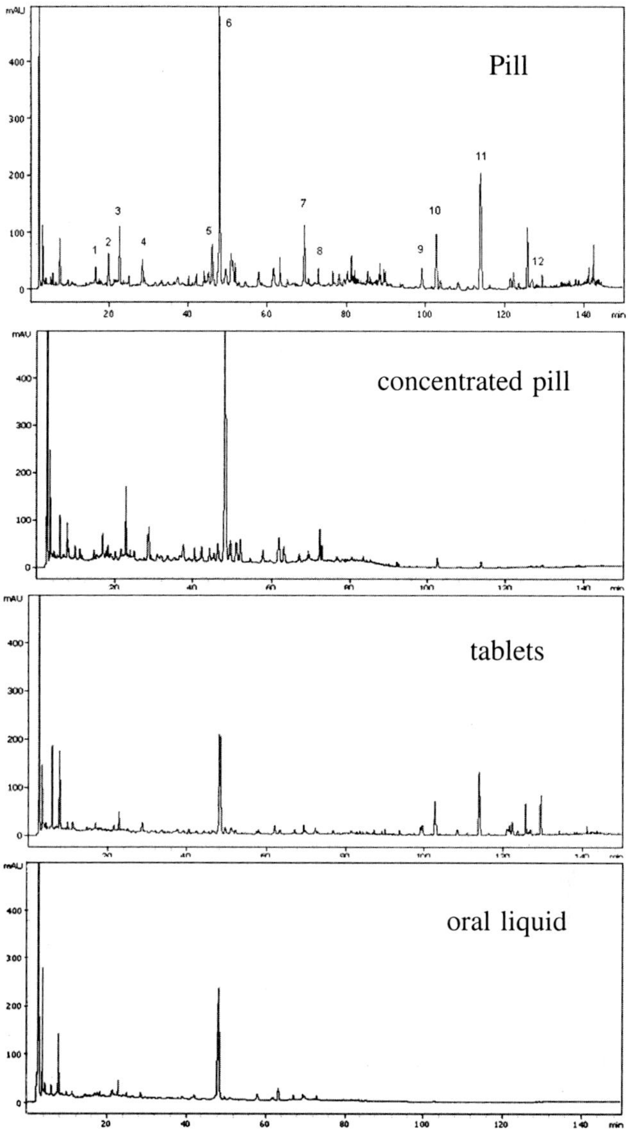

Fig. 1.5. HPLC fingerprints of various dosage forms of the same TCHM product (BJW) produced by different process techniques. Peak 1: Chlorogenic acid, peak 2: Caffeic acid, peak 3: Puerarin, peak 4: Daidazin, peak 5: 3,5-Oxy-dicaffeyl-quinic acid, peak 6: Naringin, peak 7: Luteolin, peak 8: Acacetin-7-O-β-glucoside, peak 9: Imperatorin, peak 10: Honokiol, peak 11: Magnolol, peak 12: Atractylodine.

1.5 Monitoring the Dynamic Change Due to Interaction of Mixed Herbal Drugs During Extraction

The classical empirical formula of *Sheng Mai Yin* (SMY) consisted of ginseng root (*Renshen*), Ophiopogon root (*Maidong*) and Schizandra fruits (*Wuweizi*). A quality survey of commercial SMY products in the market by means of fingerprinting revealed that the ginsenosides, the main active constituent in ginseng, had been destroyed; in some, none of the primary ginsenosides were even detected. The reason was obviously that ginsenosides in ginseng root were hydrolysed uncontrollably by the organic acids in *Wuweizi* when the mixture was subjected to extending heating in water

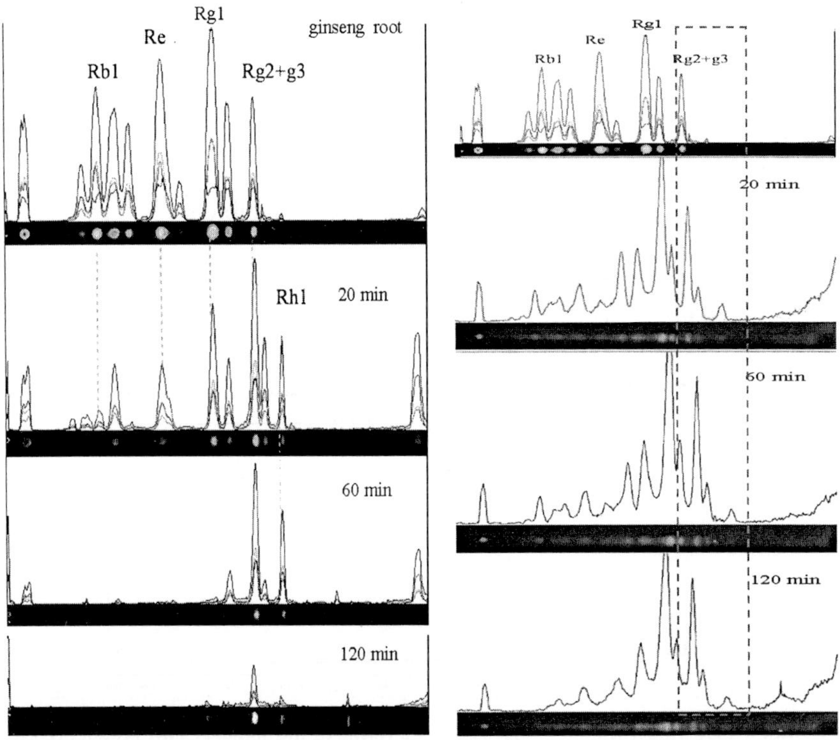

Fig. 1.6. HPTLC fingerprint of SMY decoction under rigorous heating (left) and gentle heating (right). Ginsenosides in SMY has been destroyed seriously under rigorous heating (mimic products in industry) while rather stable in a certain extent under gentle heating (home-made decoction) condition.

during manufacture. Analysis showed that the primary ginsenosides were hydrolysed rapidly when the mixed ginseng and *Wuweizi* was boiled with water under rigorous heating for only 20 minutes and destroyed gradually afterwards (Fig. 1.6, left). However, such hydrolysation behavior would stabilise under gentle heating for 120 minutes, similar to that undergone by home-made decoctions. The ginsenoside-Rb1, -Re and -Rg1 were hydrolysed into ginsenoside-Rg3 and -Rh with a rather consistent state of the hydrolysed ginsenosides pattern (Xie, 2005b) (Fig. 1.6, right). It is well known that ginsenoside-Rg3 and -Rh are active components for the cardiovascular system. The conventional home-made SMY decoction probably generated a "hidden" added positive value for preventing and curing diseases.

1.6 Conclusion

Authentication and consistent quality are the basic requirements for TCHM and its commercial products, regardless of the kind of research conducted to modernise the TCM. The complexities of TCHM challenge the current official quality control mode for which only a few markers were selected for identification and quantitative assay. Referring to too many unknown factors existed in TCHM, it is impossible and unnecessary to pinpoint qualitatively and quantitatively every single component contained in the herbal drug. Chromatographic fingerprinting is a rational option to meet the need for more effective and powerful quality assessment to TCHM. The optimised chromatographic fingerprint is not only an alternative analytical tool for identification, but also an approach to express the various patterns of chemical ingredients distribution in the herbal drugs and to preserve such wholeness-target "database" for further multi-faceted studies. Through active research and with rapid development in both analytical techniques and computer capacity, the fingerprint analysis will be constantly improved and fine-tuned. This quality assessment mode is complementary with findings from areas of pharmacology, biochemistry, clinical research and TCM philosophy. In forward-looking a viewpoint, a system to correlate fingerprinting data with the TCM efficacy can be expected and it would be the ultimate goal for developing the fingerprinting technique. However, it is important to be aware that the fingerprinting analysis also has its limitations. The active principles in herbal medicine cannot be totally detected by the current chromatographic techniques. It will be also very difficult to distinguish the active components from the inactive components in all fractions of the chromatographic fingerprint. Moreover, there may be other unpredictable questions or difficulties in the usage of fingerprinting analysis in the development process that need to be conquered. Nevertheless, the wholeness-targeted quality assessment mode achieved by fingerprinting analysis will advance the quality control of TCHM forward another progressive step in its continual development and modernisation.

References

Qian, H.Q. and Xie, P.S. (2005) *J. Instru. Anal.* **23**(5), 7–11 (in Chinese).

Xiao, P.G. (ed.) (2002) *The Chinese Materia Medica*. Chemical Industry Press, Vol. 1, pp. 962–975.

Xie, P.S. (ed.) (2005a) *The Chromatographic Fingerprint of Chinese Herbal Medicine*. People's Health Publishing House, pp. 263–372 (in Chinese).

Xie, P.S. (ed.) (2005b) *The Chromatographic Fingerprint of Chinese Herbal Medicine*. People's Health Publishing House, pp. 373–386 (in Chinese).

Chapter 2

Evidence-Based Herbal Medicine: Challenges in Efficacy and Safety Assessments

Harry H.-S. Fong, Guido F. Pauli, Judy L. Bolton, Richard B. van Breemen, Suzanne Banuvar, Lee Shulman, Stacie E. Geller & Norman R. Farnsworth

Abstract

The efficacy and safety assessments of medicines, whether modern or herbal, invariably encounter challenges or problems during the course of pre-clinical and clinical research. Some of the challenges in evidence-based herbal medicinal research are unique, and the researcher must be cognizant of them in order to safeguard the quality of the data obtained. Key challenges are: the quality of raw materials; appropriateness of biological/pharmacological activity assessment methodology, and data interpretation; standardisation methodology; pharmacokinetics and bioavailability of active constituents and metabolites; clinical dosage formulation/production; and clinical study designs and outcome measures. These challenges were encountered, and resolved, at the UIC/NIH Center for Botanical Dietary Supplements Research in Chicago, IL, USA. Although the University of Illinois at Chicago studies were directed at botanicals for women's health, the challenges and solutions encountered are also applicable to research on the efficacy and safety of herbal medicinal materials in general.

Keywords: Herbal Medicine; Efficacy and Safety Assessment; Challenges and Solutions.

2.1 Introduction

Over the past two decades, the use of alternative and complementary therapies, particularly botanical supplements, has become a topic of increasing global importance with both medical and economic implications (Mahady, 2001). According to a 1983 World Health Organization (WHO) estimate, a majority of the population in developing countries depend on traditional and herbal medicines as their primary source of health care (Bannerman *et al.*, 1983). In a 1997 survey, American consumers spent an estimated US$5.1 billion on herbal medicines, primarily in the form of dietary supplements (Eisenberg *et al.*, 1998). Even as the use of botanical products has increased dramatically in recent years, either in the form of drugs in traditional systems of medicine (TRM) such as Traditional Chinese Medicine (TCM) or as botanical dietary supplements in Complementary and Alternative Medicine (CAM), the evidence of their efficacy and safety has not been well documented. If these preparations are continued to be used in TRM or CAM therapy, they should be developed as "evidence-based medications" relative to their efficacy and safety.

Evidence of efficacy and safety of herbal medicines, like all forms of medicaments, can best be generated by clinical studies under Good Clinical Practices (GCP). Unfortunately, very few such studies on herbal products have been published. In the past two decades, most clinical studies have been conducted in Europe on single herb preparations, with very few being concerned with herbal mixtures such as those commonly found in TCM. With respect to the latter, a review of 2938 RCTs on TCM reported in 28 journals in the period of 1980–1997 (Tang *et al.*, 1999) concluded that the majority of these studies suffered from methodological defects. Additionally, these studies, as well as other clinical studies on herbal medicine have been conducted by clinicians, who, being accustomed to evaluating pure single molecule drugs, are unaware that the assessment of efficacy and safety of herbal products in basic and/or clinical studies can be severely hampered by a lack of appropriate quality assurance or quality control in the preparation of herbal extracts (Barrett, 2004; Fong, 2002; Tyler, 2004). Consequently, current evidence-based herbal medicine studies suffer from the duo challenges of GCP and quality assurance of the study product in general. However, it should be noted that even when studies are designed to incorporate GCP employing well characterised and standardised herbal preparations, other less obvious, but nevertheless, important problems or challenges abound that require attention.

2.2 UIC/NIH Center for Botanical Dietary Supplements Research

The UIC/NIH Center for Botanical Dietary Supplements Research in Chicago was established in 1999 with a multi-disciplinary team of investigators and the goal to establish the quality, standardisation, safety and efficacy of herbal supplements to alleviate the symptoms of menopause or other female disorders. Among the herbs investigated or under investigation are *Trifolium pratense* L. (Fabaceae) (red clover), *Cimicifuga racemosa* (L.) Nutt. (Syn: *Actaea racemosa* L.) (Ranunculaceae) (black cohosh), *Vitex agnus-castus* L. (Verbenaceae), (chaste berry), *Angelica sinensis* (Oliv.) Diels (Apiaceae) (dong quai), *Humulus lupulus* L. (Cannabaceae) (hops), *Vaccinium macrocarpon* Ait. (Ericaceae) (cranberry), *Viburnum prunifolium* L. (Caprifoliaceae) (black haw), *Ginkgo biloba* L. (Ginkgoaceae), *Glycyrrhiza glabra* L. (Fabaceae), *Panax ginseng* C.A. Mey. (Araliaceae) (Asian ginseng), and *Valeriana officinalis* L. (Valeriaceae) (valerian).

The research philosophy of the Center is that any botanical supplement/herbal medicine to be considered for clinical trial studies must be botanically authenticated as well as chemically and biologically standardised. Operationally, any herb to be evaluated for its safety and efficacy is subjected to an integrated, multidisciplinary study employing the following investigational steps: (1) acquire plant materials according to good agriculture and collection practices (GACP); (2) select and/or establish appropriate bioassays to determine the action mechanism for that herb; (3) perform bioassay-directed isolation and chemical characterisation of the active constituent(s) to be employed as biomarker(s); (4) standardisation of extract for subsequent preclinical and clinical studies; (5) production of the biologically and chemically standardised dosage form for clinical evaluation employing good manufacturing practice (GMP); (6) perform metabolism, pharmacokinetic, bioavailability, mechanism of action and toxicity studies on the standardised clinical dosage form; and (7) conduct phases I and II clinical studies.

Of the 11 botanicals cited above, *Trifolium pratense* and *Cimicifuga racemosa* were chosen for in-depth studies involving steps 1 to 7. Other botanicals, including *Vitex agnus-castus* (chaste berry), *Angelica sinensis* (dong quai), *Humulus lupulus* L. (Cannabaceae) (hops) and

Vaccinium macrocarpum (cranberry) have also been investigated to various depth. In studying these herbs, we encountered challenging problems in one or more of the seven steps. Some of the problems are herb-specific. In this paper, we will discuss the major problems and solutions encountered in some of these studies. Although our studies were directed at botanicals for women's health, the challenges/problems encountered and the solutions found to remedy them are also applicable to research on the efficacy and safety of herbal medicinal materials in general.

2.3 Acquisition of Quality Source Materials

The UIC/NIH Botanical Center investigators have recognised for many years that the quality of raw plant material must be assured before the commencement of any biological or chemical studies. Our advocacy of this requirement has recently been validated the World Health Organization Programme on Traditional Medicine (WHO/TRM) through its publication (WHO, 2003) of a guideline on good agriculture and collection practices (GACP) for the acquisition of quality botanicals for research, and by the National Center for Complementary and Alternative Medicine (NCCAM), NIH (USA), which established an interim guidance on product quality for grant applicants (2005). In spite of our philosophy and prior experiences in acquiring medicinal plants for our drug discovery research, we nevertheless encountered some challenging problems in the procurement of quality source materials for our botanical supplements/herbal medicine research.

For our chemical and biological studies on the flowering aerial parts of *Trifolium pratense* L. (Fabaceae), we initially obtained a sample from a commercial source. On routine macroscopic examination aided by a hand lens (10×), we noted that in addition to leaf fragments and flowering heads of *T. pratense*, there were also significant quantities of leaf and flower heads of unidentified species, as well as small amounts of *T. repens* leaf fragments, some unidentifiable flowerheads/fruits, insect and insect larvae (unpublished data). Obviously, this material was problematic and unacceptable as the source material for our studies. To solve this problem, we elected to cultivate *Trifolium pratense* under GAP conditions at our University of Illinois Pharmacognosy Field Station, a 40-acre facility, located some 40 kilometres from our laboratories in Chicago. The plant material was harvested at the flowering stage, its identity confirmed by macroscopic and microscopic means, and was further validated by DNA analysis (Xu *et al.*, 2002). To ensure the quality of the *Cimicifuga racemosa* (L.) Nutt. (*Actaea racemosa* L.) (Ranunculaceae) root and rhizome, the second candidate herb for our safety and clinical efficacy studies, samples were field collected by good field collection practices from various mountain sites of the eastern USA, including Pennsylvania, Virginia, Tennessee, and North Carolina. These materials were identified and validated by macroscopic, microscopic and DNA analysis (Xu *et al.*, 2002; Chen *et al.*, 2002). Besides ensuring quality source materials of these two herbs for our chemical, biological and clinical studies, our experiences in their procurement enabled us to assist the WHO/TRM in drafting its guideline on good agriculture and collection practices (WHO, 2003).

2.4 Selection of Appropriate Bioassays

The use of an appropriate biological/pharmacological activity assessment methodology is self-evident, whether it is employed in drug discovery research or for determining the mechanism of action of a herbal medicine. In the case of *T. pratense*, it has been well established that this herb contains oestrogenic isoflavones. Indeed, a MeOH extract of our source material was confirmed to be oestrogenic *in vitro* and *in vivo* (Liu *et al.*, 2001; Burdette *et al.*, 2002). On the other hand, the mechanism of action in reducing hot flashes by *C. racemosa* was not well understood at the time of our initial study on this herb. A review of the literature (Mahady *et al.*, 2002) cited earlier and contradictory reports of whether there was an oestrogenic effect. In our hands, a MeOH extract of our source material was not oestrogenic (Liu *et al.*, 2001; Burdette *et al.*, 2003), hence the employment of these assays would be inappropriate. Consequently, it was necessary to explore other mechanisms for its hot flash reduction effect. At the end, we discovered that a 40% 2-propanol extract inhibited serotonin receptor. Specifically, it inhibits the 5-HT_7 and 5-HT_{1A} receptors (Burdette *et al.*, 2003). The discovery of this centrally acting mechanism allowed us to overcome a major hurdle to our chemical, biological and clinical studies of black cohosh.

2.5 Bioassay-Directed Isolation Bioactive Marker(s)

The major challenge in conducting bioassay-directed isolation of bioactive marker compound or compounds lies not in the actual phytochemical isolation process itself, nor in the chemical characterisation/structure elucidation. With an array of separation techniques including adsorption, size-exclusion, counter current partition and preparative high-performance liquid chromatography, the isolation of phytochemical constituents has become a matter of routine. With the availability of increasingly more powerful nuclear magnetic resonance (NMR) and mass spectrometric (MS), and other spectroscopic instrumentation, the characterisation, structure identification and/or structure elucidation of isolated molecules can be accomplished with greater and greater ease.

Instead, the major problem encountered in our studies is a biological one. The isolation of actein, 26-deoxyactein and 23-*epi*-26-deoxyactein as the bioactive markers from *C. racemosa* (Chen *et al.*, 2002) was complicated by the time consuming process of identifying the HT_7 receptor inhibition assay as the appropriate bioassay to be used in guiding the isolation of these compounds. Once the appropriate bioassay was identified, the phytochemistry and structural identification/elucidation work proceeded without major problems.

2.6 Standardisation of Pre-clinical and Clinical Extract

As indicated above, the research philosophy of our Center is that any botanical supplement/herbal medicine to be considered for clinical trial studies must be chemically and biologically standardised. Having determined the biological mechanisms of action and through bioassay-directed isolation procedures that identified the bioactive marker compounds (Liu *et al.*, 2001; Burdette *et al.*, 2002 and 2003), the next step was to chemically analyse and standardise these extracts to contain the appropriate concentrations of the active compounds for subsequent pre-clinical and clinical studies. Procedures for the quality control analysis of active marker chemical compounds can be accomplished by colourimetric, spectroscopic and/or chromatographic methods. Colourimetric and direct spectroscopic methods are older analytical procedures quantifying the absorption of structurally related compounds at a specific wavelength of light, and expressed as concentration of a reference standard (marker). Since other plant constituents possessing the same absorbance are included in the measurement, a higher concentration is usually ascribed to the test material. More modern methods for the chemical analysis of secondary chemical constituent markers in botanical products involve some form of chromatography. Thin-layer chromatographic (TLC) procedures have the advantage of being simple, rapid, can provide useful characteristic profile patterns, and are inexpensive to use. However, their resolving power is limited and quantitative data for minor constituents are difficult to obtain. Gas chromatography (GC) can provide high resolution of the more volatile complex mixtures, but is of limited value in the case of non-volatile polar compounds, especially the polar polyhydroxylated and glycosidic compounds. High-performance liquid chromatography (HPLC) is capable of resolving complex mixtures of polar and non-polar compounds, and has become the chromatographic method of choice for the qualitative and quantitative analysis of botanical extracts and products. HPLC can be coupled with a range of analytical detection techniques including ultraviolet (UV) spectroscopy, evaporative light-scattering detection (ELSD), and mass spectrometry (MS) to produce a "fingerprint" of the botanical product, and/or to quantify the concentration of one or more of the active markers. Detection by UV is readily available in most labs, and is carried out either with a single- or dual-wavelength, or a full spectrum (e.g. photo-diode array) detector, and is the most appropriate technique for the routine analysis of compounds that contain a UV-active chromophore. Combined HPLC–mass spectrometry (LC-MS) and liquid chromatography–tandem mass spectrometry (LC-MS^n) is being increasingly used. The advantage of these methods is that as each compound elutes, the mass can be determined by the mass spectrometer, elemental composition can be determined using exact mass measurement, and structurally significant fragmentions can be detected, which can provide specific identification of the eluting "peak". A third commonly used detection technique is evaporative light scattering detection (ELSD), as a vast majority of all plant secondary metabolites are detectable whether or not they contain a spectroscopically active chromophore.

In the case of the two herbs under study for safety and efficacy, the bioactive marker compounds in *T. pratense* were identified as the isoflavones formononetin (**1**), daidzein (**2**), biochanin A (**3**) and genistein (**4**). These compounds possess conjugated aromatic chromophores, which are amenable to HPLC-UV detection, and were so analysed (Booth *et al.*, 2006). The bioactive markers actein (**5**), 26-deoxyactein (**6**) and 23-*epi*-26-deoxyactein (**7**) identified in *C. racemosa*, on the other hand, contain no UV absorbing chromophores, and hence, cannot be analysed by HPLC-UV. This problem was overcome by the use of HPLC-ELSD detection (Fabricant, 2006).

Structure Drawings

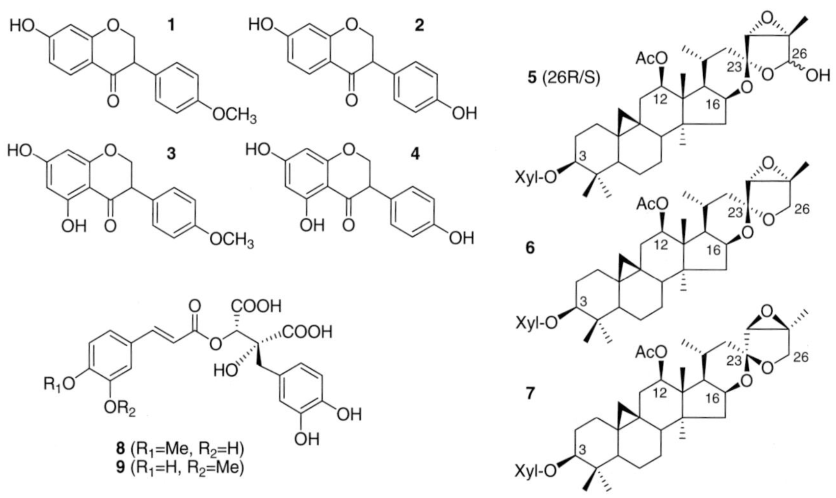

Once prototype standardised extracts were formulated, one of our industrial partners, Pureworld Botanicals, South Hackensack, NJ, a GMP certified manufacturer of botanical extracts prepared the clinical extracts per our specifications for subsequent pre-clinical and clinical studies.

2.7 Production of Biologically and Chemically Standardised Dosage Forms

In the safety and efficacy evaluation of herbal supplements/medicines, an important consideration is the dosage formulation, which can affect the bioavailability of the active chemical constituents present in the standardised clinical extract. For oral administration, one may consider the use of liquid (syrup), hard capsules (gelatin), soft gel capsules, tablets, or even powders. Each of these formulations has its unique characteristics, advantages and disadvantages. Liquid and powdered dried extract dosage forms can facilitate absorption, but the production of a placebo with the same taste and smell is most difficult. For non-polar constituents, soft gels containing an oil-based vehicle, offer greater degrees of absorption, however, this may be problematic in the case of polar compounds. Hard shell capsules and tablets are the most popular oral dosage forms. In the case of tablets, the presence of binders and excipients, plus the compacting of the mixture can lead to disintegration and dissolution problems, which in turn lead to questions of bioavailability. As an example, a study on the pharmaceutical quality of melatonin tablets by Hahm *et al.* (1999), three of five immediate release tablets (different brands) failed both the USP tablet disintegration (30 minutes) and dissolution tests, with two of them not disintegrating after more than 20 hours. There is an obvious manufacturing problem, perhaps due to excessive compacting of the tablets during production. In our own post marketing study of ginseng products as part of the American Botanical Councils Ginseng Evaluation Program (Hall *et al.*, 2001a and b), we found that the detectable content of ginsenosides was much higher in the hard gelatin capsule (> 3% total ginsenoside) than in the corresponding tablet (< 0.7%) formulations (Fitzloff *et al.*, 1998). The disparate quantifiable ginsenosides in the two formulations was probably due to the fact that in the case of the tablets, the analytes were much more tightly bound to the binders and excipients in the tablets than in the capsules, and hence might have been incompletely extracted.

Given the Hahm *et al.* report and our own ginseng evaluation experience, we concluded that the use of opaque hard gelatin capsules would be the best dosage formulation for our clinical studies. Having made this choice, we then had to decide on what excipient material to be used to formulate our clinical extracts. For many years, lactose has been the most commonly used excipients for gelatin capsules. However, it has been shown in recent years there are a number of individuals in the general population, who are lactose-intolerant. To avoid such potential problems in our study subjects, we elected to use rice powder as the excipient for our clinical dosage form.

For our clinical studies, the test materials and their corresponding placebo and positive control capsules were prepared under GMP conditions by Pharmavite, Mission Hills, CA, our other industrial partner.

2.8 Pharmacokinetic and Bioavailability

It is generally recognised that unlike single ingredient pharmaceuticals, pharmacokinetic and bioavailability studies of herbal medicine, especially

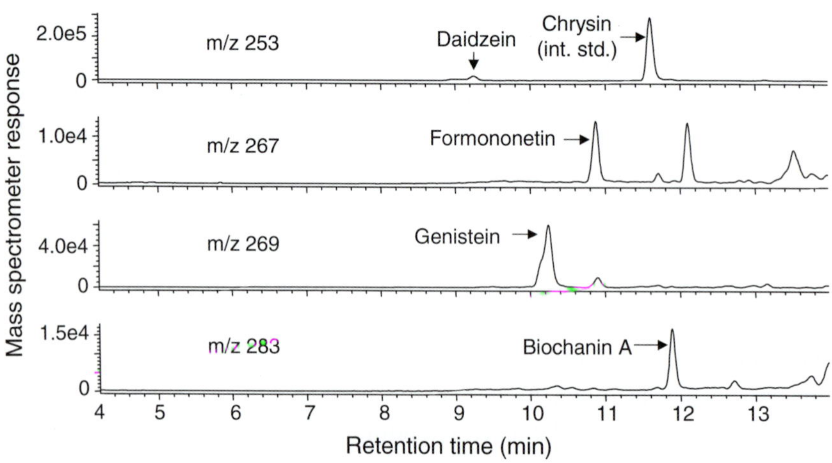

Fig. 2.1. LC-MS analysis of an extract of 30 μL of serum obtained from a healthy female volunteer 5 hours after oral administration of a standardised red clover dietary supplement containing 40 mg of oestrogenic isoflavones. Glucuronide and sulfate conjugates in the serum were hydrolysed enzymatically, 1 μg/mL chrysin was added as an internal standard, and then the sample was extracted using ethyl acetate, evaporated to dryness, and reconstituted in methanol/water. Finally, the extract was analysed using LC-MS, which consisted of reversed phase HPLC separation (Waters Xterra MS C_{18} 1.0 × 50 mm column) with a 14-minute gradient from 10–98% aqueous acetonitrile followed by negative ion electrospray mass spectrometric detection (reprinted from Piersen *et al.*).

poly-prescriptions, containing a multiplicity of chemical constituents, many of which are unknown and/or unidentifiable, are very difficult, if not impossible, to conduct. If one or more bioactive constituents are known, limited studies involving these compounds can be conducted to provide some information. In a limited pharmacokinetic study on *T. pratense*, we encountered no bioavailability problems as demonstrated by our being able to quantitatively determine the level of the bioactive markers formononetin (**1**), daidzein (**2**), biochanin A (**3**) and genistein (**4**) in the blood (Fig. 2.1) and urine samples of five health women subjects in our phase I study (Piersen *et al.*, 2004).

In the case of *C. racemosa*, two classes of compounds were found to be active in the $5HT_7$ *in vitro* bioassay. The non-polar triterpenes, actein (**5**), 26-deoxyactein (**6**) and 23-*epi*-26-deoxyactein (**7**) showed

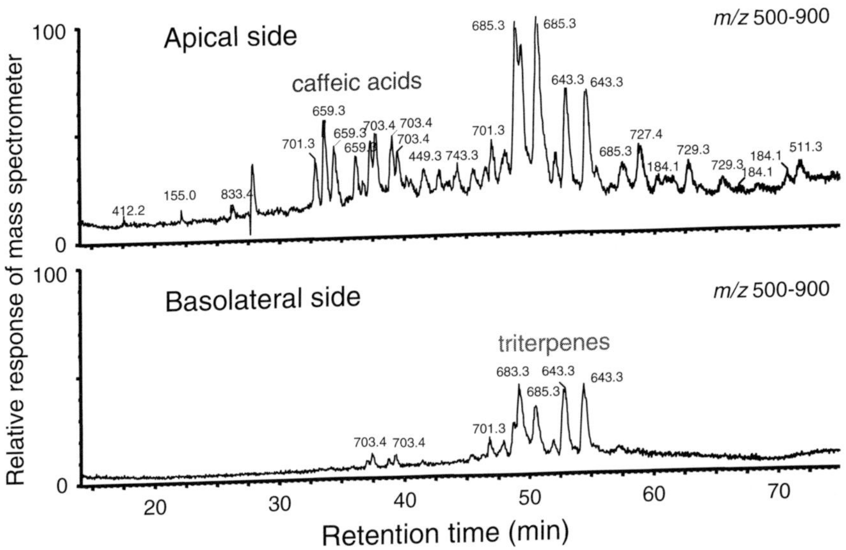

Fig. 2.2. Caco-2 cell monolayer screening of a standardised black cohosh extract (100 μg/mL initial concentration on the apical side of the monolayer) for intestinal permeability. After 2-hour incubation at 37°C, aliquots were removed from both the apical and basolateral sides of the Caco-2 cell monolayer and analysed using LC-MS with reversed phase HPLC separation (YMC AQ 2.1 × 250 mm C_{18} column with a gradient from 0.5% acetic acid to acetonitrile) and negative ion electrospray mass spectrometric detection (Micromass QTOF2 hybrid mass spectrometer).

receptor inhibition activities of 50%, 55% and 31%, respectively at 100 μg/ml, whereas the very polar caffeic acid derivatives, cimicifugic acids A (**8**) and –B (**9**) were much more active, each with an IC_{50} value of 1.2 μM (unpublished data). Unfortunately, recovery experiments showed that neither cimicifugic acids A nor B was present in the serum of women volunteers receiving a single oral dose of the clinical product. After extensive investigation, we discovered that while the caffeic acid derivatives showed a much stronger *in vitro* $5HT_7$ receptor inhibition activity than the triterpenes, the former compounds were not absorbed, and hence not bioavailable, as demonstrated by their failure to penetrate a Caco cell monolayer (Fig. 2.2) (unpublished data). Consequently, one cannot always draw a correlation between *in vitro* activity and *in vivo* pharmacological effect, without examining the bioavailability of the potential biomarker compound(s).

2.9 Clinical Studies

The final step in our evidence-based evaluation of *T. pratense* and *C. racemosa* consisted of a randomised double-blind, positive and placebo-controlled study to determine their efficacy for treatment of menopausal symptoms over a 1-year period. The study was designed to randomise each of 112 subjects into four arms: placebo, standard HRT (Prempro® 0.625 mg/2.5 mg MPA), black cohosh (4 mg), and red clover (120 mg). The primary endpoint being to determine the efficacy of black cohosh and red clover for the relief of vasomotor symptoms (hot flashes), with secondary endpoints designed to assess the relief of somatic symptoms (insomnia, joint pain, and fatigue), to determine alterations in specific biochemical markers (lipids, bone density, endometrial assessments), and the relief of sexual dysfunction (vaginal dryness, dyspareunia, libido, difficulty in achieving orgasm). To insure the validity of the results, the study design included criteria for the inclusion and exclusion of the human volunteers. Inclusion Criteria: menopausal women with intact uterus; have at least 35 hot flushes per week; have been amenorrhoea for more than 6 months, but less than 10 years duration; have FSH levels greater than 40 IU/L if > 6 months, but < 1 year amenorrhoea; the subject has a requirement for HRT; and is able to give informed consent to the study. Exclusion Criteria: subject has last menstrual period for more than 10 years duration; has positive pregnancy test or breast feeding; experiences less than 35 hot flushes per week; is obese (> 35 BMI); has previous history of endometrial hyperplasia/neoplasia; previous history of cancers of the breast or reproductive tract; history of severe recurrent depression/severe psychiatric disturbance; previous hysterectomy; history of the presence of cardiovascular incident; has severe varicose veins; has sickle cell anaemia; experiencing post-menopausal bleeding; and is a vegan.

As with many other clinical studies conducted under GCP, the major challenge that we encountered is not due to experimental design, nor the lack of study volunteers. The problem lies in our inability to enroll and randomise the desired number (112) of subjects into the study within the prescribed period. Patient recruitment was initiated in 2003, soon after the results of the Women's Health Initiative were published that showed that HT increases the risk of breast cancer and cardiovascular disease. The clinical trial started one year late due to problems with development of test article, difficulty in determining mechanism of action of active components for black cohosh, delay in standardisation and encapsulation of products, and IRB (Institutional Review Board) issues related to the need for an IND (Investigational New Drug application). As of 15 December 2005, we were able to randomise only 58 study subjects, with an additional 17 currently enrolled and undergoing evaluation for suitability for randomisation at the University of Illinois at Chicago and at the Northwestern University Feinberg School of Medicine study sites. This begot the question of why were we unable to recruit sufficient number of study subjects when so many candidates are available? An analysis of the data indicated that of 880 candidates screened, 583 were ineligible for our study due to their not meeting the inclusion and exclusion criteria. Another 222 candidates elected not to enroll in the study for a variety of reasons, including their unwillingness to be randomised into the positive HRT (Prempro®) or the placebo control groups; undergo a "wash out" period; the length of study period (1 year); not being residents of the State of Illinois; refusal to be involved in a blind study; and unspecified reasons, among others. In such a situation, what can we do to meet this challenge? One always needs to be prepared to have additional funding sources if the recruitment timeline goes beyond what was predicted and we were fortunate to secure additional funding to continue our clinical study.

2.10 Conclusion

Evidence for the efficacy and safety of herbal medicine must be established by scientifically valid research, the conduct of which is filled with challenges ranging from the pre-clinical determination of the quality of the source material; chemical and biological standardisation parameters and methodologies; choice of clinical formulations and GMP manufacturing; to the clinical evaluation of the formulated products. These challenges were encountered, and resolved, at the UIC/NIH Center for Botanical Dietary Supplements Research in Chicago. Although the UIC studies were directed at botanicals for women's health, the challenges and solutions encountered are also applicable in general to research on the efficacy and safety of herbal medicinal materials for other disease targets.

Acknowledgements

Research conducted within the UIC/NIH Botanical Center is supported by NIH grant P50 AT00155 jointly funded by the Office of Dietary Supplements ODS), the National Center for Complementary and Alternative Medicine (NCCAM), the National Institute of General Medical Sciences (NIGMS), and the Office for Research on Women's Health (ORWH). The contents are the responsibility of the authors and do not necessarily represent the views of the funding agencies.

A summary of this paper was presented by one of us (HHSF) by invitation at the Tung Wah Group of Hospitals' *1st TWGHs Eddie Wang International Symposium on Complementary Chinese and Western Medicine — Integrated Approach*, held in Hong Kong, SAR, China, 4–5 November, 2005.

References

Bannerman, R., Burton, J. and Chen, W.C. (eds.) (1983) *Traditional Medicine and Health Care Coverage.* World Health Organization, Geneva, Switzerland.

Barrett, M. (2004) Identifying and characterising botanical products. In: *The Handbook of Clinically Tested Herbal Remedies*, Vol. 1 (ed.) Barrett, M. The Haworth Herbal Press, New York, pp. 23–36.

Booth, N.L., Overk, C.R., Yao, P., *et al.* (2006) Seasonal variation of red clover (*Trifolium pratense* L., Fabaceae) isoflavones and oestrogenic activity. *J. Agric. Food Chem.* (in press).

Burdette, J.E., Liu, J., Chen, S.-N., *et al.* (2003) Black cohosh acts as a mixed competitive ligand and partial agonist of the serotonin receptor. *J. Agric. Food Chem.* **51**, 5661–5670.

Burdette, J.E., Liu, J., Lantvit, D., *et al.* (2002) *Trifolium pratense* (red clover) exhibits estrogenic effects *in vivo* in ovariectomized Sprague–Dawley rats. *J. Nutr.* **132**, 27–30.

Chen, S.-N., Li, W., Fabricant, D.S., *et al.* (2002) Isolation, structure elucidation and absolute configuration of 26 deoxyactein from *Cimicifuga racemosa* and clarification of nomenclature associated with 27-deoxyactein. *J. Nat. Prod.* **65**, 601–605.

Eisenberg, D.M., Davis, R.B., Ettner, S.L., *et al.* (1998) Trends in alternative medicine use in the United States, 1990–1997. Results of a follow-up national survey. *JAMA* **280**, 1569–1575.

Fabricant, D. (2006) *Pharmacognostic Investigation of Black Cohosh* (*Cimicifuga racemosa* (L.) Nutt.). Ph.D. Dissertation, University of Illinois at Chicago.

Fitzloff, J.F., Yat, P., Lu, Z.Z., *et al.* (1998) Perspectives on the quality assurance of ginseng products in North America. *Proceedings of the 7th Internal Ginseng Symposium*, 22–25 September 1998, Seoul, Korea.

Fong, H.H.S. (2002) Integration of herbal medicine into modern medical practices: issues and prospects. *Integr. Cancer Ther.* **1**, 287–293.

Hall, T., Lu, Z.-Z., Yat, P.N., *et al.* (2001a) An introduction to the ginseng evaluation program. *HerbalGram* **52**, 27–30.

Hall, T., Lu, Z.-Z., Yat, P.N., *et al.* (2001b) Evaluation of consistency of standardised Asian ginseng products in the ginseng evaluation program. *HerbalGram* **52**, 31–45.

Liu, J., Xu, H., Gu, C., *et al.* (2001) Evaluation of oestrogenic activity of plant extracts for the potential treatment of menopausal symptoms. *J. Agric. Food Chem.* **49**, 2472–2479.

Mahady, G.B. (2001) Global harmonization of herbal health claims. *J. Nutr.* **131**(Suppl. 3), 1120–1123.

Mahady, G.B., Fabricant, D., Chadwick, L.R., *et al.* (2002) Black cohosh: an alternative therapy for menopause? *Nutr. Clin. Care* **5**, 283–289.

Mahady, G.B., Fong, H.H.S. and Farnsworth, N.R. (2001) *Botanical Dietary Supplements: Quality, Safety and Efficacy.* Swets & Zeitlinger, Lisse, Netherlands.

NCCAM (2005) *http://grants.nih.gov/grants/guide/notice-files/NOT-AT-05-004.html*

Piersen, C.E., Booth, N.L., Sun, Y., *et al.* (2004) Chemical and biological characterization and clinical evaluation of botanical dietary supplements: a phase I red clover extract as a model. *Curr. Med. Chem.* **11**, 1361–1374.

Tang, J.L., Zhan, S.Y. and Ernst, E. (1999) Review of randomized controlled trials of traditional Chinese medicine. *B. Med. J.* **319**, 160–161.

Tyler, V.E. (2004) Product definition deficiencies in clinical studies of herbal medicines. In: *The Handbook of Clinically Tested Herbal Remedies*, Vol. 1 (ed.) Barrett, M. The Haworth Herbal Press, New York, pp. 13–22.

WHO (1998) *Regulatory Situation of Herbal Medicines. A Worldwide Review.* World Health Organization, Geneva, Switzerland.

WHO (2003) *WHO Guidelines on Good Agricultural and Collection Practices (GACP) for Medicinal Plants.* World Health Organization, Geneva, Switzerland.

Xu, H., Fabricant, D.S., Piersen, C.E., *et al.* (2002) A preliminary RAPD-PCR analysis of *Cimicifuga* species and other botanicals used for women's health. *Phytomedicine* **9**, 757–762.

Chapter 3

Good Agricultural Practice — GAP Does it Ensure a Perfect Supply of Medicinal Herbs for Research and Drug Development?

Ping-Chung Leung

Abstract

While users of herbal formulae have been disappointed with the lack of uniformity in the quality of herbs provided by the herb suppliers of different standings, they do not have better guarantee apart from relying on the more reputable ones. The tradition of identifying special geographic sites as being specific for the supply of certain herbal items is no longer reliable since the high demand for large quantities of quality supply would have drained any traditional supply dry. Since the European Union started to advocate a quality supply of the first manufacturing material for herbal products by introducing a comprehensive recommendation of practices: from seedling, planting, fertilising, harvesting, storage and distribution, the idea of good agricultural practice becomes an attractive reality. There is good prospect of an excellent supply of quality herbal products with uniformity, if Good Agricultural Practice (GAP) could be enforced. The substantiation of GAP will be a great blessing for both the manufacturers and consumers of herbal products.

Although the need for GAP is urgent, and Japan, China and the World Health Organization have, one after the other, written up their recommendation, to put GAP into real practice would take time. GAP in China is particularly difficult, not only because the herbal items involved are in great numbers but also because the current practice of growing medicinal herbs, their marketing and distribution, have been counter-productive to the introduction of the new system of GAP.

Unless the demand for herbal supply was limited, otherwise, GAP will not be able to satisfy the extensive need for uniformity. Short of the knowledge of the exact, accurate nature of the active component within a herb, there will be no perfect guarantee on the quality supply. Henceforth, even when GAP becomes a mature practice, what is required for quality control, *viz*, different levels of authentication, from chemical fingerprinting to molecular, DNA identification, will remain necessary as cross-checking mechanisms to make sure that uniformity in scientific experiments and drug development is not violated.

Keywords: Agriculture; Chinese Medicine; Herb Quality.

3.1 Introduction

Medicinal herbs used in Chinese Medicine are traditionally gathered from wild resources with the exception of edible, vegetable categories. With the rising demand from users over the ages, more and more popularly used items are grown in agricultural fields. It is estimated that over 10% of the plant species in the world can be found in China, including 240 peculiar genera. National survey done in the past 30 years indicated that China had a total of 12,807 species of medicinal materials (Huang *et al.*, 2002b; Gao *et al.*, 2002) of which there are 383 families, 2309 genera and 11,146 species. Most of these items, of course, are originally obtained from wild sources. Those that are in popular use have already followed the natural course of turning to agricultural production.

The natural force of supply and demand has initiated the agricultural production of commonly used medicinal herbs, particularly for the precious, expensive items. The over-harvest of wild medicinal plants is frequently observed and thus threatens the extinction of the species and might lead to the eventual loss of biodiversity of the wild resources. The only way to prevent this process of ecological disaster is to introduce agricultural growth of these wild species (Wang and Xiao, 2000).

The Chinese botanical and medicinal plant experts are aware of the urgent need for the promotion of agricultural production of herbal plants and the first national meeting on this issue was held in 1998 (Wang and Lin, 1999), and Good Agricultural Practice (GAP) for medicinal plants was put on the agenda. Drafting of the guidelines therefore was started and the first document for trial use was ready by 2002 (Zhan and Lin, 2002).

Although China might be the country that commands the greatest need for medicinal plants, obviously related to the popular use and regular prescriptions from Chinese Medicine Practitioners, Europe also owns a tradition for the use of medicinal plants. Hence, at about the same time in 2002, the European Union responded to the needs and issued the "New European Union Good Agricultural and Collection Practice Rules" (Scholten, 2003).

The World Health Organization (WHO) has always been supportive on native medicine. It gave a timely response in 2003 to the general need for agricultural guidelines that would lead to the healthy development of the supply of medicinal herbs, based on the recommendations of the Chinese and European guidelines (WHO, 2003).

This chapter will take a critical look at GAP for medicinal herbs, and discuss its requirements, the present state of practice and measures that are required to go parallel with the acquisition of herbs for research and drug development. References are taken mostly from journals of Chinese language (Shiu *et al.*, 2005).

3.2 The Need for G.A.P.

In China, there is an urgent need to deal with the over-exploitation of medicinal herbs. In a narrow sense, to protect the medicinal plant resources means just to maintain an adequate supply. In the broader sense, it refers to the conservation of biodiversity. While China could be proud of its richness in biodiversity, being the champion in the Northern hemisphere and the eighth in the world, China should be aware of the fact that its biodiversity is being seriously challenged (Yuan *et al.*, 2000; Zou, 2001). Around 200 species of plants in China have already become extinct and another 1000 others are under imminent threat.

Due to the over-exploitation, the reserves and output of wild medicinal plants are rapidly decreasing. Examples of these plants are given below:

Acanthopanax senticosus
Atractylodes lancea
Anemarrhena asphodeloides
Asarum sieboldii
Cistanche salsa
Cynomorium songaricum
Dichroa febrifuga
Ephedra sinica

Gastrodia elata
Gentiana macrophylla
Gentiana scabra
Glycyrrhiza uralensis
Lithospermum erythrorhizon
Notopterygium incisum
Paris polyphylla
Phellodendron amurense
Pinellia ternate
Rheum officinale
Saposhnikovia divaricata
Scutellaria baicalensis
Stellaria gypsophiloides
Tripterygium wilfordii
Uncaria rhynchophylla
Vitex trifolia
Ziziphu jujube

A very commonly used medicinal herb, *radix glycyrrhiza*, for example was originally found in Inner Mongolia. Its reserve and output in this province has decreased so much that its annual yield is only 40% of its 1950 production. The main supply for this plant, therefore, was shifted to Xinjiang Province (Yuan *et al.*, 2000).

Another popular medicinal plant item, *Radix Astragalus*, is experiencing the same fate. The wild Astragulus output in the 1960s had amounted to 2000 tons in Inner Mongolia, but recently, it dropped to less than 100 tons (Wang and Xiao, 2000).

In the Chinese medicinal plant market, the quality of the supply is hinged closely with the origin of the herb. Practitioners who prescribe the herbs also specify the origin that is firmly believed to be crucial for the quality. Indeed, a special term has been traditionally used to qualify the best supply as the *Daodi* (道地) product. As the supply from classical origins of production shrinks, *Daodi* supply either becomes extremely expensive or it does not mean much at all if the genuine supply of good origin has already become minimal.

As long as the nature of the *Daodi* species is known, there is no reason why they cannot be reproduced in agricultural fields, so as to ensure a constant supply of the best quality *Daodi* choice. It will be a blessing for both the herb dealers and users.

It might appear just a simple practice of planting the herbs in the traditional area of production, so that the best quality supply of herbs could be maintained. However, the issue is much more complicated. A herb might appear identical to what is described in the Chinese Materia Medica or in Botanical Classics, and yet the chemical and biological qualities expressed in its extract might not be what are desired. The traditional use of herbs rely on quality suppliers that ensure quality origins, i.e. *Daodi* origin. The current users cannot rely on *Daodi* origin anymore, for reasons already discussed. Modern technology has also revealed that *Daodi* quality should be related to special chemical and might be molecular biological profiles as are expressed in DNA patterns, which could be identified with chemical and biological tests. The supply of quality herbs, therefore, refers to not necessarily the origin of supply but to the innate chemical and molecular qualities. With full recognition of the modern interpretation of the *Daodi* supply of herbs, GAP is aimed at the production of herbs that are not only of identical morphological characteristics, but also of ideal chemical and biological profiles.

Planning for GAP, therefore, is not only confined to the place of cultivation, but involves the genetic conditions of the seeds, the field environment, the growing and harvest procedures, storage, etc.

The complex requirements for GAP, in actual fact, have arisen from a more complex need apart from that of a quality supply and a good sale for the supplier. The supply of herbs with detailed qualities has become a practical issue because of the multiple needs of safety, effectiveness and research uniformity.

While herbal preparations for health can no longer be assumed to be safe, in cases where adverse effects were encountered, the chemical and biological nature of the herbs need to be immediately known, so that the adverse effects could be explained as soon as possible. Indeed, the assumption that natural healing causes no harm and that herbal treatment is a form of natural healing should be challenged. Adverse effects could occur as a result of an inaccurate supply of herbs, adulteration from either the supplier or prescriber, or problems arising from the consumer himself as he might be developing allergic reactions. Interactions with other drugs being consumed might be the other reasons behind adverse effects. Situations of such nature are happening more and more frequently, creating professional problems or sometimes, even legal challenges. To avoid such mishappenings, GAP measures could greatly help (Lo and Pun, 2005).

On the research side, the need for a quality supply of herbs is of vital importance. Until the exact active components with their chemical characteristics are known, or better still, until the chemical structure and chemical equation responsible for its pharmacological action are known, using a herb or a combination of herbs enjoys no guarantee for its safety and quality. The availability of a quality supply from a GAP therefore will not totally relieve the concerns about safety and quality, but it will significantly simplify the complexity of the procedures required for the related authentication.

The need for GAP, is therefore of multiple purposes, not only with regard to the practice standards, but also to the research requirements in a basic demand for uniformity and repeatability. GAP could be considered as an essential step towards the modernisation of Chinese Medicine.

3.3 China Recommendations

3.3.1 *Good Agricultural Practice (GAP) in China for medicinal herbs*

The Rules and Regulations concerning GAP drafted in 2002 by the State Administration of Traditional Chinese Medicine of China (SATCM), State Drug and Food Administration of China (SFDA) and China National Group Corporation of Traditional and Herbal Medicine (Qin *et al.*, 2001; Zhou, 2001) cover wide areas, from the environment and soil, germplasm and breeding, cultivation, transport and storage, to quality control, as well as record keeping.

A summary of the recommendations are given as follows:

Chapters	Items	Main Contents
Chap 1	General principles	Purpose and significance.
Chap 2	The environment of the cultivation area	The detail request for the ecological environment such as air, water, and soil conditions in the cultivation area.
Chap 3	The germplasm and breeding material	The plant or animal species should be identified correctly and the quality of the germaplasm resource should be controlled.

Chapters	Items	Main Contents
Chap 4	The management of cultivation	The cultivation process, such as how to use fertiliser, soil, water and how to control the insect pest and plant diseases, should be controlled by standard operating procedure (SOP) principles.
Chap 5	The harvest and process at the harvest place	The optimal harvest time should be studied and fixed. The specific request for process, drying conditions, etc. is clearly written in this chapter.
Chap 6	Package, transport and storage	It should be clearly recorded for each batch of the drug materials. The request for the transport, such as using clean container, for the storage, such as light, temperature, and humidity, is clearly provided in this chapter.
Chap 7	Quality control	The specific request for quality control, such as the items to be checked, the request for the characteristic, foreign matter, water, and ash content, is clearly provided in this chapter.
Chap 8	The equipment and operator	This chapter provides the request for the trained operators, the request about the product and process place, and equipment.
Chap 9	The document management	It should be recorded in every detail and particular for the whole process of cultivation, process, transport and storage, etc. The document should be kept properly at least five years.
Chap 10	Supplement	Supplementary explanation.

While the draft recommendations might appear quite comprehensive, explanations might still be deficient. A better conceptual account could be obtained from the World Health Organization, which obviously has made use of the Chinese Recommendations as the backbone of its own document concerning GAP. A summary of the WHO document is supplied below.

3.4 World Health Organization Recommendations

3.4.1 *World Health Organization GAP guidelines*

3.4.1.1 Background

Some reported adverse events following the use of certain herbal medicines have been associated with a variety of possible explanations, including the inadvertent use of the wrong plant species, adulteration with undeclared other medicines and/or potent substances, contamination with undeclared toxic and/or hazardous substances, over-dosage, inappropriate use by health care providers or consumers, and interaction with other medicines, resulting in an adverse drug interaction. Among those attributable to the poor quality of finished products, some clearly result from the use of raw medicinal plant materials that are not of a sufficiently high quality standard.

The safety and quality of raw medicinal plant materials and finished products depend on factors that may be classified as intrinsic (genetic) or extrinsic (environment, collection methods, cultivation, harvest, post-harvest processing, transport and storage practices). Inadvertent contamination by microbial or chemical agents during any of the production stages can also lead to deterioration in safety and quality. Medicinal plants collected from the wild population may be contaminated by other species or plant parts through mis-identification, accidental contamination or intentional adulteration, all of which may have unsafe consequences.

At a WHO Informal Meeting on Methodologies for Quality Control of Finished Herbal Products, held in Ottawa, Canada from 20–21 July 2001, the entire process of production of herbal medicines, from raw materials to finished herbal products, was reviewed. It was recommended that WHO should give high priority to the development of globally applicable guidelines so as to promote the safety and quality of medicinal plant materials through the formulation of codes for good agricultural practices and good collection practices for medicinal plants.

3.4.1.2 Objectives

The main objectives of these guidelines are to

- Contribute to the quality assurance of medicinal plant materials used as the source for herbal medicines, which aims to improve the quality, safety and efficacy of the finished herbal products;
- Guide the formulation of national and/or regional Good Agricultural and Collection Practices (GACP) guidelines and GACP monographs for medicinal plants and related standard operating procedures; and
- Encourage and support the sustainable cultivation and collection of medicinal plants of good quality in ways that respect and support the conservation of medicinal plants and the environment in general.

These guidelines should be considered in conjunction with the existing documents and publications relating to the quality assurance of herbal medicines and to the conservation of medicinal plants.

Selection of medicinal plants

Where applicable, the species or botanical variety selected for cultivation should be the same as that specified in the national pharmacopoeia or recommended by other authoritative national documents of the end-user's country. In the absence of such national documents, the selection of species or botanical varieties specified in the pharmacopoeia or other authoritative documents of other countries should be considered.

Botanical identity

The botanical identity — scientific name (genus, species, subspecies/variety, author, and family) — of each medicinal plant under cultivation should be verified and recorded.

Specimens

In the case of the first registration in a producer's country of a medicinal plant or where reasonable doubt exists as to the identity of a botanical species, a voucher botanical specimen should be submitted to a regional or national herbarium for identification. Where possible, a genetic pattern should be compared to that of an authentic specimen. Documentation of the botanical identity should be included in the registration file.

Seeds and other propagation materials

Seeds and other propagation materials should be specified, and suppliers of seeds and other propagation materials should provide all necessary information relating to the identity, quality and performance of their products, as well as their breeding history, where possible.

Cultivation

The conditions and duration of cultivation required vary depending on the quality of medicinal plant materials required. If no scientific published or documented cultivation data are available, traditional methods of cultivation should be followed, where feasible. Otherwise a method should be developed through research.

Site selection

Medicinal plant materials derived from the same species can show significant differences in quality when cultivated at different sites, owing to the influence of soil, climate and other factors. Risks of contamination as a result of pollution of the soil, air or water by hazardous chemicals should be avoided.

Ecological environment and social impact

The cultivation of medicinal plants may affect the ecological balance and, in particular, the genetic diversity of the flora and fauna in surrounding habitats. The quality and growth of medicinal plants can also be affected by other plants, other living organisms and by human activities. The social impact of cultivation on local communities should be examined to ensure that negative impacts on local livelihood are avoided.

Climate

The duration of sunlight, average rainfall, average temperature, including daytime and night-time temperature differences, influence the physiological and biochemical activities of plants, and prior knowledge should be considered.

Soil

Optimal soil conditions, including soil type, drainage, moisture retention, fertility and pH, will be dictated by the selected medicinal plant species and/or target medicinal plant part. The use of fertilisers is often indispensable in order to obtain large yields of medicinal plants. It is, however, necessary to ensure that correct types and quantities of fertilisers are used through agricultural research. Human excreta must not be used as a fertiliser owing to the potential presence of infectious microorganisms or parasites.

Irrigation and drainage

Irrigation and drainage should be controlled and carried out in accordance with the needs of the individual medicinal plant species during its various stages of growth.

Plant maintenance and protection

The timely application of measures such as topping, bud nipping, pruning and shading may be used to control the growth and development of the plant, thereby improving the quality and quantity of the medicinal plant material being produced. Integrated pest management should be followed where appropriate. When necessary, only approved pesticides and herbicides should be applied at the minimum effective level.

Harvest

The time of harvest depends on the plant part to be used. Detailed information concerning the appropriate timing of harvest is often available in national pharmacopoeias, published standards, official monographs and major reference books. It is well known that the concentration of biologically active constituents varies with the stage of plant growth and development.

Personnel

Growers and producers should have adequate knowledge of the medicinal plant concerned. This should include botanical identification, cultivation characteristics and environmental requirements (soil type, soil pH, fertility, plant spacing and light requirements), as well as the means of harvest and storage.

Good collection practices for medicinal plants should be included. These include permission to collect, technical planning, selection of medicinal plants for collection and collection procedures.

It is appropriate to point out this time that GAP, apart from giving general principles of growing medicinal herbs, attempts also to recommend standard operating procedures. However, no matter how comprehensive the recommendations could be meant, they are only general conceptual guidelines that specific cultivations need to take reference, and each and every different herb should ideally develop its own guidelines (Huang *et al.*, 2002a).

3.5 European Union Recommendations

The European Union has taken equivalent concerns over the cultivation of medicinal herbs, and basing on different country's past experience, the union drafted its own recommendations that bear different emphasis.

Good Agricultural and Collection Practice (GACP) for Starting Materials of Herbal Origin was released by the European Agency for the Evaluation of Medicinal Products (EMEA) in May 2002 after providing interested parties with the opportunity to comment (EMEA, 2002). The rules were prepared by EMEA's Working Party on Herbal Medicinal Products starting in January 1999. They were written on the basis of a draft made by the European growers association, Europam.

GAP applies to the first part of the production, for which Good Manufacturing Practice (GMP) does not apply, that is, growing the plant material and primary processing. From that point on, the starting material is ready for the pharmaceutical production process, and GMP applies.

Applying GAP eliminates or reduces the risks of microbiological or chemical contamination, mistaken identity and adulteration, and deterioration during primary processing and storage. Eliminating and reducing these risks enhances the reliability of the starting materials used in the production of herbal medicines.

If a set of GAP rules would provide for measures to increase the reproducibility of the starting material, it could help increase the reproducibility and reliability of herbal medicines made from the plant materials. In a certain way, the European Union GAP does so by preventing the use of low-quality starting materials, such as rotten plants, cross-contaminated material, or the use of other species by adulteration.

However, variations within one species can be very high if no special measures are taken to standardise the plant material. This variation can lead to batch-to-batch variation of the plant material, which, in most cases, could influence the batch-to-batch activity of the herbal medicine made from it. Such variation in activity will have a negative impact on the reliability and the good name of herbal therapy.

Korthout *et al.* compared the constituents of ginkgo biloba at sunrise and sunset (Korthout *et al.*, 2002). They harvested ginkgo leaf at sunrise and sunset and compared the extracts with thin layer chromatography. They used specific colouring for ginkgolides and bilobalides, for flavonoids, and for biflavonoids and measured the colour intensity of each as a function of the Rf value. They found a difference in ginkgolide and bilobalide composition between sunset and sunrise. Ginkgolide A and B levels and bilobalide levels increased, while other substances in this group remained almost unchanged.

The usual way to deal with batch-to-batch variation in the present herbal medicine production is to standardise the primary extract or the end-product by diluting and/or mixing it with other batches. However, in many situations, this kind of adjustment might not be sufficient to obtain a product of optimal reliability.

Measures to standardise the starting material depend upon whether the material is cultivated or collected. Since cultivation provides more possibilities for standardisation, it is preferred.

Medicinal cannabis in the Netherlands has been quoted as an example. The Netherlands has a policy of developing a licensed medicinal product based on cannabis (Scholten, 2000). To supply pharmaceutical companies developing such products with reliable starting material, the government has contracted with several growers. They operate under contract and have a controlled substance license under the condition that they apply an extended version of European Union GAP. Apart from security measures to prevent diversion, there are rules for standardised cultivation.

It is clear from the European Union's Recommendations that Europe is concerned more with drug production arising from the use of plant substances. The term "starting material" is firmly adopted. Different "starting materials" requires different sets of recommendations and regulation. The scope of concern in Europe, therefore, is within narrower boundaries as compared with the wide use of herbs in Asia. Examples quoted like cannabis and ginkgo biloba serve well the unique nature of separate consideration (Itenov *et al.*, 1999). In contrast, although the general rules are set for GAP in China and the recommended date of implementation is November 2003, there will be a long way before the commonly used items will set their own recommendation in order to ensure guaranteed qualities, when used either in treatment procedures or as "starting material". There should be no assumption, that since the GAP recommendation are set, the supply of herbal products would enjoy better or uniform quality immediately. One needs to realise at the same time that the establishment of so-called GAP farms or foundations refers to the cultivation of one medicinal plant only. The following section is taking a realistic look into the current GAP situation in China.

3.6 The Current Situation of GAP in China

The establishment of GAP recommendations is a world trend basing on practical needs. China had a quick response to the need and drafted its own recommendations in 2002. It has been said that China's timely response must be related to trade considerations. According to world statistics, there is an annual sales value of US$15 billion for traditional medicine in the world market. However, China receives only a sales value of US$600 million, i.e. only 3% in the international market. In fact, a good proportion of these sales is related to health supplements, vitamins, food items and herbal products, which actually find their origin in Europe. However, it is still logical to assume that China, with its strong tradition on alternative medicine, could have done better. The loss in the race for herbal products sales value, has been attributed to the improper efforts given on quality control and standardisation. Hence, a quick redemption might be possible with quick measures to boost up the proper standardisation of medicinal herbs. This consideration must have formed a strong support to the GAP establishment (Bai, 2002).

While Europe's need for medicinal herbs has been understood mainly as "starting materials" in drug manufacturing and the items of concern are much less compared with the popular herbs used in Chinese Medicine, one would expect that the European recommendations might be too simplistic for China. It has been said that GAP recommendations in China are essentially stimulated by the Japanese and European experience (Guo, 2004). If it were true, the implementation in China would follow a much more complicated course.

Since the announcement of the GAP recommendations in China in 2002, another draft "Chinese Medicinal Plant GAP Evaluation Standards" was issued in September 2003. This document outlined the details of GAP, the what-to-do's and what not-to-do's, the eligible parties and those not eligible. In fact, many GAP bases have been established, pending evaluation. The following table contains some of the known bases (SFMB, 2002).

GAP Bases	Cultivated Medicinal Plants
Anhui province	*Paeonia suffruticosa*
Chongqing	*Pinellia ternata*
Gansu province	*Angelica sinensis*
Guangxi province	*Momordica grosvenorii*
GuiZhou province	*Dendrobium candidum*; *Eucommia ulmoides*; *Ginkgo biloba*
Hebei province	*Angelica dahurica*; *Scutellaria baicalensis*
Heilonjiang province	*Panax ginseng*
Henan province	*Rehmannia glutinosa*
Hubei province	*Lespedeza cyrtobotrya*
Hunan province	*Eucommia ulmoides*
Inner Mongolia	*Glycyrrhiza uralensis*
Jiangsu province	*Chrysanthemum morifolium*
Jiling province	*Panax ginseng*; *Panax quinquefolium*
Liaoning province	Panax ginseng
Ningxia province	*Lycium chinensis*
Shandong province	*Lonicera japonica*
Shanghai	*Crocus sativus*
Shanxii province	*Salvia miltiorrhiza*
Sichuan province	*Crocus sativus*; *Ligusticum chuanxiong*
Tibet province	*Rhodiola rosea*
Yunnan province	*Dracaena draco*; *Panax notoginseng*

Some GAP bases of Chinese Materia Medica in China (2003).

List of GAP (Good Agricultural Practice) Bases and Companies in China

Company	Species	Producing Areas	Condition	Announcement Date
1. Shanxi TASLY Plants Pharmaceutical Co., Ltd. 陝西天士立植物藥業有限責任公司	*Radix Salviae Miltiorrhizae* 丹參	Shan Xi Province, Shangluo City 陝西省商洛市	Pass	16 March 2004
2. Daphnenotoginseng Pharmaceutical Co., Ltd. 雲南特安吶三七產業股份有限公司	*Radix Notoginseng* 三七	Yunnan Province, Wenshan, Mashan, Yanshan County 雲南省文山縣、馬關縣、硯山縣	Pass	16 March 2004
3. Henan Wanxi Pharmaceutical Co., Ltd. 南陽張仲景山茱萸有限責任公司	*Fructus Corni* 山茱萸	Henan Province, Xixia County 河南省西峽縣	Pass	16 March 2004

List of GAP (Good Agricultural Practice) Bases and Companies in China

Company	Species	Producing Areas	Condition	Announcement Date
4. Sichuan Yanan Sanjiu Material Medica Co., Ltd. 四川雅安三九中藥材科技產業化有限公司	*Herba Houttuyniae* 魚腥草	Sichuan Province, YaAn City 四川省雅安市雨城區	Pass	16 March 2004
5. Sichuan Yanan Sanjiu Material Medica Co., Ltd. 四川雅安三九中藥材科技產業化有限公司	*Radix Ophiopogonis* 麥冬	Sichuan Province, YaAn City 四川省雅安市雨城區	Pass	16 March 2004
6. Anhui Province Yangbaishan Isatis Technical Development Co., Ltd. 安徽省陽白山板藍根技術開發有限公司	*Radix Isatidis* 板藍根	Anhui Province, Taihe County 安徽省太和縣	Pass	16 March 2004
7. Jilin Province American Ginseng Group Co., Ltd. 吉林省西洋參集團有限公司	*Radix Panacis Quinquefolii* 西洋參	Jilin Province, Jingyu County 吉林省靖宇縣	Pass	16 March 2004

List of GAP (Good Agricultural Practice) Bases and Companies in China

Company	Species	Producing Areas	Condition	Announcement Date
8. Beijing Tongrentang Co., Ltd. 北京同仁堂吉林人參有限責任公司	*Radix Ginseng* 人參	Jilin Province, Jingyu, Linjiang County 吉林省靖宇縣、臨江縣	Pass	16 March 2004
9. Shanghai Hua Yu Pharmaceutical Co., Ltd. 上海華宇藥業有限公司	*Stigma Croci* 西紅花	Shanghai Baoshan County, Chanxing, Chongming Island 上海市寶山區長興島、崇明島	Pass	29 December 2004
10. Jiangxi Huiren Tang Traditional Chinese Medicine Co. Ltd. 江西匯仁堂中藥飲片有限公司	*Fructus Gardeniae* 梔子	Xinggan County, Zhangshu City, Jiangxi Province 江西省樟樹市新干縣	Pass	29 December 2004
11. Chongqing Huayans Natural Sources Developing Co. Ltd. 重慶市華陽自然資源開發有限責任公司	*Herba Artemisiae Annuae* 青蒿	Youyang County, Chongqing 重慶市酉陽縣	Pass	29 December 2004

List of GAP (Good Agricultural Practice) Bases and Companies in China

Company	Species	Producing Areas	Condition	Announcement Date
12. Gansu Province Agricultural Cultivation Group Co. Ltd. 甘肅省農墾集團有限責任公司	*Pericarpium Papaveris* 罌粟殼	Wuwei City, Zhangye City, Jinchang City and Baiyin City, Gansu Province 甘肅省武威市、張掖市、金昌市、白銀市	Pass	29 December 2004
13. Chongqing Shizhu Coptis Rhizome Co. Ltd. 重慶石柱黃連有限公司	*Rhizoma Coptidis* 黃連	Shizhu Tujia Tribe, Autonomous County, Chongqing 重慶市石柱土家族自治縣	Pass	29 December 2004
14. Beijing Tong Ren Tang Traditional Chinese Medicinal Materials Co. Ltd. (Zhejiang Branch) 北京同仁堂浙江中藥材有限公司	*Fructus Corni* 山茱萸	ZhunAn County, Linan City, Zhejiang Province 浙江省臨安市，淳安縣	Pass	29 December 2004

List of GAP (Good Agricultural Practice) Bases and Companies in China

Company	Species	Producing Areas	Condition	Announcement Date
15. Jilin Changbai Shenlong Group Co. Ltd. 吉林長白參隆集團有限公司	*Radix Ginseng* 人參	Chengbai County, Jelin Province 吉林省長白縣寶泉山參場種植區、尼粒河參場種植區、馬鹿溝參場種植區	Pass	29 December 2004
16. Qingyuan Bai Yun Shan Creation Technical Developing Co. Ltd. 清遠白雲山穿心蓮技術開發有限公司	*Herba Andrographis* 穿心蓮	Yinde City, Qing Yuan, Guangdong Province 廣東省清遠英德市	Pass	29 December 2004
17. Honghe Qian Shan Biotechnics Co. Ltd. 千山生物工程有限公司	*Herba Erigerontis* 燈盞花	Luxi County, Yunan Province 雲南省瀘西縣	Pass	29 December 2004

List of GAP (Good Agricultural Practice) Bases and Companies in China

Company	Species	Producing Areas	Condition	Announcement Date
18. Foping Hanjiang Cornel Scientific & Technical Developing Co. Ltd. 佛坪漢江山茱萸科技開發有限責任公司	*Fructus Corni* 山茱萸	Foping County, Shanxi Province 陝西省佛坪縣	Pass	29 December 2004
19. Guizhou Province Qian Dong Nan Xingban Traditional Chinese Medicine Co. Ltd. 貴州省黔東南州信邦中藥飲片有限責任公司	*Radix Polygoni Mulitiflori* 何首烏	Shibin County, Chongjian County, Guangdong Town, Jingping County, Tongqu Town, Danzhai Town, and Kaili City, Guizhou Province 貴州省施秉縣，從江縣、貫洞鎮，錦屏縣、銅鼓鎮、敦寨鎮，凱裏市	Pass	22 June 2005

List of GAP (Good Agricultural Practice) Bases and Companies in China

Company	Species	Producing Areas	Condition	Announcement Date
20. Guizhou Province Qian Dong Nan Xingban Traditional Chinese Medicine Co. Ltd. Jiangzhong Pseudostellaria Root Branch 貴州省黔東南州信邦中藥飲片有限責任公司江中太子參分公司	*Radix Pseudostellariae* 太子參	Shibin County, Maxi Township, Baidao Township Huangping County, Leishan County and Kaili City, Guizhou Province 貴州省施秉縣、馬溪鄉、白垛鄉，黃平縣，雷山縣，凱裏市	Pass	22 June 2005
21. Shangdong DingLi Traditional Chinese Medicinal Materials Sciences & Technology Co. Ltd. 山東鼎立中藥材科技有限公司	*Radix Platycodonis* 桔梗	Qi Yuan County, Shan Dong Province 山東省沂源縣三岔鄉	Pass	22 June 2005

List of GAP (Good Agricultural Practice) Bases and Companies in China

Company	Species	Producing Areas	Condition	Announcement Date
22. Beijing Tong Ren Tang Lingchuan Radix Codonopsis Co. Ltd. 北京同仁堂陵川黨參有限責任公司	*Radix Codonopsis* 黨參	Linquan Town, Chongwen Township Linshuan County Province, Shanxi 山西省陵川縣六泉鄉、崇文鎮	Pass	22 June 2005
23. Zhejiang Kang Lai Te Group Co. Ltd. 浙江康萊特集團有限公司	*Semen Coicis* 薏苡仁	Guihu Town, Shiyang Town, Taishun County Zhejiang Province 浙江省泰順縣龜湖鎮、仕陽鎮	Pass	22 June 2005
24. An Kang Beiyida Pingli Fireleaf Gynostemma Co. Ltd. 安康北醫大平利絞股藍有限公司	*Gynostemma pentaphyllum* 絞股藍	Chengan Town, Pingli Country, An Kang Shanxi Province 陝西安康平利縣長安鎮	Pass	22 June 2005

List of GAP (Good Agricultural Practice) Bases and Companies in China

Company	Species	Producing Areas	Condition	Announcement Date
25. Zhejiang Tiantai Institute of Traditional Chinese Medicine 浙江省天臺縣中藥藥物研究所	*Herba Dendrodii Officinalis* 鐵皮石斛	Tiantai County, Zhejiang Province 浙江天臺縣麗澤基地、田洋陳基地、西方洋基地、後洋基地	Pass	22 June 2005
26. Quality Traditional Chinese Medicinal Materials Breeding Co. Ltd., Yunnan Baiyao Group 雲南白藥集團中藥材優質種源繁育有限責任公司	*Radix Notoginseng* 三七	Matong Town, Wenshan, Yunnan Province 雲南省文山州文山縣馬塘鎮、德厚鄉，馬關縣夾寒鄉	Pass	22 June 2005

Note: GAP list is increasing with more and more approved items.

Since April 2004, there had been three State Food and Drug Administration (SFDA) reports (http://www.sfda.gov.cn) in which 26 medicinal plant producers were qualified for GAP evaluations. These items were selectively chosen from a bigger group of GAP bases.

As a matter of fact, a total of 600 medicinal plantations have already been established since 1999, out of which 60 standard plantations of important medicinal plant species were registered and official recognition gradually followed (Guo, 2004).

Looking at the GAP Evaluation Standards, the checklist appears strict and demanding. However, academics and professional in the field are critical about their suitability for China. The GAP Evaluation Standards contain 104 items of inspection, 19 of which are crucial; a single failure to reach the standard would mean disqualification. Of the other items of inspection, 85 are less demanding and could be selectively spared. Standards are obviously vague.

In China, it is estimated that there are currently over one million families growing medicinal plants as their main source of income. They own small plots of land, and their harvests are collected by traders; 95% of farm land cultivating herbal plants are served by these peasants, and the remaining 5% of land are developed by about 2000 medicinal plant dealers. The GAP evaluation is available to the registered dealers only. That means only 5% of the medicinal plantations are qualified for GAP development, whereas the majority, i.e. 95% are deprived of GAP opportunities (Zhou, 2003; Zhou *et al.*, 2004).

The GAP initiative is not enjoying harmony with some other policies implemented since 1985. For example, there are 17 Chinese medicinal material trade markets endorsed in different provinces. Medicinal plant growers have been encouraged to sell their products in those markets. How does the new GAP initiative harmonise with the practical trading venues that are enjoying good businesses? If most of the medicinal material trading to-date goes through the 17 markets, how does GAP contribute towards the medicinal plant market in China?

There is another dilemma. The Department of Health in China has, since decades ago, categorised about 100 plant items as both food and medicine. Examples include *semen coicis*, *rhizoma dioscoreae*, *radix angelicae dahuricae*, *radix codonopsis*, and *radix glyeyrrhizae*. These items are recommended to be consumed as food or medicine, and they compose of over 30% of medicinal plants artificially cultivated. How does the GAP initiative harmonise with this established practice?

It is therefore observed that when over 80% of cultivation land for medicinal plants and 95% of farmers involved in the plantation are not included under the GAP initiative, the outcome would be worrying. When the majority of peasants involved in the medicinal herbs are not included under the GAP initiative, only a small number of items of herbs could go through the evaluation processes. In fact, visitors returning from the few GAP farms growing special items reported that, indeed, registered firms still have to rely on individual peasants to supply the specific products. The peasants do receive special instructions on the essential agricultural requirements, both general and specific to the special item, but how the required standard is being practiced and evaluated are still uncertain.

Concerned professionals in China have expressed their views and made observations:

(1) The GAP initiative will not be able to elevate the quality standard of medicinal herbs because the coverage is too limited. In contrast, poor quality products might hide under the protection of the GAP principles and unfairly win marketing priorities.
(2) GAP-evaluated products might enjoy unqualified benefits. GAP-evaluated products enjoy the hallmark of certified quality which they may not deserve. The cost for evaluation, however, would be added to the primary costs, thus pushing the price up.
(3) The monopoly of GAP-evaluated products might lead to new problems. The popular items will enjoy priority in the GAP evaluation. A state of monopoly is likely to appear in no time. A perfect guarantee to the supply will be required.
(4) Discrepancies between the conventional ways of cultivation well familiar with the peasants and the GAP recommendations might be too critical to be born by the peasants.
(5) When the main crop growers in China are well subsidised by the state with the new national agricultural policy, medicine plant growers might give up their familiar commitment and shift over to the growing of main crops.

(6) The GAP qualification is really too much of an attraction so that malpractice is highly likely in an immature system (Ma *et al.*, 2002).

Other concerned professionals have made constructive suggestions:

(1) Establish a National Bureau for the control of medicinal plant production.
(2) Train more professional experts in the field of medicinal plants, and
(3) Strengthen the already existing 17 trading markets for herbal medicinal material and introduce systems of quality control there (Zhou *et al.*, 2004).

It is becoming clear that the GAP initiative in China is encouraging a tripartite co-operation, which involves the registered dealers, the agricultural production site owners and the medicinal plant growers. The leader is the registered dealer who controls the production processes and thence the products. Traditionally, all three areas are not closely linked. The new requirements will have to go through long processes of adaptation, re-organisation and investment (Li, 2005; Wai *et al.*, 2004).

3.6.1 *How long will it take?*

The first few years of GAP in China, did not appear to have brought breakthroughs in the expectation of better quality control of medicinal plants. With the complexity of the large varieties of medicinal herbs, the slow advances might be expected. Whatever the immediate outcome and irrespective of any negative effects coming out from the initiatives, one has no doubt that the direction is a right one. The need to maintain reliable quality is the universal direction towards the supply of medicinal plants. The message will be clear and sound to all levels involved: suppliers, collectors, traders and peasants alike. Immediate solid improvement might be seen only after some time, but the benefits are sure to come; perhaps more rapidly with more facilitations from the state level.

3.6.2 *Short of GAP, what need to be done?*

Before the good days will come, we need to be aware of the deficiencies and do our best to get the best possible supply of herbal samples. *Daodi* samples were supplied in the old days as reliable quality material. *Daodi* supplies are still understood as the best and are genuine if the production sites have not changed and the quality of supply has not changed in the past decades under the ruthless insults of weather changes, soil loss, pollutions, over-harvesting and other mischievance practices. The best supplier 20 years ago might no longer be the best today. The old *Daodi* concept relies on trust and historical reputation. Now that the *Daodi* concept might have to be given up, we could only rely on science and technology. Until the maturation of GAP, which guarantees to a large extent a quality supply, we have to set our own quality data bank. The most commonly used medicinal herbs should possess a reliable record of its chemical profile, i.e. indications of its main chemical components that are considered to be responsible for the main biological activities of the herbs. Any new supply of the same herb, be it from a *Daodi* source, reputable supplier, with special arrangement or off the street purchase, could be subjected to qualitative chemical evaluation (spectrometry) to establish the chemical profile. This profile will be cross-checked with reliable standards and the data will be stored up for future references, in the case research needs to be replanned or repeated. The progression onto drug production would naturally require such information as well.

Chemical profiling is only a basic test. For further in-depth investigation, DNA profiles will serve as additional safeguards on quality authentication. In fact, until the active components from a medicinal plant becomes known, extracted and used as active treatment agents, when uniformity becomes inevitable, authentication and establishment of the identity profiles will remain mandatory. GAP, therefore, is undoubtedly a great advance, but will need to be supported by authentication on all levels, currently and in the coming years.

References

Bai, H.L. (2002) People's Daily on-line, http://english.peopledaily.com.cn/20020514.

European Agency for the Evaluation of Medicinal Products (2002) Points to consider on Good Agricultural and Collection Practice for Starting Materials of Herbal Origin. May 2002, EMEA/HMPWP/31/99 rev.3.

Gao, W., Jia, W. and Duan, H. (2002) Good Agricultural Practice (GAP) and Sustainable Resource Utilisation of Chinese Materia Medica. *J. Plant Biotechnol.* **4**(3), 103–107.

Good Agricultural Practice for Chinese Crude Drugs (2002) State Food and Medicine Bureau of Control and Regulations. State Drug Administration, Order 32 of SDA.

Guo, G.K. (2004) GAP of Chinese herbs — research and development. *China New Med.* **3**(9), 84.

Huang, L.Q., Cui, G.H. and Chen, M.L. (2002a) Study on complex system of Chinese Materia Medica GAP fulfilling, the situation, problems and prospects. *China J. Chin. Mater. Med.* **27**, 481–483.

Huang, L.Q., Cui, G.H. and Dai, R.W. (2002b) Study on complex system of Chinese Materia Medica GPP fulfilling. *China J. Chin. Mater. Med.* **27**, 1–3.

Itenov, K., Molgaard, P. and Nyman, U. (1999) Diurnal fluctuations of alkaloid concentration in latex of poppy Papaver. *Phytochemistry* **52**, 1229–1234.

Korthout, H.A.A.J., Benkelman, C.J. and Wang, M. (2002) *Varieties in Samenstelling Secundaire Metabolieten in Ginkgo Biloba.* Internal Report Netherlands Organisation for Applied Scientific Research TNO, Leiden.

Li, Y. (2005) *The Practicality of GAP Evaluation in China*. Evaluation Forum 03, pp. 51–53.

Lo, L. and Pun, G.K. (2005) The importance of GAP in the modernisation of Chinese medicine. *Chin. Arch. Tradit. Chin. Med.* **23**(4), 716–719.

Ma, S.J., Chen, S.L. and Sung, J.Y. (2002) Difficults in GAP implementation for Chinese medicinal plants. *GAP Res. Pract.* **2**(4), 3–6.

Qin, L.P., Huang, B.K. and Zheng, H.C. (2001) Background, present situation, problem and tactics of GAP of Chinese Materia Medica. *Yaoxue Shijian Zachi* **19**, 67–70.

Scholten, W.K. (2000) Legal aspects on medicinal use of hemp. *Drug Info. J.* **34**(1), 329–332.

Scholten, W.K. (2003) The New European Union Good Agricultural and Collection Practice Rules. *Drug Info. J.* **37**, 321–327.

Shiu, T.C., Shen, Y.H. and Dai, Y. (2005) GAP for medicinal plants — publications and analysis. *Chin. J. Med. Libr. Inf. Sci.* **14**(2), 59–61.

Wai, J.H., Chan, S.L. and Guo, K.S. (2004) Implementation of GAP in China. *Res. Info. Tradit. Chin. Med.* **6**(9), 4–8.

Wang, L.X. and Xiao, L.L. (2000) Significance of medicinal botany to the conservation of endangered species. In: *Conservation of Endangered Medicinal Wildlife Resources in China* (eds.) Zhang, E.D. and Zheng, H.C. Second Military Medical University Press, Shanghai, China, pp. 83–86.

Wang, W.Q., Lin, C.S. and Sun, Z.R. (1999) The study of GAP and its application in TCM. *Tradit. Chin. Med.* **3**(10), 14–16.

World Health Organization (2003) *WHO Guidelines on Good Agricultural and Collection Practices (GACP) for Medicinal Plants*. WHO publication.

Yuan, C.Q., Wang, N.H. and Lu, Y. (2000) Conservation of endangered medicinal plants in China. In: *Conservation of Endangered Medicinal Wildlife Resources in China*. (eds.) Zhang, E.D. and Zheng, H.C. Second Military Medical University Press, Shanghai, China, pp. 25–32.

Zhan, N.P. and Lin, R.C. (2002) The establishment of SOP for different Chinese Materia Medica in China. *Res. Info. Tradit. Chin. Med.* **3**(3), 15–17.

Zhou, C.M. (2003) Foundations of Chinese medicinal plants cultivation. *Mod. Res. Pract. Chin. Med.* **17**(2), 8–10.

Zhou, C.M., Kun, K.K. and Fu, K.Q. (2004) Thoughts and suggestions on the evaluation of GAP of Chinese medicinal plants. *World Sci. Technol./ Modern. Tradit. Chin. Med. Mater. Med.* **6**(5), 66–75.

Zhou, R.H. (2001) Improve the process of GAP application in TCM in China. *Foreign Med. Plant Drug* **16**, 5–7.

Zou, T.C. (2001) Studies on investigation and utilisation of medicinal plant germ plasma resources for sustainable development in Guizhou. China *J. Guizhou Normal Univ.* **19**, 1–11.

Chapter 4

Supply and Cultivation of Medicinal Plants in Japan

Zhongzhen Zhao, Zhijun Yang & Osamu Iida

Abstract

The supply of Chinese herbal medicine has evolved from wild to mainly cultivation-oriented. In order to ensure sufficient supply and reliable quality, it is very important to carry out Good Agricultural Practice (GAP) of medicinal plants. This article summarises the market status of *Kampo* medicines in Japan, the general status of cultivation of medicinal plants in Japan, the main content of technical guidelines on cultivation of medicinal plants in Japan, and Japan Good Agricultural Practices (J-GAP). The content offers some references for other countries to bring GAP into practice.

Keywords: Cultivation of Medicinal Plants; Japan; GAP; J-GAP; Chinese Herbal Medicine; Quality Control.

Japan is one of the foremost countries that produces and uses Chinese herbal medicine, where they are known as "*Kampo*". Since September 1976, when part of the formulated preparations of *Kampo* medicine were officially adopted for medical insurance, the demand for crude drugs has dramatically increased (Dai and Zhao, 1998). In 1988, Japan initiated a project named "Investigation of the actual situation, and preparation of the guidelines for quality evaluation of the cultivation of medicinal herbs", which has already standardised the cultivation of 67 kinds of the herb. In April 2005, Japan Good Agricultural Initiative called the first seminar of Japan Good Agricultural Practice (J-GAP); and, the benchmark of manufacturing management of the J-GAP was constituted before the seminar (J-GAP, 2005). During this period, Japan has invested considerable effort in developing cultivation techniques and standardisation of medicinal plants that are very successful, and has accumulated rich experience. Japan is an herb consumer and also a highly developed, densely populated country; there is no doubt that Japanese GAP experience on the herb should be valuable as a global reference for herbal cultivation.

4.1 The Market Status of *Kampo* Medicines in Japan

Japan has a big market for traditional medicine. Since 1976, 210 formulated preparations of *Kampo* medicine have been gradually adopted in Japan's national health assurance system. Then, the cultivation of medicinal plants, production industry of *Kampo* medicine have quickly developed in Japan, making it the other great nation of natural medicine besides China (Zhao and Hu, 1996).

The Japan Society for Oriental Medicine has grown nearly 100-fold from the original 98 founding members to 9165, of whom 7416 are medical doctors. The people treating patients with *Kampo* are required by Japan's medical system to be qualified as physicians. It explains why *Kampo* therapy has become such a rapidly growing part of health care in Japan today. The development of extract forms of *Kampo* prescriptions in the 1950s greatly simplified the use of *Kampo* medicine and adapted it to modern life. Then, in 1967, four *Kampo* prescriptions were, for the first time, approved for reimbursement under Japan's national health insurance. An additional 42 prescriptions were added to the approved list in 1976, and the number expanded thereafter to reach 148. Valued at 9.5 billion yen in 1976, *Kampo* medicine production has grown to reach 1.2 trillion yen (about US$1 billion) in 1999. Beginning in 1991, Japan's Ministry of Health and Welfare initiated a programme of re-evaluating *Kampo* prescriptions, and a series of double-blind studies is being undertaken to corroborate their effectiveness. Three prescriptions have already been verified as effective for the indications specified: *Daio-kanzo-to* (constipation), *Sho-seiryu-to* (allergic rhinitis) and *Sho-saiko-to* (chronic hepatitis). *Kampo* prescriptions have proved particularly valuable for treating the multiple illnesses and complaints of the elderly, and have the additional attraction of playing a role in health maintenance. Thus, *Kampo* can be expected to

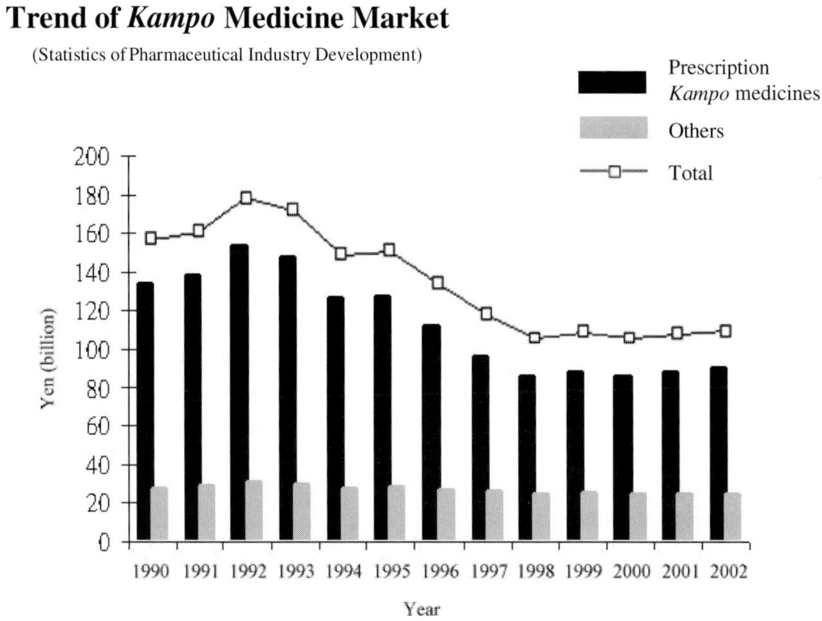

Fig. 4.1. Trend of *Kampo* Medicine Market (Japan *Kampo* Medicine Manufacturers Association, 2004).

play an increasingly important role in advancing health care for older people in Japan, where the population is ageing faster than in any other country (Tokyo International Forum, 1999).

The use of crude drugs in 1974 was 7094 tons; 20 years later, this number increased about 7.4 times to 52,817 tons. Despite the incident involving *Xiaochaihu* decoction, which led to a drop in the demand for crude drugs, the situation has become stable after some adjustments. Figure 4.1 shows the trend in the *Kampo* medicine market (Japan *Kampo* Medicine Manufacturers Association, 2004).

The Japanese Pharmacopoeia (14th Edition) recorded 130 crude drugs in 2001 (Table 4.1) (Japan Pharmaceutical Affairs Bureau, 2001). They are the official common crude drugs in Japan and are the highlights of research and cultivation as well. Currently, there are 390 crude drugs that circulate within Japan; among these, 361 are sourced from plants, making up 92.6% of the whole.

Table 4.1. List of crude drugs in *Japanese Pharmacopoeia* (14th Ed.).

Scientific Latin Name	Scientific Latin Name
1. *Acacia senegal* Willdenow	33. *Atropa belladonna* Linné
2. *Achyranthes bidentata* Blume	34. *Bupleurum falcatum* Linné (= *Bupleurum scorzonerifolium*)
3. *Achyranthes fauriei* Leveillé et Vaniot	
4. *Aconitum carmichaeli* Debeaux	35. *Caesalpinia sappan* Linné
5. *Aconitum japonicum* Thunberg	36. *Cannabis sativa* Linné
6. *Akebia quinata* Decaisne	37. *Capsicum annuum* Linné
7. *Akebia trifoliata* Koidzumi	38. *Carthamus tinctorius* Linné
8. *Alisma orientale* Juzepczuk	39. *Cassia acutifolia* Delile
9. *Aloe africana* Miller	40. *Cassia angustifolia* Vahl
10. *Aloe ferox* Miller	41. *Cassia obtusifolia* Linné
11. *Aloe spicata* Baker	42. *Cassia tora* Linné
12. *Alpinia officinarum* Hance	43. *Catalpa bungei* C.A. Meyer
13. *Alpinia oxyphylla* Miquel	44. *Catalpa ovata* G. Don
14. *Amomum xanthioides* Wallich	45. *Cephaelis acuminata* Karsten
15. *Anemarrhena asphodeloides* Bunge	46. *Cephaelis ipecacuanha* (Broterol) A. Richard
16. *Angelica acutiloba* Kitagawa	
17. *Angelica acutiloba* Kitagawa var. *sugiyamae* Hikino	47. *Chrysanthemum indicum* Linné
	48. *Chrysanthemum morifolium* Ramatulle
18. *Angelica dahurica* Bentham et Hooker	49. *Cimicifuga dahuriea* (Turcz.) Maximmowicz
19. *Arctium lappa* Linné	
20. *Arctostaphylos uva-ursi* (Linné) Sprengel	50. *Cimicifuga foetida* Linné
	51. *Cimicifuga heracleifolia* Komarov
21. *Areca catechu* Linné	52. *Cimicifuga simplex* Wormskjord
22. *Artemisia capillaris* Tunberg	53. *Cinnamomum cassia* Blume
23. *Asiasarum heterotropoides* F. Maekawa var. *mandshuricum* F. Maekawa	54. *Citrus aurantium* Linné
	55. *Citrus aurantium* Linné var. *daidai* Makino
24. *Asiasarum sieboldii* F. Maekawa	56. *Citrus natsudaidai* Hayata
25. *Asparagus cochinchinensis* Merrill	57. *Citrus reticulata* Blanco
26. *Astragalus gummifer* Labillardière	58. *Citrus unshiu* Markovich
27. *Astragalus membranaceus* Bunge	59. *Clematic hexapetala* Pallas
28. *Astragalus mongholicus* Bunge	60. *Clematis chinensis* Osbeck
29. *Atractylodes chinensis* Koidzumi	61. *Clematis manshurica* Ruprecht
30. *Atractylodes japonica* Koidzumi ex Kitamura	62. *Cnidium monnieri* Cusson
	63. *Cnidium officinale* Makino
31. *Atractylodes lancea* De Candolle	64. *Coix lacryman-jobi* Linné var. *ma-yuen* Stapf
32. *Atractylodes ovata* De Candolle	

Table 4.1. (*Continued*)

Scientific Latin Name	Scientific Latin Name
65. *Coptis chinensis* Franchet	96. *Forsythia viridissima* Lindley
66. *Coptis deltoidea* C.Y. Cheng et Hsiao	97. *Fritillaria verticillata* Willdenow var. *thunbergii* Baker (= *Fritillaria thunbergii* Miq.)
67. *Coptis japonica* Makino	
68. *Coptis teeta* Wallich	98. *Gardenia jasminoides* Ellis
69. *Cornus officinalis* Siebold et Zuccarini	99. *Gastrodia elata* Blume
	100. *Gelidium amansii* Lamouroux
70. *Corydalis turtschaninovii* Basser forma *yanhusuo* Y.H. Chou et C.C. Hsu	101. *Gentiana lutea* Linné
	102. *Gentiana manshurica* Kitagawa
	103. *Gentiana scabra* Bunge
71. *Crocus sativus* Linné	104. *Gentiana triflora* Pallas
72. *Curcuma longa* Linné	105. *Geranium thunbergii* Siebold et Zuccarini
73. *Curcuma zedoaria* Roscoe	
74. *Cyperus rotundus* Linné	106. *Glehnia littoralis* Fr. Schmidt ex Miquel
75. *Digenea simplex* C. Agardh	
76. *Dioscorea batatas* Decaisne	107. *Glycyrrhiza glabra* Linné
77. *Dioscorea japonica* Thunberg	108. *Glycyrrhiza uralensis* Fisher
78. *Elettaria cardamomum* Maton	109. *Houttuynia cordata* Thunberg
79. *Ephedra equisetina* Bunge	110. *Hydrangea macrophylla* Seringe var. *thunbergii* Makino
80. *Ephedra intermedia* Schrenk et C.A. Meyer	
	111. *Jateorhiza columba* Miers
81. *Ephedra sinica* Stapf	112. *Lindera strychnifolia* F. Villars (= *Lindera aggregata*)
82. *Epimedium brevicornum* Maximowicz	
	113. *Lithospermum erythrorhizon* Siebold et Zuccarini
83. *Epimedium grandiflorum* Morren var. *thunbergianum* Nakai	
	114. *Lonicera japonica* Thunberg
84. *Epimedium koreanum* Nakai	115. *Lycium barbarum* Linné
85. *Epimedium pubescens* Maximowicz	116. *Lycium chinense* Miller
86. *Epimedium sagittatum* Maximowicz	117. *Magnolia biondii* Pampanini
87. *Epimedium sempervirens* Nakai	118. *Magnolia denudata* Desrousseaux
88. *Epimedium wushanense* T.S. Ying	119. *Magnolia kobus* De Candolle
89. *Eriobotrya japonica* Lindley	120. *Magnolia obovata* Thunberg
90. *Eucommia ulmoides* Oliver	121. *Magnolia officinalis Rehder* et Wilson
91. *Evodia bodinieri* Dode	
92. *Evodia officinalis* Dode	122. *Magnolia officinalis* Rehder et Wilson var. *biloba* Rehder et Wilson
93. *Evodia rutaecarpa* Bentham	
94. *Foeniculum vulgare* Miller	
95. *Forsythia suspensa* Vahl	123. *Magnolia salicifolia* Maximowicz

Table 4.1. (*Continued*)

Scientific Latin Name	Scientific Latin Name
124. *Magnolia sprengeri* Pampanini	153. *Prunella vulgaris* Linné var. *lilacina* Nakai
125. *Mallotus japonica* Mueller Arg.	154. *Prunus armeniaca* Linné
126. *Marsdenia cundurango* Reichenbach fil.	155. *Prunus armeniaca* Linné var. *ansu* Maximowicz
127. *Mentha arvensis* Linné var. *piperascens* Malinvaud	156. *Prunus persica* Batsch
128. *Morus alba* Linné	157. *Prunus persica* Batsch var. *davidiana* Maximowicz (= *Prunus davidiana*)
129. *Notopterygium forbesii* Boissieu	158. *Pueraria lobata* Ohwi
130. *Notopterygium incisum* Ting ex H.T. Chang	159. *Rehmannia glutinosa* Liboschitz
131. *Nuphar japonicum* De Candolle	160. *Rehmannia glutinosa* Liboschitz var. *purpurea* Makino
132. *Ophiopogon japonicus* Ker–Gawler	161. *Rheum coreanum* Nakai
133. *Paeonia lactiflora* Pallas	162. *Rheum officinale* Baillon
134. *Paeonia suffruticosa* Andrews (*Paeonia moutan* Sims)	163. *Rheum palmatum* Linné
135. *Panax ginseng* C.A. Meyer (*Panax schinseng* Nees)	164. *Rheum tanguticum* Maximowicz
136. *Panax japonicus* C.A. Meyer	165. *Rosa multiflora* Thunberg
137. *Papaver somniferum* Linné	166. *Saposhnikovia divaricata* Schischkin
138. *Perilla frutescens* Britton var. *acuta* Kudo	167. *Saussurea lappa* Clarke
139. *Perilla frutescens* Britton var. *crispa* Decaisne	168. *Schisandra chinensis* Baillon
140. *Pharbitis nil* Choisy	169. *Schizonepeta tenuifolia* Briquet
141. *Phellodendron amurense* Ruprecht	170. *Scopolia carniolica* Jacquin
142. *Phellodendron chinense* Schneider	171. *Scopolia japonica* Maximowicz
143. *Picrasma quassioides* Bennet	172. *Scopolia parviflora* Nakai
144. *Pinellia ternata* Breitenbach	173. *Scutellaria baicalensis* Georgi
145. *Plantago asiatica* Linné	174. *Sinomenium acutum* Rehder et Wilson
146. *Platycodon grandiflorum* A. De Candolle	175. *Smilax glabra* Roxburgh
147. *Polygala senega* Linné	176. *Sophora flavescens* Ation
148. *Polygala senega* Linné var. *latifolia* Torrey et Gray	177. *Strychnos nux-vomica* Linné
149. *Polygala tenuifolia* Willdenow	178. *Styrax benzoin* Dryander
150. *Polygonum multiflorum* Thunberg	179. *Swertia japonica* Makino
151. *Polyporus umbellatus* Fries	180. *Syzygium aromaticum* Merrill et Perry (*Eugenia caryophyllata*)
152. *Poria cocos* Wolf	181. *Tribulus terrestris* Linné
	182. *Trichosanthes bracteata* Voigt
	183. *Trichosanthes kirilowii* Maximowicz

Table 4.1. (*Continued*)

Scientific Latin Name	Scientific Latin Name
184. *Trichosanthes kirilowii* Maximowicz var. *japonica* Kitamura	190. *Zanthoxylum piperitum* De Candolle
185. *Uncaria gambir* Roxburgh	191. *Zingiber officinale* Roscoe
186. *Uncaria macrophylla* Wallich	192. *Zizyphus jujuba* Miller var. *inermis* Rehder
187. *Uncaria rhynchophylla* Miquel	193. *Zizyphus jujuba* Miller var. *spinosa* (Bunge) Hu ex H.F. Chou
188. *Uncaria sinensis* Haviland	
189. *Valeriana fauriei* Briquet	

*Oils, starches, animals and minerals are excluded. Crude drugs described on 1st Supplement (2002) and 2nd Supplement (2004) are included in this list.

4.2 General Status of Cultivation of Medicinal Plants in Japan

As there are many concerns on the safety of medicinal plants, cultivation is the starting step to assure Chinese herbal medicine is produced in safe and good quality. Due to the rise of medicinal plant use, from Japan government to the public, more and more attention has been paid to the cultivation of Chinese medicine.

The National Institute of Health Sciences has five cultivation ranches from north to south: Hokkaido, Tsukuba, Wakayama, Izu and Tanegashima.

The crude drugs of Japan's *Kampo* medicines are mostly imported for preparation. As demand for production rises, implementation of setting up guidelines for cultivation techniques is essential in order to assure stable quantity and quality of the *Kampo* medicine.

Since the late 1980s, Japan has compiled a series of *Cultivation of Medicinal Plants and Quality Reviews*, which give guidelines on species selection and cultivation techniques, and serves as a guideline for GAP. Participants include experts from the National Institute of Health Sciences, scholars from universities, people from the *Kampo* industry and the *Kampo* Medicine Manufacturers Association. After more than ten years of work, 11 volumes have finally been published (Ministry of Health and Welfare, 1992–2005).

4.3 The Main Content of Technical Guidelines on Cultivation of Medicinal Plants in Japan

The published *Cultivation of Medicinal Plants and Quality Review* has 65 types, which can be seen in Table 4.2.

Its content prescribes the items as follows:

(1) Plant name: Japanese name (in Japanese Katakana), crude drug name (in Chinese character notation with Japanese pronunciation by Katakana) and Latin scientific name.
(2) Medicinally used parts: root, rhizome, stem, leave, flower, fruit and seed, etc.
(3) Morphological description: original species or imported species, habitat, geographical environment, morphology and systematic classification.
(4) Feature and place of origin: authentication feature and distribution area.
(5) Feature of cultivation: feature of plant during different growing stages, amount of active ingredients among different production area, distribution area and soil, climate criteria such as sun, soil, drainage and adaptability.
(6) Method of cultivation: breeding method, seeding and seedling, fertiliser, management, prevention from pest, harvest and manufacturing, seed storage and harvest rate. The contents of nitrogen, phosphorous, potassium in fertiliser are also recorded.
(7) Quality assessment: principally based on *The Japanese Pharmacopoeia*. Also prescribes the items about property, weight loss after dry, ash content, undissolved ash content. Marker of main active ingredients.
(8) Characteristic classification: classification based on seedlings and cultivating conditions.
(9) Diary of cultivation.
(10) Related information: background of seed, reference for cultivation methods, clinical application and formulation.

Table 4.2. Guidelines of cultivated medicinal plants in Japan (Ministry of Healh and Welfare, 1992–2005).

Scientific Latin Name	Scientific Latin Name
1. *Achyranthes bidentata* Blume	32. *Sinomenium acutum* Rehder et Wilson
2. *Achyranthes fauriei* Leveillé et Vaniot	33. *Foeniculum vulgare* Miller
3. *Aconitum carmichaeli* Debeaux	34. *Patrinia scabiosaefolia* Fischer
4. *Angelica acutiloba* Kitagawa	35. *Pinellia ternate* Breitenbach
5. *Arctostaphylos uva-ursi* (Linné) Sprengel	36. *Angelica dahurica* Bentham et Hooker
6. *Artemisia capillaris* Thunberg	37. *Lithospermum erythrorhizon* Siebold et Zuccarini
7. *Asiasarum sieboldii* F. Maekawa	38. *Lycium barbarum* Linné
8. *Astragalus membranaceus* Bunge	39. *Lycium chinense* Miller
9. *Atractylodes lancea* De Candolle	40. *Matricaria chamomilla* Linné
10. *Atractylodes ovata* De Candolle	41. *Paeonia lactiflora* Pallas
11. *Bupleurum falcatum* L.	42. *Paeonia suffruticosa* Andrews
12. *Carthamus tinctorius* Linné	43. *Panax ginseng* C.A. Meyer
13. *Cassia acutifolia* Delile	44. *Perilla frutescens* Britton var. *acuta* Kudo
14. *Cassia angustifolia* Vahl	45. *Phellodendron amurense* Ruprecht
15. *Cassia obtusifolia* Linné	46. *Plantago asiatica* L.
16. *Cnidium officinale* Makino	47. *Platycodon grandiflorum* A. De Candolle
17. *Coix lacryma-jobi* Linné var. *ma-yuen* Stapf	48. *Plectranthus japonicus* (Burm.) Koidzumi
18. *Coptis japonica* Makino	49. *Polygala senega* Linné var. *latifolia* Torrey et Gray
19. *Crocus sativus* Linné	50. *Poria cocos* Wolf
20. *Curcuma longa* Linné (= *Curcuma domestica* Valeton)	51. *Prunella vulgaris* Linné var. *lilacina* Nakai
21. *Curcuma zedoaria* Roscoe	52. *Rauwolfia serpentina* Bentham
22. *Ephedra sinica* Stapf	53. *Rehmannia glutinosa* Libosch. var. *purpurea* Makino
23. *Fritillaria verticillata* Willd. var. *thunbergii* Baker	54. *Rehmannia glutinosa* Libosch.
24. *Gardenia jasminoides* Ellis	55. *Rheum coreanum* Nakai
25. *Gentiana lutea* Linné	56. *Rheum officinale* Baillon
26. *Geranium thunbergii* Siebold et Zuccarini	57. *Rheum palmatum* L.
27. *Glycyrrhiza glabra* Linné	58. *Rheum tanguticum* Maxim.
28. *Glycyrrhiza uralensis* Fisher	59. *Saposhnikovia divaricata* Schischkin
29. *Houttuynia cordata* Thunberg	60. *Saussurea lappa* Clarke
30. *Lindera strychnifolia* F. Villars	61. *Schizonepeta tenuifolia* Briquet
31. *Foeniculum vulgare* Miller	

Table 4.2. (*Continued*)

Scientific Latin Name	Scientific Latin Name
62. *Scutellaria baicalensis* Georgi	65. *Uncaria rhynchophylla* Miquel
63. *Swertia japonica* Makino	66. *Valeriana fauriei* Briquet
64. *Trichosanthes bracteata* Voigt	67. *Zanthoxylum piperitum* De Candolle

4.4 Japan Good Agricultural Practices (J-GAP)

Because producing herbs is very closely related to agriculture, so here, the J-GAP is introduced (Scheme 4.1). In April 2005, the Japan Good Agricultural Initiative called the first seminar of Japan Good Agricultural Practice (J-GAP), and the benchmark of manufacturing management of the J-GAP was established before the seminar.

J-GAP enumerated four chapters as the concepts of J-GAP, the introduction of J-GAP, about the manufacturing management benchmark, and the manufacturing management benchmark. The main parts are the manufacturing management benchmark. As a reference of the cultivating of the herbs, here, the J-GAP manufacturing management benchmark is correspondingly introduced.

The J-GAP manufacturing management benchmark regulates the following ten sections:

(1) The manufacture management benchmark: This benchmark prescribes the items about the producing process, benchmark of the quality, the environments for the labouring, and the waste.
(2) The risk analysis benchmark: This benchmark prescribes the items about the background of the cropland, the barnyard manure, the water quality, the essential protection measures for the crop, the sanitation during the ingathering, the sanitation for the harvest, the health and safety of the labourers, and the contamination of the agriculture to the environment.
(3) The seeds and saplings management benchmark: This benchmark prescribes the guidelines about the seeds and saplings, management of seeds, and growing seedlings.

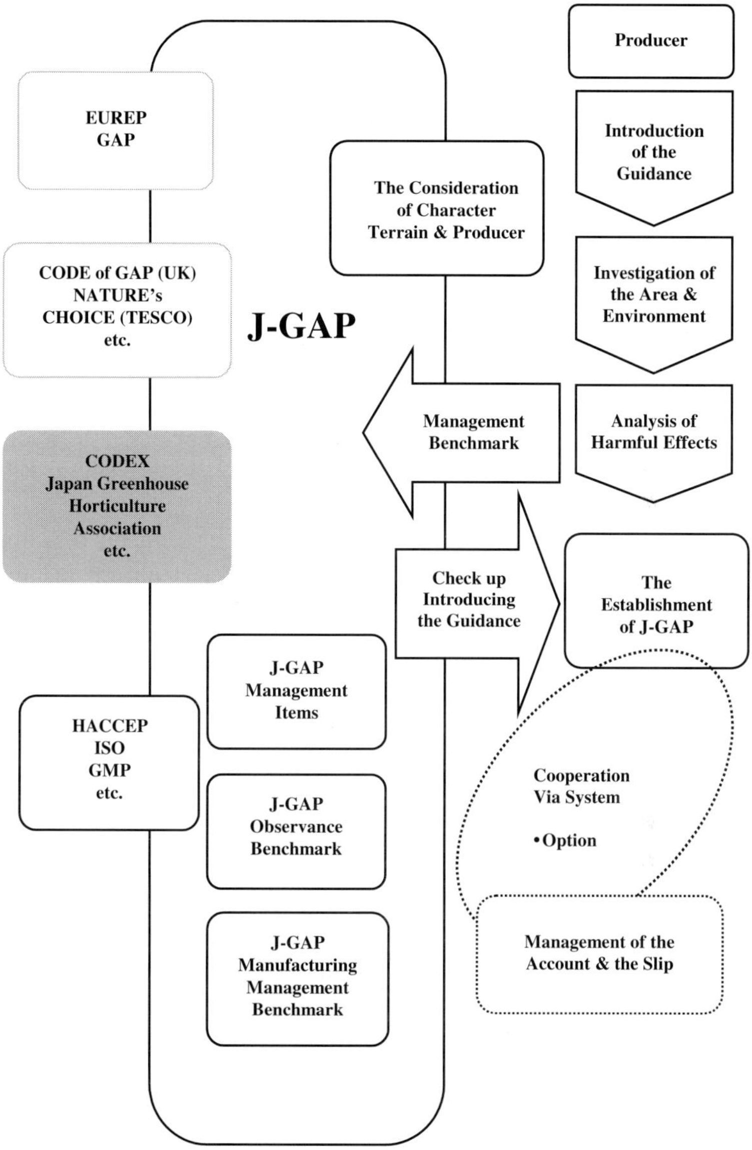

Scheme 4.1. The outline of Japan Good Agricultural Practice.

(4) The managements of agricultural chemicals and the benchmark of the usage: This section prescribes the items about the IPM (Integrative Protective Managements of crops), the usage of agricultural chemicals, the usage of additional agricultural chemicals out of the list of the appointed agricultural chemicals, the revision and validation of the list of appointed agricultural chemicals, the agricultural chemicals spent containers, the disposal of the washing water, the management of the machinery for sprinkling agricultural chemicals, and the education for the users of the agricultural chemicals.
(5) The managements of fertiliser and the benchmark of the usage: This section prescribes the items about the management of the fertiliser, the usage of the fertiliser, the disposal of the spent containers, the machinery for sprinkling fertiliser, the usage of the barnyard manure and organic fertiliser, and the education for the users of the fertiliser.
(6) The agricultural machinery and the weighing instruments benchmark: This section prescribes the items about the agricultural machinery and the weighing instruments.
(7) The information management benchmark.
(8) The manufacture management benchmark: This section prescribes the items about the manufacturing process and managing points, as well as the list of the negative effects.
(9) The barnyard manure benchmark.
(10) The guidelines for carrying out the J-GAP.

From the above items, it is obvious that J-GAP is very practical and feasible. As the J-GAP is carried out, the herb must also be cultivated according to the J-GAP in Japan. It could be imagined that the Japanese *Kampo* industry will import the crude drug materials, which should require that the cultivation must measure up to J-GAP in the future, no matter the area or country. If so, because Japan *Kampo* occupies over 70% of the international herbal medicinal industrial product market, the crude drug trade rules may be changed. Surely, it is of no doubt that the quality of the herbs must be controlled at a relative constant level by the implementation of GAP in cultivating the herbs. This is a valuable action to improve the practice of Chinese medicine globally.

4.5 Summary

Under the current state where the production material of crude drugs is shifting from wild to cultivated plants, useful resources, crude drugs, and cultivation techniques should be shared among countries (Osamu, 2005). The content of *The Guidelines for Cultivation Techniques of Japan Medicinal Plants* is rich, with detailed references and highly applicable instructions. It is a convenience reference for technicians who do cultivation of Chinese herbal medicine.

Some drugs such as *Danggui* (當歸) in China refers to *Angelica sinensis* (Oliv.) Diels but *Angelica acutiloba* Kitagawa in Japan; *Huanglian* (黄連) in China refers to *Coptis chinensis* Franch. but *C. japonica* Franchet in Japan; *Houpo* (厚樸) in China refers to *Magnolia officinalis* Rehd. et Wils. but *M. obovata* Thunberg in Japan; and *Chuanxiong* (川芎) in China refers to *Ligusticum chuanxiong* Hort. but *Cnidium officinale* Makino in Japan. These drugs have the same names in China and Japan, but in fact refer to different species. As the cultivation industry develops, the above-mentioned crude drugs can satisfy its own demand in Japan; therefore, the relative Chinese species are no longer listed in Japan's selection range.

Japan's GMCP is now being implemented. It is suggested that every country should develop GAP that enhances interaction among the world. Japan is a country that imports most crude drugs from China; it also shares similar geographical, climatic conditions with China. Therefore, the work of Japan can serve as a reference which China can learn from.

Concerning the J-GAP and constituting the GAP for the herb in each country is imperative under the situation. Cultivating the herbs according to the requirements of GAP not only keep the markets clean, but also improve and provide the evidence and the quality of Chinese Medicine effects.

References

Dai, Z.Y. and Zhao, Z.Z. (1998) *Current Situation and Trend of Japan Traditional Medicine.* Huaxia Press, Beijing.

J-GAP (2005) http://www.jgai.jp/Introduction/PDF/jgap.pdf

Japan *Kampo* Medicine Manufacturers Association (2004).

Japan Pharmaceutical Affairs Bureau (2001) *The Japanese Pharmacopoeia*, 14th ed. Society of Japanese Pharmacopoeia, Tokyo.

Ministry of Health and Welfare (1992–2005) *Cultivation of Medicinal Plants and Quality Review*, Part 1–11. Yakuji Nippo, Tokyo.

Osamu, I. (2005) *New Trial of Producing of Good Quality Herbal Medicine.* International Trends on Harmonization of Herbal Drugs Conference, Cheong-Ju, Korea.

Tokyo International Forum (1999) http://www.tsumura.co.jp/english/kampo/today/03/3-3-01.htm

Zhao, Z.Z. and Hu, M. (1996) Current cultivation of Japan's medicinal plants. *Zhongguo Zhongyao Zachi* **7**, 400–402.

Chapter 5

Organic Produce of Medicinal Herbs in Australia

S.J. Sheng, C.L. Xue, E. Pang, D.F. Story & C.G. Li

Abstract

Good Agricultural Practice (GAP) guidelines have been developed internationally to ensure consistency of practice and Australian National Standard for Organic and Bio-dynamic Produce has broader implications. Both of them have been applied to the production of herbal medicines including Chinese herbal medicines. This paper compares the similarities and differences of these two set of standards and illustrated the application of these standards in a Chinese herbal medicine farming project funded by the Australian Government and RMIT University, Australia through an effective collaboration of academic institution with local government, farmers' association as well as the industry. This collaboration will contribute to the development of herbal medicine as a responsible industry and provide means to ensure quality of herbal medicines for safe use.

Keywords: Organic Produce; Good Agricultural Practice (GAP); Australian National Standard for Organic and Bio-dynamic Produce; Medicinal Herbs.

5.1 Introduction

The past two decades has witnessed a rapid growth in the consumption of medicinal herbs worldwide. This trend is in-line with the significant increase in using complementary and alternative medicines (CAM) in the general population. For example, in Australia, approximately 52% of the national population use CAM therapies, and 21.6% used herbal medicines, which translated into expenditure on alternative therapies of

AUD$2.3 billion in 2000, nearly four times as much as the public contribution to all pharmaceuticals (MacLennan *et al.*, 2002). Specifically, there is also substantial use of Chinese herbal medicine in Victoria, Australia (Xue *et al.*, 2005a; 2005b). Similarly, a recent study in US found that the greatest relative increase in CAM use was herbal medicine between 1997 and 2002 (12.1% versus 18.6%, respectively), representing over 38 million US adults (Eisenberg *et al.*, 1998). The current world market for medicinal botanicals was estimated at about US$60 billion in 2003 and has been increasing steadily (World Health Organization, http://www.who.int/mediacentre/factsheets/fs134/en/, accessed 31 December 2005).

The increasing demand of herbal consumption has created new challenges for the government and industry in developing policies, regulations and standards on related natural products, including quality control of raw herbs and proper evaluation of the safety and efficacy of herbal therapies (Li *et al.*, 2003, Expert Committee on Complementary Medicines in the Health System, Commonwealth of Australia 2003). The quality assurance (QA) in cultivation and collection of herbal raw materials is among the most challenging tasks facing the industries and governments, as the consistent and reproducible quality of herbal materials is not only paramount for clinical efficacy, but also important in determining the consumer's safety. For example, heavy metals and pesticide levels have been associated with some adverse reactions of herbal consumption (Li *et al.*, 2003).

One way forward is to introduce the so-called Good Agricultural Practice (GAP) in the process of production of medicinal herbs. There are different definitions of what constitutes "Good Agricultural Practices", so whether a practice can be considered "good" will depend on the standards you are applying (Food and Agriculture Organization (FAO) of the United Nations, 2003). To address this issue, the WHO released "WHO Guideline on Good Agricultural and Collection Practices (GACP) for Medicinal Plants" (World Health Organization, 2003) in February 2004. In the European Union, the Guidelines for Good Agricultural Practice (GAP) of Medicinal and Aromatic Plants has been applied to the growing and primary processing of all such plants traded and used in European Union (European Union, 1998). The Chinese State Food and

Drug Administration (SFDA) also introduced a guideline for Good Agricultural Practice (GAP) for Chinese Crude Drugs in 2002 and a number of herbal companies in China have now been certified (Chinese State Food and Drug Administration, 2002, 2004 and 2005).

In Australia, standards and guidelines have been developed for crop organic produce, e.g. *Guideline for On-Farm Food Safety for Fresh Produce* (2nd ed.) (Australia Government, Department of Agriculture, Fisheries and Forestry, 2004), *National Standard for Organic and Bio-dynamic Produce* (3rd ed.) (Organic Produce Export Committee, Australian Quarantine and Inspection Service, 2002), and *Organic Standard* (ver. 6) (Australian Certified Organic, 2003). These standards or guidelines have also been referred in the organic produce of medicinal herbs in Australia. This article briefly reviews and highlights some features of the Australian Organic Standard with a comparison with certain existing GAP guidelines for medicinal herbs.

5.2 The Organic Produce Standard in Australia

By definition, organic refers to the application of practices that emphasise the use of renewable resources; conservation of energy, soil and water; and recognition of livestock welfare needs; and environment maintenance and enhancement, while producing optimum quantities of produce without the use of artificial fertilisers or synthetic chemicals (Organic Produce Export Committee, Australian Quarantine and Inspection Service, 2002). *The Australian National Standard for Organic and Bio-dynamic Produce* (3rd ed.) was published by the Australian Quarantine Inspection Service (AQIS) in December 2002. This Standard aims to provide transparency and credibility for the industries with a framework of food production covering production, processing, transportation, labelling and importation. It also aims to ensure conditions of fair competition in the market by distinguishing those products produced according to this Standard from those produced by other traditional methods, to protect the consumers against deception and fraud. It is important to note that requirements in this Standard are complementary and additional to other health, agricultural and food standards or regulatory requirements recognised or enacted by the Commonwealth, States or Territories, and operators are responsible for the use of inputs and must also follow relevant Commonwealth, State or Territory laws.

The Standard covers general principles that apply to organic and bio-dynamic activities, the specific conditions that must be met by an operator of an organic or bio-dynamic unit, as well as exceptions. Production requirements are vital procedures for the quality and safety of produced products. For example, there are minimum criteria that must be met by operators before their products can be labeled as in-conversion, organic or bio-dynamic. There are 14 chapters in the Standard, including Scope of the Standard; Definitions; Production requirements; Processing, packaging, storage and transport; Inspection and certification; Labelling and advertising; Imported products; Retail, wholesale, and export; Farming inputs-introduction and requirements for use; Substances permitted for sanitation, storage and handling; Processing inputs; Criteria to evaluate input substances for inclusion in this Standard; Criteria to evaluate additives and processing aids for inclusion in this standard; and Application to alter the national standard.

In Australia, the Australian Quarantine Inspection Service (AQIS) is the regulator of the national organic standard. All certifying bodies must be approved by AQIS and must comply with the national standard. Currently, seven private organic certifying organisations are registered and accredited with AQIS as certification bodies for the organic industries in Australia. They also developed their own organic standards under the principles of the National Standard for Organic and Bio-dynamic Produce. For example, Australian Certified Organic (ACO) is registered with AQIS as certifying body for the organic industries. ACO claimed that it currently certifies about 55% of the Australian organic industry. The peak body for the organic industries is the Organic Federation of Australia (OFA), who is responsible for the contact between governments and the relevant industries.

5.3 Australian Organic Standard and GAP

As far as medicinal herbs are concerned, the Australian National Standard for Organic and Bio-dynamic Produce and GAP are two different agriculture standards, although certain principles between them are similar

Table 5.1. Principles outlined in production requirements of National Standard for Organic and Bio-dynamic Produce (AQIS, 2002).

Items	Principles description
Farm	1. The basic aim of an operator to meet this requirement is to achieve optimum quantities of quality produce while enhancing the sustainability of natural agricultural resources. 2. Operators should develop an Organic Management Plan and ensure the enhancement of biological activities in its farming system; maintain or improve soil fertility using crop rotation; minimise the use of non-renewable resources; avoid the contaminations such as non-permitted imputes, genetic engineering products, pesticides, which result from agricultural practices; and protect its environment. 3. An organic certified operator must not routinely switch back and forth between organic and conventional production.
Conversion of land	1. An in-conversion production system should be implied before certified as organic or bio-dynamic. 2. An operator has practiced this Standard for at least one year, and then the second-year produced products may be labeled as in-conversion. 3. Systems certified as in-conversion shall progress to organic status within a timeframe, which cannot be less than three years from the date to commence organic management practices.
Landscape management and biodiversity	1. Operators must include landscape management and biodiversity within Organic Management Planning. 2. Operators should develop 5% of their property as buffer zone such as treed areas, grasslands or other reserves within five years from the attaining in-conversion status.
Soil management	1. The maintenance or improvement of soil structure, fertility and nutrient cycling is fundamental to all procedures adopted in organic farming system. 2. Off-farm inputs are not encouraged by this Standard. 3. An appropriate rotation program should be adopted using of legumes, green manure crops or perennial deep-rooting plants. Animal manures may be used as sheet composting, but these areas should grow two green manure crops firstly, then the area can be planted to crops for human consumption.

Table 5.1. (*Continued*)

Items	Principles description
	4. Fully composted organic matter that listed in the selected sources can be applied in this Standard. 5. Application of bio-dynamic preparations and methods, husbandry measures such as tillage techniques, and incorporation of livestock into the farming system may be adopted.
Water management	1. Recycling of water should be applied in this standard. 2. On-site harvest of water for agricultural use must allow for maintenance of on-farm ecosystem. 3. Water from off-farm sources requires appropriate and regular testing to determine if some contaminations exist. 4. Raw animal liquid waste must be from a certified organic production system and can only be applied to green manure crops and never be directly used to edible crops for human consumption.
Plant production	1. The crops and varieties grown in an organic system are those best suited to local conditions; the least susceptible to pest and disease; and of a good nutritional and physiological quality. 2. Organic plants must be grown from organic seed or organic plant propagation material. 3. The genetically modified/engineered seed and transgenic plants or plants treaded with genetically modified organism (GMO)-derived substances are prohibited.
Plant protection	1. Pests, diseases and weeds must be controlled by any combination of the following: choice of appropriate species and varieties; biological control such as protection of natural enemies of pests and grazing of livestock, appropriate rotation programmes, specific bio-dynamic measures; mechanical control such as traps, barriers; light and sound; mechanical cultivation; mulching and mowing, and flame/steam weeding. 2. Mulches should be of natural materials, and solid non-woven plastic or synthetic material sheets are prohibited.
Harvest of plants from natural environments	1. Products must be sourced from a clearly defined collection area and have been under an approved certifying organisation inspection system for at least 12 months. 2. The collection of plants or parts thereof does not disturb the stability of the natural habitat.

Table 5.2. Comparison of principles between National Standard for Organic and Bio-dynamic Produce and Good Agricultural Practice (GAP).

Items	National Standard for Organic and Bio-dynamic Produce	Good Agricultural Practice (GAP) (WHO and SFDA's GAP for Chinese Crude Drugs)
Farm	The Standard must have been applied to the land for at least three years before products can be labelled as organic or bio-dynamic.	The environment conditions of production sites should meet the requirements of the related national standards such as Atmospheric Conditions Standard, Soil Quality Standard and Farm Irrigation Water Standard.
Conversion of land	An in-conversion production system is adopted.	n/a
Landscape management and biodiversity	Operators should develop 5% of their property as buffer zone such as treed areas, grasslands or other reserves within five years from the attaining in-conversion status.	n/a
Soil management	1. An appropriate rotation programme should be adopted. 2. Animal manures may be used as sheet composting, but cannot be used for human consumption crops directly. 3. Fully composted organic matter listed can be applied.	1. Farmyard manures should be thoroughly composted before used. 2. Organic manures should be main fertilising agent. 3. Chemical fertilisers could be applied sparingly.
Plant production	The genetically modified/engineered seed and transgenic plants or plants treaded with GMO (genetically modified organism)-derived substances are prohibited.	1. Species, sub-species, varieties or cultivars should be clearly identified and recorded. 2. The selection of fine varieties should be enhanced.

Table 5.2. (*Continued*)

Items	National Standard for Organic and Bio-dynamic Produce	Good Agricultural Practice (GAP) (WHO and SFDA's GAP for Chinese Crude Drugs)
Plant protection	Pests, diseases and weeds must be controlled by any combination of measures listed and subsequently have no contamination on products and its produced environment.	If necessary, minimum effective input of pesticides with high efficacy, hypo-toxicity and low residue could be used.
Harvest	1. Products have been under an approved certifying organisation inspection system for at least 12 months. 2. The collection of plants or parts thereof does not disturb the stability of the natural habitat.	Appropriate collection time and method should be determined in accordance with the quality and yield of the plants.
Processing	1. Products received by certified processors must be clearly identified as in-conversion, organic or bio-dynamic. 2. Irradiation is not permitted in this procedure.	1. The contamination of Chinese crude drugs should be prevented and degradation of their active constituents should be avoided. 2. Geo-authentic (*Di Dao*) crude drugs should be processed according to traditional methods.
Packaging, storage and transport	The use of packaging containing polyvinyl chloride (PVC) is prohibited.	n/a
Quality management	Soil, water and/or product sampling and analytical testing will be conducted as part of the certification process.	The producer should establish a quality management department, which is responsible for the quality control of entire production.

Table 5.2. (*Continued*)

Items	National Standard for Organic and Bio-dynamic Produce	Good Agricultural Practice (GAP) (WHO and SFDA's GAP for Chinese Crude Drugs)
Inspection and certification	1. Certifying organisations conduct inspection and certification activities; 2. Operators will be subject to at least one annual inspection to determine their compliance to this Standard. 3. An operator must apply to a certifying organisation for certification. 4. An operator will retain all records that relate to the certified operation for a period of at least five years.	1. SFDA conducts GAP certification of herbal industries in China. 2. The validation of GAP certification is five years; and one annual inspection for certification will be applied. 3. The certified herbal industries should keep the original records for at least five years.
De-certification	When an operator is de-certified by the approved certifying organisation, all marks, logos and descriptive terms should be removed, defaced or stenciled over on all products/packaging materials.	When infringements against this Standard happen, a de-certified will be applied to its herbal industry by SFDA.
Labelling and advertising	1. The words in-conversion, organic may only appear on the labelling of products which is in accordance with this Standard. 2. Product labels must be authorised by the certifying organisation.	n/a

and overlapping. Basically, the Organic Standard aims to operate by organic practice and to ensure both inputs and outputs are organic, while GAP mainly focuses on the standard operation procedure (SOP) of growing process and aims to ensure the consistent quality of the raw materials. Tables 5.1 and 5.2 highlights the principles involved in Australian Organic Standard in comparison with GAP.

5.4 Produce of Organic Medicinal Herbs in Australia

Currently, more than ten medicinal herbs, including *Ginseng*, *Radix Astragali*, *Echinacea*, *Goldenseal* and *Skullcap*, have been commercially grown in Australia (Rubin, 2001). Some of these herbs are available with organic authentication such as *St John's Wort*, *Aloe*, *Ginseng*, *Echinacea*, *Astragali* and *Licorice*. The Australian government has provided research funds for studies on organic produce of medicinal herbs. The Rural Industries Research and Development Corporation (RIRDC) have supported a variety of research projects on medicinal herbs in Australia, and published reports regarding herbal organic production, e.g. *Ginseng* (Wills and Stuart, 2001), *Echinacea purpurea* (Stuart *et al.*, 2004) and *Skullcap* (Wills and Stuart, 2004).

5.4.1 *Ginseng*

A project on Production of High Quality Australian Ginseng was funded by RIRDC and completed by The University of Newcastle, Center for the Advancement of Food Technology and Nutrition in 2001. The research objectives focused on reliable methods for the analysis of ginsenosides, changes in ginsenosides in plant parts during plant growth and maturation, effect of post-harvest handling and processing operations on ginsenosides, survey the situation and practices of *Australian Ginseng* farms. Currently, several commercial identities have organic authentication of *Ginseng* production and provide their organic products to national and international herbal market.

5.4.2 *Echinacea*

The cultivation of *Echinacea* and its annual production have been significantly increased in recent years in Australia, largely due to the growing world market for *Echinacea*. The Australian growers have concentrated on production from *Echinacea purpurea* with the utilisation of both the aerial ant root sections of this plant. The quality standard for *Echinacea* changes in different countries, with the caffeyl phenols used in the US, and either the alkylamides or caffeoyl used in Australia. In Europe, however, the products have been standardised on the polysaccharide content. The research carried out in the past decade was aimed at developing quality parameters and associated tests to enable growers to harvest and handle *Echinacea purpurea* to maintain optimum polysaccharide content, and to identify efficient processing techniques that ensure polysaccharides are transferred through to the end-products (Stuart *et al.*, 2004).

5.5 Recent Developments on GAP for Medicinal Herbs in Australia

There are a number of recent developments in Australia for developing GAP for Chinese medicinal herbs. For example, over the last three years, we have applied principles of National Standard for Organic and Bio-dynamic Produce in our herbal medicine trial project funded by the Australian Commonwealth Department of Transportation and Regional Services (DoTARS) and RMIT University through its Division of Chinese Medicine. The RMIT Chinese Medicine Research Group, in conjunction with the City of Whittlesea and Victoria Farmer's Federation conducted a research project on Chinese herbal farming in Victoria. With more than 100 Chinese herbs, including Radix Salviae Miltiorrhizae (*Danshen*), Radix Astragali (*Huangqi*) and Radix Glycyrrhizae (*Gancao*), have been grown in the Whittlesea area, based on the principles of organic produce. Furthermore, this study has also focused on the development of standard operation procedure (SOP) and ensured consistent and reproducible quality of grown Chinese medicinal herbs. For example, the growth features of different varieties of Salviae Miltiorrhizae (*Danshen*) have been investigated, and fertiliser trials, density trials and variety comparison trials have been undertaken, and optimised harvesting time has been investigated through various field trials. A series of standard operation procedures (SOPs) of *Danshen* farming are being established based on the National Standard for Organic and Bio-dynamic Produce (AQIS) and GAP principles consistent with the WHO guidelines (Sheng *et al.*, 2005a). Furthermore, HPLC fingerprinting and a number of quantitative marker compounds have been developed, analyzed and validated, and will be used for quality assessment of local grown *Danshen* varieties (Sheng *et al.*, 2005b).

5.6 Conclusion

The escalating use of herbal products requires introduction of regulations and standards to improve the quality and safe use of these products. An important aspect of quality assurance of cultivation and collection of herbal raw materials is the adoption of certain standards such as Good Agricultural Practice (GAP) and Standard for Organic and Bio-dynamic Produce. In Australia, the Organic Standard (the National Standard for Organic and Bio-dynamic Produce) has been adopted for agriculture production of certain medicinal herbs. This standard differs from the standard GASP in that it deals more with the operation by organic practice, while GAP involves more on the standard operation procedure (SOP) of growing process. Several medicinal herbs have been grown in Australia with organic authentications. There is a recent development in combining GAP and organic produce standards to aim for a consistent and reproducible production of quality of medicinal herbs in Australia.

Acknowledgements

The authors would like to thank the funding support for this project by the Australian Department of Transportation and Regional Services (two grants in 2002 and 2004 with Professor Charlie Xue as Project Leader) and an RMIT University Research Investment Fund (VRII Project 43, from 2004–2006, Professor Charlie Xue as Project Team Leader). We also would like to thank our partners for their contribution to this project: Mr. John Francis and Mr. Brian May, The City of Whittlesea; Mr. Graeme Taylor, Northern Melbourne Institute of TAFE; Mrs. Jane Edwards, The Nothern Consultative Committee; and Mrs. Judy Clements, Victorian Farmers' Federation.

References

Australian Certified Organic (2003) *Organic Standard* (ver. 6).

Australia Government, Department of Agriculture, Fisheries and Forestry (2004) *Guidelines for On-farm Food Safety for Fresh Produce.*

Chinese State Food and Drug Administration (SFDA) (2002) *Good Agricultural Practice for Chinese Crude Drugs* (Interim).

Chinese State Food and Drug Administration (SFDA) (2004 and 2005) *GAP Certification for Chinese Crude Drugs* (Nos. 1 to 3).

Eisenberg, D., Davis, R., Ettner, S., *et al.* (1998) Trends in alternative medicine use in the United States, 1990–1997: results of a follow-up national survey. *JAMA* **280**(18), 1569–1575.

European Union (1998) *Guidelines for Good Agriculture Practice (GAP) of Medicinal and Aromatic Plants.*

Expert Committee on Complementary Medicines in the Health System, Commonwealth of Australia (2003) *Complementary Medicines in the Australian Health System.*

Food and Agriculture Organization (FAO) of the United Nations (2003) *Good Agricultural Practices (GAPs).*

Li, C.G., Moyle, K. and Xue, C.C. (2003) Problems and challenges with Chinese herbal medicine. In: *A Comprehensive Guide to Chinese Medicine*, 1st ed. (eds.) Leung, P.C., Xue, C.C. and Cheng, Y.C., World Scientific Publishing Co., Singapore, pp. 85–112.

MacLennan, A.H., Wilson, D.H. and Taylor, A.W. (2002) The escalating cost and prevalence of alternative medicine. *Prevent. Med.* **35**(2), 166–173.

Organic Produce Export Committee, Australian Quarantine and Inspection Service (2002) *National Standard for Organic and Bio-dynamic Produce*, 3rd ed..

Rubin, H. (2001) *Supporting the Growth of the Australian Herb Growing Industry.* RIRDC Publication No. 01/24.

Sheng, S.J., Xue, C.C., Pang, E. and Li, C.G. (2005a) *Growth Profile of Radix Salviae Miltiorrhizae in Whittlesea, Victoria.* Paper presented (Invited Speaker) at the International Symposium of Harmonisation of Traditional and Modern Medicine, 12–14 December 2005, Melbourne, Australia.

Sheng, S.J., Xue, C.C., Pang, E. and Li, C.G. (2005b). *Quality Assessment of Radix Salviae Miltiorrhizae*. Paper presented at the Australian Society for Clinical and Experimental Pharmacology and Toxicology, 4–7 December 2005, Melbourne, Australia.

Stuart, D.L., Wills, R.B.H. and Dickson, T.M. (2004) *Optimisation of Polysaccharides in Processed Echinacea Purpurea*. RIRDC Publication No. 04/118.

Wills, R.B.H. and Stuart, D.L. (2001) *Production of High Quality Australian Ginseng*. RIRDC Publication No. 01/170.

Wills, R.B.H. and Stuart, D.L. (2004) *Generation of High Quality Australian Skullcap Products*. RIRDC Publication No. 04/020.

World Health Organization (2003). *WHO Guidelines on Good Agriculture and Collection Practices (GACP) for Medicinal Plants*. World Health Organization, Geneva, Switzerland.

Xue, C.C., Lee, C., Karagiannis, J., Li, C.G., Yang, A.W.H., Zhang, L. and Story, D.F. (2005a) Public attitudes towards Chinese medicine in Melbourne, Australia, *J. Complement. Integr. Med.* **2**(1), Article 8, http://www.bepress.com/jcim/vol2/iss1/8

Xue, C.C., Zhang, L., Story, D., Lin, V. and Da Costa, C. (2005b). *Current Usage of Complementary Medicines in Australia: A National Study*. Paper presented (Invited Speaker) at the International Symposium of Harmonisation of Traditional and Modern Medicine, 12–14 December 2005, Melbourne, Australia.

Chapter 6

Quality Control of Herbs: Principles and Procedures, Using *Panax* as an Example

Aik-Jiang Lau & Hwee-Ling Koh

Abstract

As a result of the growing popularity of herbal medicines, the need for the assessment of quality, safety and efficacy of these products is increasingly important. Compared to conventional preparations, herbal products present a number of unique problems when quality aspects are considered. These arise due to the complex mixtures of constituents which can vary considerably with a large number of factors. Research in this area is increasing and with modern analytical techniques becoming widely available, there are numerous methods for the quality control of herbal medicines. This paper reviews the various methods that have been used for the quality control of herbal medicines, using *Panax* species and *P. notoginseng* products as an example.

Keywords: Quality; *Panax* Species; Notoginseng; Herbal Medicine.

6.1 Safety, Quality and Efficacy of Herbal Medicine

According to the World Health Organization (WHO, 2003), the global market for herbal medicines currently stands at over US$60 billion annually and this figure is growing steadily, with a projected US$400 billion market by 2010 (Wang and Ren, 2002). It is estimated that 65–80% of the world's population use traditional medicine as the primary form of healthcare (WHO, 2003). In the United States, 158 million of the adult population use complementary medicines and according to the USA Commission for Alternative and Complementary medicines, US$17 billion was spent on traditional remedies in 2000 (WHO, 2003). These statistics showed the growing worldwide importance of herbal medicine in both developing and industrialised countries.

Despite the common misconceptions that herbal medicines are safer than western medicines, there are many problems associated with herbal medicines. The adverse effects or toxicities can be classified into two main categories. The first category is the intrinsic or plant-associated health risks due to active ingredients in the plant. The second category is extrinsic or non-plant-associated, which include factors such as contamination (with heavy metals, pesticides, microorganisms, etc.), misidentification, substitution, and adulteration (accidental or deliberate). More scientific evidence using *in vitro*, *in vivo* studies and clinical trials to prove the efficacy of herbal medicine is also needed to support their traditional uses and claims. As both the efficacy and safety are based mainly on their constituents, quality control of the preparations has to be carried out and proper regulations are needed to ensure the compliance to the quality standards. Quality control is, therefore, an essential prerequisite for ensuring their safety and efficacy.

6.2 Methods of Quality Control

Unlike western medicines, herbal medicines present some unique problems in quality standardisation. These variables are caused by intrinsic and extrinsic factors such as species difference, organ specificity, seasonal variation, age, cultivation, harvest, storage, processing methods or manufacturing practices (Mahady *et al.*, 2001). Furthermore, there is a general lack of expertise in quality control of herbal medicines among national drug regulatory authorities (WHO, 2003), as well as lack of stringent regulations. The current lack of uniform quality undermines consumer and healthcare professional confidence in herbal medicine. Total quality assurance of herbal medicines would require multiple methods. Similar to western medicines, Good Manufacturing Practices (GMP) for manufacturing of herbal preparations should be imposed. However, this requirement would not be sufficient as the source of the botanicals greatly affects its quality. Good Agricultural Practices (GAP), which ensures that the whole cultivation process from field collection to post-harvest processing is standardised, is the first step in ensuring the quality of the raw materials and this should be implemented.

To standardise and control the quality of herbal samples, chemical analysis methods will be needed to ensure product authenticity and potency. The literature is replete with numerous analytical methods for herbal medicines. The challenge to the industry is the harmonisation of standards and methods to ensure the consistent quality of herbal medicines and their products. Some of the methods used include macroscopic, microscopic, and organoleptic analyses, DNA fingerprinting, analysis of active or marker compounds, and chromatographic fingerprinting. A few markers or active components have been commonly used to evaluate quality of medicinal herbs or preparations. However, this does not give a complete picture as multiple components may work together to give its therapeutic effects (Liang *et al.*, 2004). Therefore, in recent years, the use of chromatographic fingerprinting for the identification and quality control of medicinal herbs has attracted a lot of interest. Analysis of chromatographic profiles, generally with the goal of making a classification, is known as "fingerprinting" and it provides a macro-analytical approach to evaluate the complex characteristics of medicinal herbs and products (Xie and Wong, 2005). Chromatographic fingerprinting is also one of the requirements proposed by the US FDA (2004) for botanicals and The European Agency for the Evaluation of Medicinal Products (2000) for herbal preparations. Chromatographic fingerprints are unique and represent powerful tools for the comparison, classification, identification and evaluation of samples.

6.3 *Panax* Species

Several *Panax* species are originally found in the northern hemisphere, from the Eastern Himalayas onward through China and Japan to North America. There are several *Panax* species such as *Panax ginseng* (*P. ginseng* or Chinese and Korean Ginseng), *P. quinquefolium* (American ginseng), *P. notoginseng* (Sanqi/Tianqi), *P. japonicus*, *P. vietnamensis*, and *P. pseudoginseng*, that are used as medicinal plants. In fact, more than ten *Panax* species reported in the world are valuable medicinal resources in traditional Chinese medicine as well as in folk medicine

(Zhu *et al.*, 2004a). *P. ginseng* and *P. quinquefolium* are probably the most well-known and widely used species in this genus. The market for ginseng in the United States is estimated to be about US$300 million annually. With such widespread usage, extensive research has been done on *P. ginseng*. The variability of the contents in ginseng preparations was found to be considerably large and standardisation may be necessary for quality assurance of the products (Harkey *et al.*, 2001). Another *Panax* species of focus in this paper is the dried root of *Panax notoginseng* (Burk.) F. H. Chen, which is also a highly valued and important Chinese medicinal herb with a long history of use. It is mainly cultivated in the Yunnan province in China.

6.3.1 *Chemical constituents of P. notoginseng*

Panax species contain triterpene saponins, essential oils, polysaccharides, peptidoglycans, as well as ubiquitous compounds such as fatty acids, etc. The main characteristic constituents in the *Panax* species contributing to its pharmacological effects are the saponins. Up to now, more than 80 saponins have been isolated from the *Panax* species and most of them belong to one of the four types of aglycone moieties, mainly, protopanaxadiol, protopanaxatriol, oleanolic acid and ocotillol types. A number of saponins known as notoginsenosides have been isolated from *P. notoginseng* and notoginsenoside R1 is found to be one of the major notoginsenosides present. The chemical structures of some saponins present in *P. notoginseng* are shown in Fig. 6.1.

6.3.2 *Pharmacological studies on P. notoginseng*

Numerous studies have been done on the pharmacology of *P. notoginseng* and its individual saponins. It was found that bioactivities of ginsenosides varied depending on different types of aglycones and various sugar moieties. The pharmacological actions of individual ginsenosides may also work in opposition.

P. notoginseng is available in two different forms — the raw and steamed forms. Traditionally, the raw form is widely used in Chinese medicine for its haemostatic and cardiovascular properties to arrest

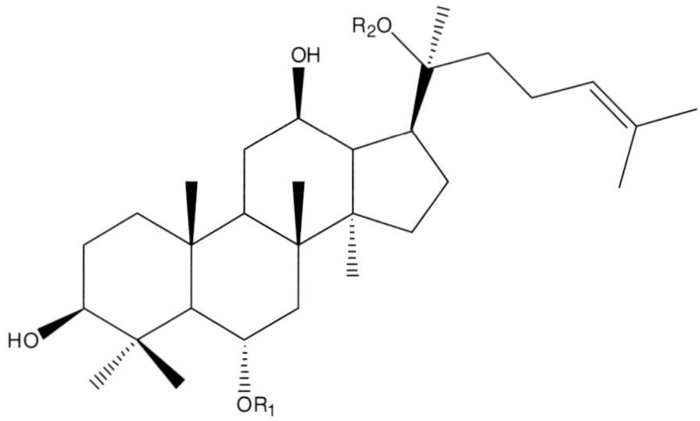

Saponins	R_1	R_2
Re	–Glc[2]–Rha	–Glc
Rg1	–Glc	–Glc
R1	–Glc[2]–Xyl	–Glc
Rh1	**–Glc**	**–H**

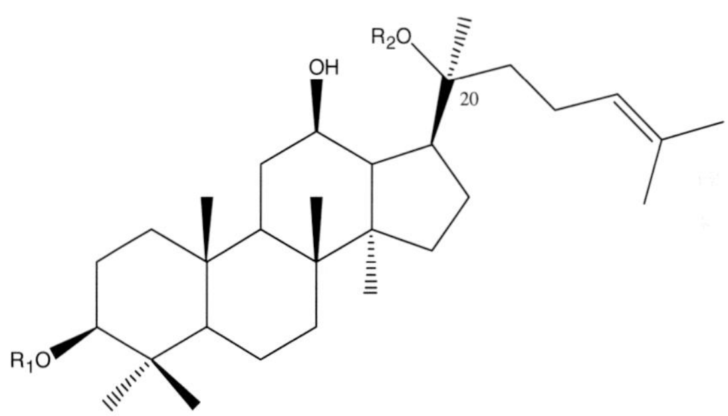

Saponins	R_1	R_2
Rb1	–Glc–Glc	–Glc–Glc
Rc	–Glc–Glc	–Glc–Ara(f)
Rd	–Glc–Glc	–Glc
Rg3	**–Glc–Glc**	**–H**

Fig. 6.1. Chemical structures of some saponins.

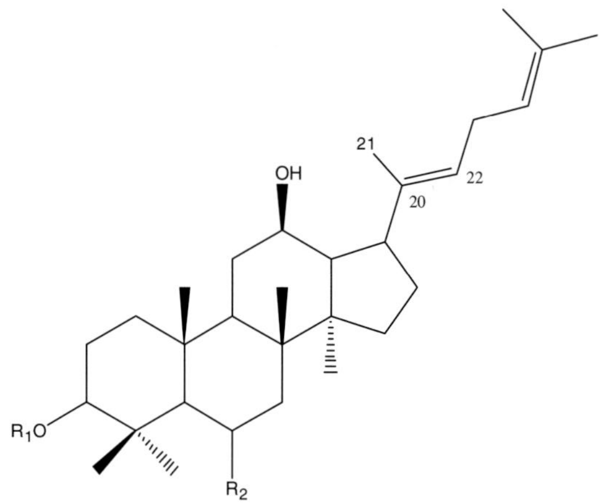

Saponins	R_1	R_2
Rg5	**–Glc–Glc**	**–H**
Rh4	**–H**	**–O–Glc**

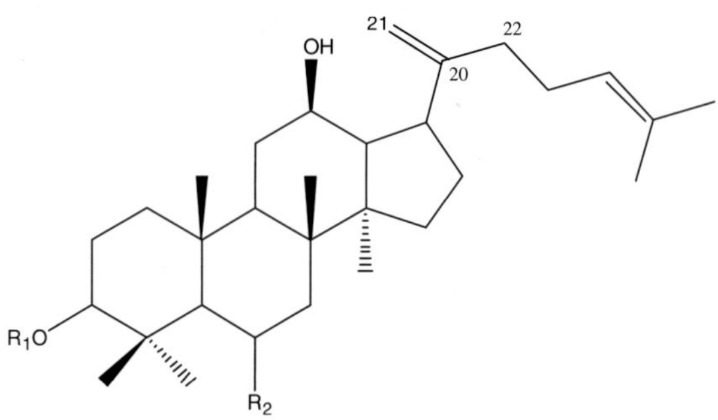

Saponins	R_1	R_2
Rk1	**–Glc–Glc**	**–H**
Rk3	**–H**	**–O–Glc**

Fig. 6.1. (*Continued*)

bleeding, disperse blood clots, improve blood circulation, disperse bruises, and alleviate swelling and pain (Zhu, 1998; State Pharmacopoeia Commission of PR China, 2000; Tang and Eisenbrand, 1992). Animal studies have also shown that *P. notoginseng* extract decreases blood pressure and peripheral vascular resistance. It can also be used for experimental heart ischaemia and may have anti-arrhythmic effects (Tang and Eisenbrand, 1992). On the other hand, the steamed *P. notoginseng* has been claimed to be a tonic used to "nourish" blood, to increase production of various blood cells in anaemic conditions and is traditionally said to be for weaker patients who cannot tolerate the raw form (Guo *et al.*, 1996) Currently, most of the research is focused on raw *P. notoginseng* as this is more commonly used for therapeutic purposes. Few studies have been done on steamed *P. notoginseng*. Due to their slightly different pharmacological actions and clinical indications, using the wrong form of herb may lead to undesirable results. There is no standard method of steaming the raw *P. notoginseng*.

6.4 Quality Control of *P. notoginseng* Roots and Its Products

Quality control of *P. notoginseng* includes authentication of the roots from its numerous similar species, as well as methods to determine the contents of the roots and its products. As raw and steamed *P. notoginseng* have different pharmacological contents, it is important to differentiate between these two forms in the products.

6.4.1 *DNA fingerprinting and molecular biological methods*

Traditional macroscopic and microscopic evaluation of plant materials with reference materials for the purposes of quality control and standardisation is subjective and highly dependent on the skills of the evaluator. Substitutes or adulterants that closely resemble the genuine material may not be detected. Some of the *Panax* species, especially, are very similar morphologically and microscopically. Herbal products in the form of powder or slices also render their authentication by such methods difficult. DNA fingerprinting has become a popular choice to identify and differentiate between different species. Unlike chemical fingerprinting methods, it is not affected by many extrinsic factors such as conditions of cultivation, sources, age and processing methods. Therefore, genetic analysis has been frequently used to accurately identify the origin of herbal medicines and provide a more objective method of differentiating species from their adulterants.

Arbitrarily-primed polymerase chain reaction (AP-PCR) and randomly amplified polymorphic DNA (RAPD) techniques have been applied (Shaw and But, 1995) to differentiate the three *Panax* species from one another and their common adulterants. *P. ginseng* is more closely related to *P. quinquefolium* than to *P. notoginseng*. Both methods were equally successful but the amount of DNA required for RAPD was ten-fold less than AP-PCR and the primers for RAPD are commercially available. Six *Panax* species as well as two common adulterants (Ngan *et al.*, 1999) were successfully differentiated using restriction fragment length polymorphism (RFLP). Using different enzymatic digestion, more than one distinctive RFLP profiles can be generated, thus providing more markers for identification. 5S-rRNA spacer domains were also isolated (Cui *et al.*, 2003) from *P. notoginseng* and other *Panax* species. The spacer domains showed 75% DNA identity among all *Panax* species, but not the adulterants. In addition to the comparison of spacer domains, RAPD analysis was also performed to distinguish the different species as well as morphological variants of *P. notoginseng*. Recently, Multiplex Amplification Refractory Mutation System (MARMS) was developed (Zhu *et al.*, 2004b) and it allowed the detection of many sites of nucleotide difference at one time. A set of specific primers was designed and synthesised for each species on the basis of species-specific sequences of two genes. This assay provided reliable authentication of five *Panax* species due to the simultaneous detection of four sites of nucleotide differences on two completely different genes.

DNA is frequently destroyed at high temperatures. However, with the advancement of molecular biological methods, it has been possible to amplify only specific genes and verify their identities based on these genes in food products subjected to heat treatments. Identifying a herb within a complex matrix of numerous herbs in the final products is challenging. Recently, a Ginseng marker primer (SIM2) that specifically amplified fragment from the DNA of *Panax* species, was also identified

(Shim *et al.*, 2005). A gradient PCR method using the SIM2 primer was used to uniquely identify *Panax* species in herbal medicines and herbal preparations containing diverse components. This study suggests the possibility of developing a *Panax* species identification kit for herbal medicinal plants as well as their preparations. This technique may be applied to many other herbs in the future and a new simultaneous identification method for many herbal medicines may be possible, thus providing a new level of quality control for herbal preparations.

An interesting combination of enzyme-linked immunosorbent assay (ELISA), western blotting and immunoaffinity concentration using an anti-ginsenoside Rb1 monoclonal antibody was used to for the qualitative and quantitative analysis of ginsenosides in *Panax* species and traditional Chinese herbal medicines (Fukuda *et al.*, 2000). It showed good correlation with the standard HPLC methods.

6.4.2 *Chemical fingerprinting*

Within each species, the quality differences in terms of contents, however, may not be detected using DNA fingerprinting or molecular biological methods. Chemical fingerprinting would therefore supplement the information provided by DNA fingerprinting.

6.4.2.1 Analysis of saponins

Saponins are the main bioactive components in *Panax* species, including *P. notoginseng*. Compared to the analysis of *P. ginseng* and *P. quinquefolium*, reports describing the methodology for the quality control of raw *P. notoginseng* were less abundant. HPLC methods are the most commonly used methods for their quality control. The qualitative profiling of the raw *P. notoginseng* roots compared to other *Panax* species had been reported (Zhou *et al.*, 2001; Zhai *et al.*, 2001). The ratios of ginsenoside Rg1 to Re is different for *P. ginseng* (10:13), *P. quinquefolium* (10:65) and *P. notoginseng* (65:10). Profiling of these three *Panax* species was also carried out in our laboratory. Figure 6.2 shows the chromatograms of the three species. Besides the differences in ratio of the ginsenosides Rg1 to Re, *P. notoginseng* contained the notoginsenoside R1, which

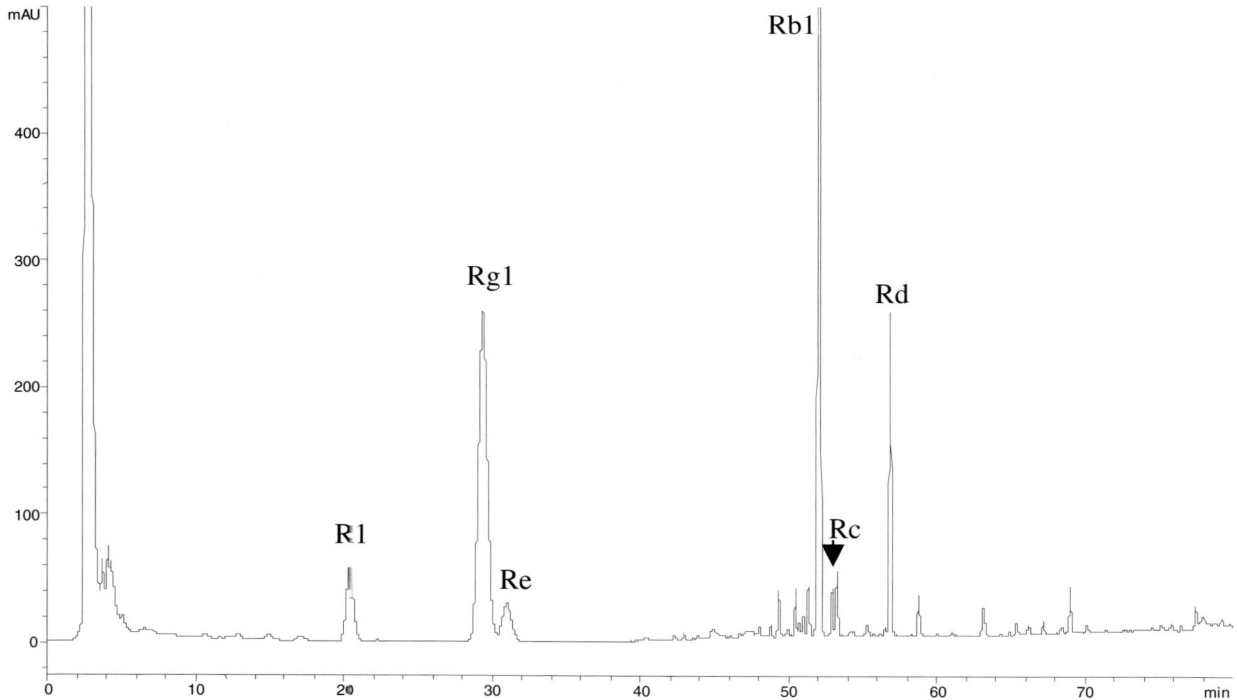

(A)

Fig. 6.2. Typical HPLC chromatograms of (A) *Panax notoginseng*, (B) *Panax ginseng*, and (C) *Panax quinquefolium*.

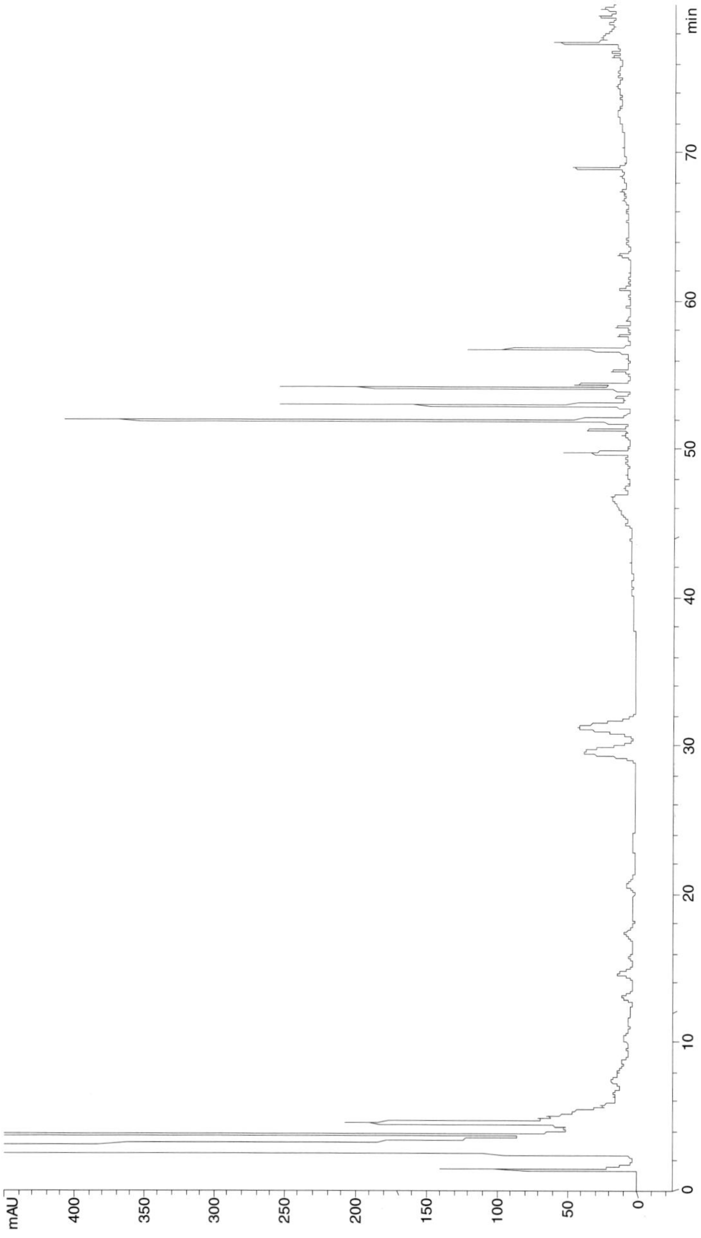

(B)

Fig. 6.2. *(Continued)*

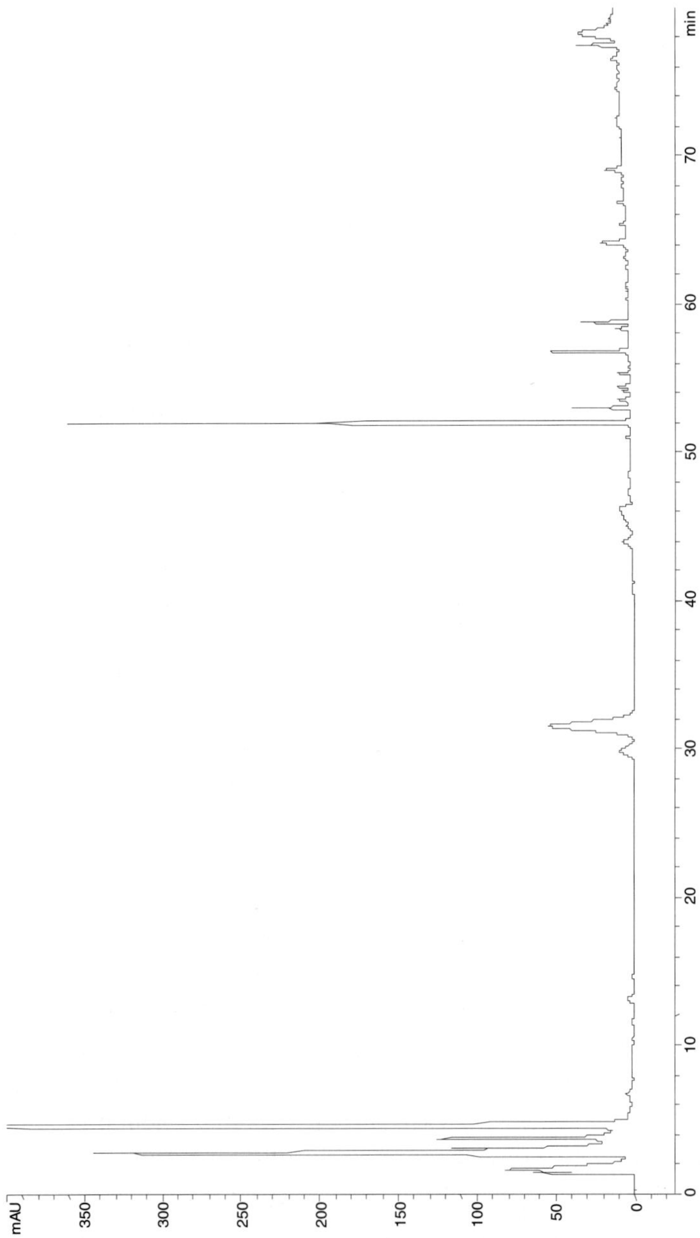

(C)

Fig. 6.2. *(Continued)*

can help to differentiate *P. notoginseng* from the other two species. Furthermore, HPLC fingerprints of *P. notoginseng* were analysed using cluster analysis, allowing classification of the roots into four different qualities (Wang and Bi, 2003).

Due to the complexity of the chemical components and the similarity of the numerous saponins, the simultaneous analysis of all the saponins is difficult. Wang *et al.* (2000) and Jiang *et al.* (2000) quantified up to three saponins present in the raw herbs using HPLC. However, Chuang *et al.* (1995) has managed to simultaneously analyse nine ginsenosides Rb1, Rb2, Rc, Rd, Re, Rf, Rg1, Rg2, R0, mRb1, mRb2, mRc in raw *P. notoginseng* and compared them to the other *Panax* species. The saponin contents in *P. notoginseng* and *P. quinquefolium* were generally higher than in *P. ginseng*. Using the chemical data and external appearance, the quality as well as postulate the origin of the herb can be obtained or postulated. Similarly, Yamaguchi *et al.* (1988) analysed 12 acidic and neutral saponins, namely, ginsenosides R0, mRb1, mRb2, mRc, mRd, Rb1, Rb2, Rc, Rd, Re, Rf, Rg1, and found differences in their contents in five *Panax* species. *P. notoginseng* does not contain saponins of the oleanolic acid prototype unlike *P. ginseng* and *P. japonicus*, but instead, the contents of ginsenosides Rb1, Rg1 and Rd are high. In the study, *P. notoginseng* was found to have large amount of mRb1, but not Rc, mRb2 and mRd. Six ginsenosides in raw *P. notoginseng* were also quantified using HPLC-ELSD (Li and Fitzloff, 2001). ELSD, a mass detector, was found to be a suitable detector for saponins that have weak UV absorbance and had the advantage of quantifying all the saponins proportionally. It eliminates the problem of high baseline noise and poor sensitivity in the use of UV detectors. An improved method (Li *et al.*, 2005) simultaneously quantified six major saponins in 23 *notoginseng* samples within a shorter run time of 30 minutes and this assay method can be utilised as a rapid quality control method. Sha and Zhang (2005) collected and analysed 23 *P. notoginseng* samples from different locations found that there was no absolute linkage between the content of saponins and the traditional grade of the root. A comprehensive study (Zhu *et al.*, 2004a) involving 47 samples from 12 *Panax* taxa was conducted. Eleven ginsenosides were quantified by HPLC to characterise the chemical constituent pattern of each *Panax* species and the relationship between genetic varieties and chemical constituent pattern. Each *Panax* taxon showed its own characteristic chromatographic profile, which also appeared as a specific shape in an 11-direction radar graph constructed on the basis of the quantitative results. This technique provides a simple visually apparent method of discrimination between *Panax* samples. The 12 *Panax* species were also grouped into two main groups based on their components. Different grades (called "*tou*" in Chinese) of *P. notoginseng*, ranked according to their dried size and weight, were analysed. It was traditionally believed that the bigger the size (the smaller the "*tou*"), the higher the quality. Results showed that there was a small increase in saponin content with the increase in size. However, the differences were not significant. The absence of oleanolic acid saponins also distinguished this taxon from other kinds of *Panax* species.

Besides the widely used chromatographic methods, near infrared spectroscopy (Chen and Sorensen, 2000) has been demonstrated to have the potential for rapid quality control of crude herbal plant materials such as *P. notoginseng*. The results obtained were satisfactory for the classification of crude herbs into low, medium and high qualities within a few minutes and the technique is non-destructive. The main drawback of this near infrared method is the calibration step, which requires analysis of several natural samples covering the spectral variation of the samples. However, when speed is important for large number of samples on a routine basis, this technique can be a useful quality control tool.

LC-MS, being a more sensitive and specific analytical technique, is increasingly used for a wide variety of applications including authentication and analysis of complex samples. *P. ginseng* and *P. quinquefolium* can be differentiated based on their ginsenosides using LC-MS techniques. LC-MS-MS (Kite *et al.*, 2003) with negative ion electrospray conditions can be used to profile the malonylated and acetylated ginsenosides in *P. notoginseng*, *P. ginseng* and *P. quinquefolium*. Analyses revealed different profiles of malonyl-ginsenosides in the three *Panax* species and this method assists in the quality control and standardisation of the *Panax* species. Xiao *et al.* (2004) also employed LC-MS to identify *P. notoginseng* roots as well as its presence in complex Chinese patented medicines containing Danshen. Extracted ion chromatograms with *m/z* of 800 and 946, which correspond to Rg1 and Re respectively, were selected to differentiate *P. notoginseng* from other herbs including *P. ginseng* and *P. quinquefolium*. These studies showed the potential of LC-MS for quality control of herbal samples.

Using HPLC and spectrophotometry, four saponins, dencichine, flavonoids and polysaccharides in raw *P. notoginseng* roots from different regions of growth in China, as well as from different seasons of harvest and market grades, were analysed (Dong *et al.*, 2003). It was found that the roots from southwestern parts of Wenshan are of the best quality. The best season for harvest is September to October. This information is important for the quality control and development of good agriculture practice standards for *P. notoginseng*. Recently, our group analysed individual roots of *P. notoginseng* of the same quality (30 "tou") harvested at the same time from a GAP farm by HPLC. Interestingly, some of the roots were found to have different profiles with different proportions of saponins, showing the lack of consistency in the roots from the same location and season. This diversity highlighted the need for better quality control and standardisation of the agricultural practices.

In contrast to the many analytical studies on raw *P. notoginseng*, to date, only two studies reported the saponins content in steamed *P. notoginseng* and compared their contents with the raw samples. One study (Yang *et al.*, 1985) isolated and identified some saponins from both raw and processed *P. notoginseng* using open column chromatography. Their contents were estimated from the yields of saponins isolated. It was found that the ginsenosides Rb1, Rd, Re, Rg1, Rh1 and notoginsenosides R1, R4 were lower in concentration in the steamed form compared to the raw root. Notoginsenoside R2, ginsenosides Rg2 and Rg3, however, were higher in concentration in the steamed root. An improved, validated high performance liquid chromatographic method with diode array detection (Lau *et al.*, 2003) for the quantification of six saponins in raw and steamed *P. notoginseng* was subsequently reported. The chromatograms of steamed samples showed several distinctive peaks around 63–76 minutes, which were absent or in very low quantities in raw samples. As the duration of steaming increased, notoginsenoside R1, ginsenosides Rg1, Re, Rb1, and Rd were reduced significantly, while the less polar peaks around 63–76 minutes were increased. A greater decrease in the content of ginsenosides corresponded to samples that were steamed

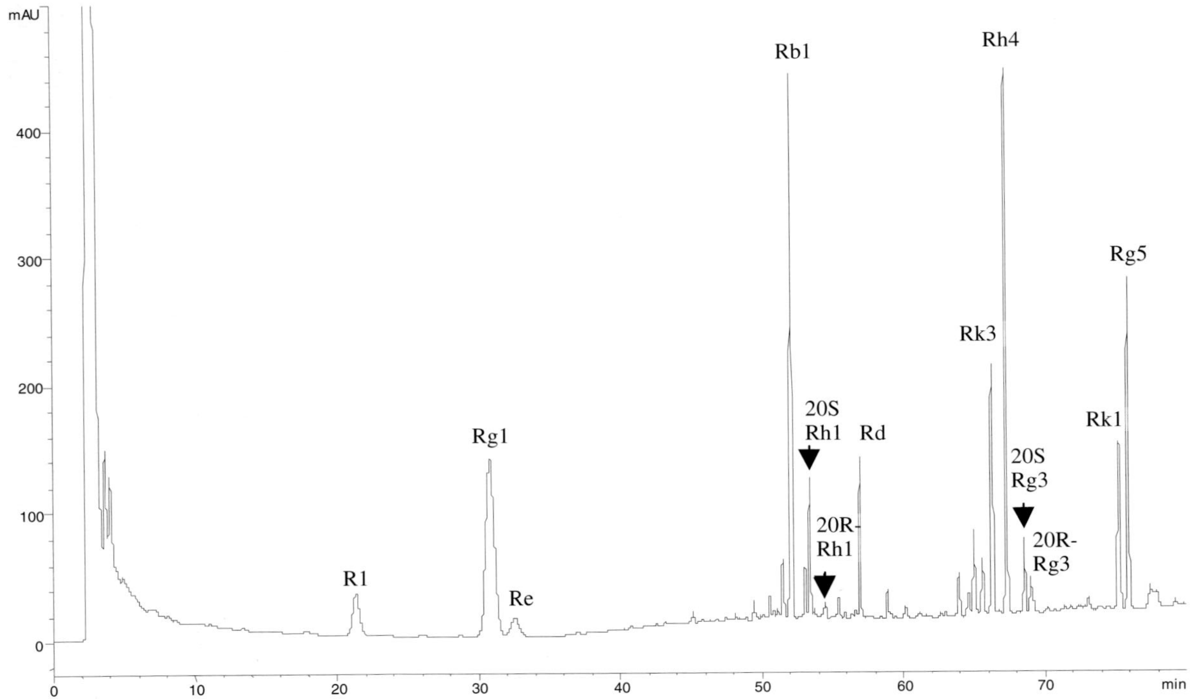

(A)

Fig. 6.3. (A) HPLC chromatogram of a typical steamed *Panax notoginseng* Chinese Proprietary Medicine, and (B) HPLC chromatograms of an atypical pair of raw (above) and steamed (below) product.

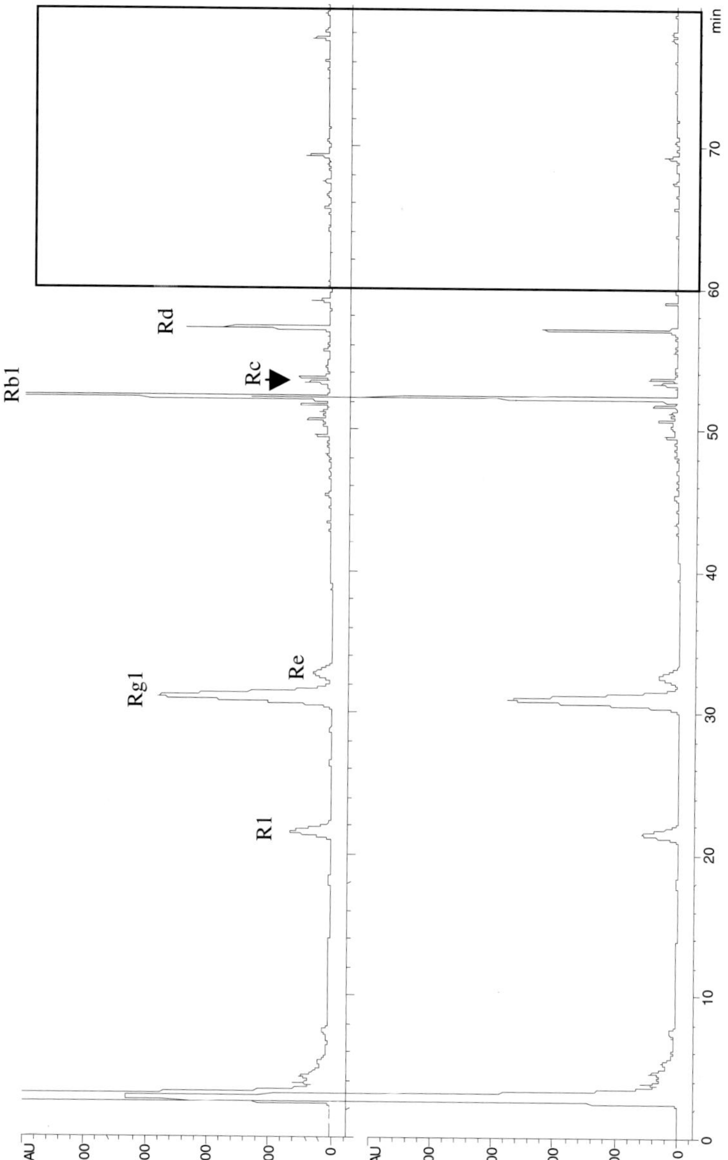

(B)

Fig. 6.3. *(Continued)*

to a greater degree. Out of 11 pairs of raw and steamed *P. notoginseng* products that were analysed, three pairs were found to have chromatograms that resembled their counterpart products instead (Fig. 6.3).

The major peaks in the chromatograms of steamed *P. notoginseng*, which can serve to differentiate raw and steamed forms, were subsequently isolated and identified. The eight major marker peaks in steamed samples were identified to be 20(S)-ginsenoside Rh1, 20(R)-ginsenoside Rh1, 20(S)-ginsenoside Rg3, 20(R)-ginsenoside Rg3, ginsenoside Rk3, ginsenoside Rh4, ginsenoside Rk1, ginsenoside Rg5. These changes in chemical constituents were due to conversion of some of the thermolabile ginsenosides to new components during the steaming process. It has been postulated that these ginsenosides were formed due to the loss of glycosyl moiety at C-20 position (Yang *et al.*, 1985). Ginsenoside Rg3 is most likely produced by the loss of the glycosyl moiety at the C-20 position of protopanaxadiol type saponins such as ginsenosides Rb1, Rb2, Rd. Ginsenoside Rg5 is proposed to be formed by the further dehydration of ginsenoside Rg3 at the C-20 position (Kim *et al.*, 2000).

6.4.2.2 Analysis of dencichine

Dencichine (β-N-oxalyl-L-α,β-diaminopropionic acid, β-ODAP) (Fig. 6.4) is a neuro-excitatory amino acid first found in the seeds of *Lathyrus sativus* (Rao *et al.*, 1964). It was reported to cause neurolathyrism (Quereshi *et al.*, 1977), when consumed in large quantities. However, this compound is also a bioactive haemostatic in *P. notoginseng* (Zhao and Wang, 1986), responsible for its therapeutic effects. As an important active constituent in *P. notoginseng*, it can also serve as a quality control marker. As dencichine has poor UV absorbance and high polarity, it is a difficult component to

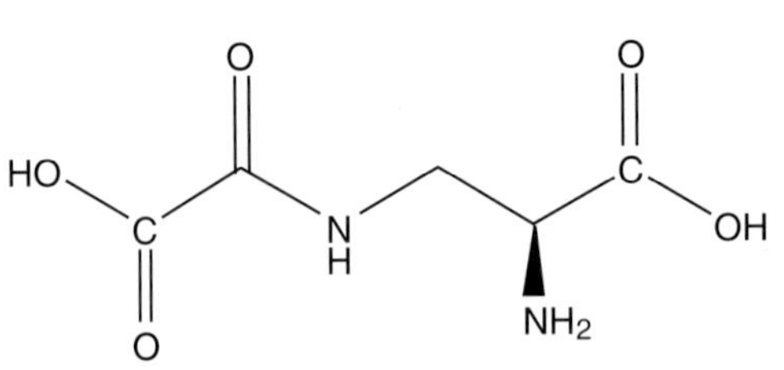

Fig. 6.4. Chemical structure of dencichine.

analyse using HPLC or LC-MS. Using anion-exchange column chromatography (Long *et al.*, 1996), HPTLC (Zhang *et al.*, 1990), amino acid analyser and HPLC with phenylisothiocyanate derivatisation (Kuo *et al.*, 2003) methods, dencichine was found to be present in *Panax* species. However, such methods requiring derivatisation of samples prior to analysis are time-consuming, inconvenient and may have potential derivative instability or reagent interference problems. Unlike saponins that differ greatly in roots obtained from different sources, the contents of dencichine in *P. notoginseng* roots from different regions and seasons did not vary significantly (Dong *et al.*, 2003). The direct HPLC-UV method employed in the study was rapid, but sensitivity was low due to weak UV absorbance of the compound.

LC-MS is highly sensitive and selective for analysis of complex samples. Recently, a novel hydrophilic interaction chromatography with tandem mass spectrometry method was first developed for the analysis of underivatised dencichine and validated for quality control of raw and steamed *P. notoginseng* (Koh *et al.*, 2005a). Steamed *P. notoginseng* root samples were found to contain significantly less dencichine than the corresponding raw samples. As the duration of steaming increase, the content of dencichine decreased accordingly. Hydrolysis of dencichine to diaminopropionic acid at high temperatures may be one of the reasons for the decrease in content in the steamed samples. The contents of dencichine were determined in 11 pairs of raw and steamed *P. notoginseng* products. Most of the samples typically showed that the raw form had higher dencichine content than the steamed form, except for two pairs. For one pair, the content of dencichine was comparable in both the raw and steamed product, showing that the steamed product may not have been steamed sufficiently. On the other hand, the content of dencichine in the raw product of another pair was found to be low, comparable to the average amount in steamed samples, implying that the raw product may have been subjected to some heat treatment. These results were consistent with the results obtained from the quantitative analysis of saponins.

6.4.2.3 Chromatographic pattern matching

Accurate analysis and interpretation of the complex chromatographic fingerprints of herbal samples pose a great challenge to analysts. One method to compare complex fingerprints is by visual comparison. This traditional method of visual chromatographic comparison is simple, but it is very subjective and non-quantitative. For complex chromatograms with incomplete separation of peaks, visual comparisons can be difficult and may miss subtle differences. Moreover, chromatography always varies from run-to-run due to pump, temperature, sample injection variations as well as changes in mobile phase and column chemistries. The resulting run-to-run chromatographic variations such as retention time drift and baseline drift, make the visual comparison method more ambiguous. In some cases, these variations also make the methods analyzing simple difference or variance of the chromatographic response non-applicable. Therefore, there is a need for a simple, valuable tool (Gorenstein, 2004) to objectively compare the entire chromatograms, detect real sample differences between them and measure the degree of differences quantitatively.

Our group employed a HPLC-chromatographic pattern matching method (Lau *et al.*, 2004) as a novel approach to study complex medicinal herbs. Raw and steamed *P. notoginseng* were objectively and quantitatively differentiated. The method takes into account five parameters of chromatographic variations to align the chromatograms, and it does not require the characterisation of peaks or other chromatographic features that are required by other known techniques. After chromatographic alignment and comparison, a quantitative value showing the relative difference between the raw and steamed samples will be generated and it is used as a criterion to differentiate between raw and steamed samples.

For a pair of identical sample, the pattern match standard deviation value (PMSD) was small. From the results obtained, a value below 0.0006 may imply that the samples were identical. This PMSD value increased when the chromatograms of raw and steamed samples were compared using this approach. The greater the difference between the chromatograms, the larger the value will be. This is therefore useful for the quality control of raw and steamed *P. notoginseng*. For a pair of raw and steamed *P. notoginseng* root sample (steamed for two hours), the PMSD was significantly higher (six times) than that of an identical pair of sample. As the duration of steaming was increased, the differences between the raw and steamed samples increased. This trend can be shown quantitatively by the increasing PMSD values.

Eleven pairs of raw and steamed *P. notoginseng* products (tablets or powder dosage forms) were also analysed using this approach. Eight pairs of raw and steamed *P. notoginseng* products showed chromatograms typical of their labels and their PMSD values were higher (> 0.0006) than those of identical samples. However, the PMSD values of these eight pairs were found to range widely from 0.0009 to 0.0050, showing that the quality of the different products in the market varies. Three pairs of the products were found to have similar chromatographic patterns and their PMSD values were less than 0.0006. The chromatograms of steamed samples in two pairs resembled their corresponding raw samples. These "steamed" samples may not be steamed sufficiently in terms of temperature or length of time or not subjected to heat treatment at all. For another pair, the raw sample showed the distinct marker peaks found in steamed sample. The raw sample may have been subjected to some steaming or heat treatment during the post-harvesting process. There may also be a possibility of mislabelling these products. The degree and method of steaming have not been standardised. A consensus on the degree of steaming needs to be reached for the standardisation raw and steamed *P. notoginseng*, otherwise, the quality of these steamed products may vary widely and this will result in a variation in efficacy of such products. For example, ginsenoside Rg3, which is a component found in the steamed sample but not in the raw sample, has been reported to have anti-tumour activities (Kim *et al.*, 2004) and one may envisage that this activity may be correlated to its concentration in the samples.

The use of this chromatographic pattern matching method for quality control is advantageous as it is able to compare the entire chromatographic fingerprints quantitatively, instead of selecting certain peaks for comparisons. The whole chromatogram provides a larger amount of data and can be used even when baseline resolution between the numerous peaks is difficult to achieve. This approach will be useful and applicable for quality control of other herbs. It can potentially give an index of the similarity between a pair of samples. An unknown sample may be compared with an authentic sample to determine its authenticity. The drawback of this method is that the two chromatograms to be compared have to be quite similar for the alignment to be successful before the quantitative comparison.

6.4.2.4 Semi-volatile components

Although most work has been carried out on the non-volatile components of the *Panax* species, fingerprinting of the semi-volatile components also provides good differentiation of the various species (Shellie *et al.*, 2003). Comprehensive two-dimensional gas chromatography (GC × GC) chromatograms revealed the presence of numerous common components as well as some species-specific components. The 2D bubble plot presentations of the data allowed rapid qualitative and semi-quantitative comparisons of the extracts. Furthermore, the use of GC × GC-quadrupole mass spectrometry permits the identification of some major components. This method would also be useful for authentication and quality control of other herbs (Di *et al.*, 2004).

6.5 Examples of Quality Control of Other Herbs

6.5.1 *Stephania tetrandra (Fangji) and Aristolochia fangchi (Guang Fangji)*

Stephania tetrandra (Fangji) and *Aristolochia fangchi* (Guang Fangji) have been used traditionally as diuretics and for rheumatic conditions. However, their chemical constituents are different. The main active constituents in *Stephania tetrandra* are tetrandrine and fangchinoline while *Aristolochia fangchi* contains aristolochic acid, which is a toxic component known to cause nephrotoxicity and renal failure. Recently, quality control methods using HPLC and LC-MS to simultaneously analyze tetrandrine, fangchinoline and aristolochic acid I were able to differentiate between the two herbs and to detect potential adulterations or substitutions. Nine out of the ten herbal samples bought in Singapore as "Fangji" were found to contain the toxic aristolochic acid I (Koh *et al.*, 2005b). *Stephania tetrandra* (Fangji) should not contain aristolochic acids. Non-aqueous capillary electrophoresis was another recent method developed for the rapid analysis of fangchinoline and tetrandrine in *Stephania tetrandra*. Its good sensitivity made it promising for quality control of the two main components in the complex herbal preparations (Gao *et al.*, 2005).

6.5.2 *Angelica sinensis (Danggui)*

Angelica sinensis (Danggui) is widely used in Chinese medicine for invigorating blood circulation. Molecular genetics approach can be used to differentiate three common species of Angelica roots in Asia (Zhao *et al.*, 2003). Diversity in DNA sequences was found in their 5S-rRNA spacer domains, which serve as markers for their identification. HPLC analyses of their ferulic acid and Z-ligustilide contents can also be used to distinguish *A. sinensis* from two other species (*A. acutiloba* and *A. gigas*) (Zhao *et al.*, 2003). In another study, HPLC fingerprints were used to distinguish *A. sinensis* from 13 related umbelliferae herbs and this is important for its authentication (Lu *et al.*, 2005b). The activities of *A. sinensis* have been linked to its ferulic acid content. Ferulic acid is present in the free form or as conjugates or esters. LC-APCI-MS has been employed recently to study both the free and total ferulic acid contents. The total ferulic content would serve as a better marker for the quality assessment of *A. sinensis*, as the total ferulic content includes both the free ferulic acid as well as those hydrolyzed from the various ferulic conjugates (Lu *et al.*, 2005a).

6.5.3 *Salvia miltiorrhiza (Danshen)*

Salvia miltiorrhiza (Danshen) is an important Chinese herbal medicine for promoting blood flow and treating cardiovascular diseases. According to the specifications in the Chinese Pharmacopoeia, the concentration of tanshinone IIA should not be less than 0.20%. However, the quantification of tanshinone IIA alone may not be sufficient for comprehensive evaluation of its quality. Besides tanshinone IIA, there are other important active marker components which can be used for its quality assessment. HPTLC fingerprinting of the water-soluble phenolics and the non-polar tanshinones have been developed for rapid analysis and identification of *S. miltiorrhiza* samples (Hu *et al.*, 2005b). Recently, simultaneous separation of the phenolics and diterpenes in the herbal medicine using several HPLC and LC-MS fingerprinting methods have also been developed for its quality control (Hu *et al.*, 2005a and b; Zhao *et al.*, 2005; Zhang *et al.*, 2005).

High-speed countercurrent chromatography has been compared with HPLC and non-aqueous capillary electrophoresis (Gu *et al.*, 2004) and it was found to be a feasible and cost effective method for fingerprinting of this herb.

6.5.4 *Isatis indigotica (Ban lan gen)*

Isatis indigotica (Ban lan gen) has anti-inflammatory, anti-bacterial, anti-viral properties and has been used for conditions such as influenza and epidermic hepatitis. Recently, HPLC with hierarchical clustering analysis (Zou *et al.*, 2005) has been developed for the quality evaluation of 18 *Isatis indigotica* samples, showing the feasibility of using hierarchical clustering for quantitative comparisons of the chromatograms.

6.6 Conclusion

In recent years, awareness of the need for quality control of herbal medicine has increased tremendously. With many factors influencing its quality, total quality management is definitely complex and an uphill task, requiring several regulations such as Good Agricultural Practices and Good Manufacturing Practices. The quality of medicinal herbs and the variation of their contents may affect their safety and efficacy. This paper stresses the importance of quality control of herbal medicine, highlights the general lack of consistent quality among *selected* species and gives an up-to-date review of various analytical methods to ensure the quality of these herbs and their products. A combination of different complementary technologies may be necessary. Although chemical and DNA fingerprinting help to ensure consistent quality, they may not ensure the consistency of efficacy. Therefore, this intricate relationship between the chemical fingerprints, DNA fingerprints and the efficacy of medicinal herbs will need to be further elucidated. To fully exploit the potential benefits of medicinal herbs and minimising potential adverse effects, more resources for and greater efforts on quality control of botanical medicine are warranted.

References

Chen, Y. and Sorensen, L.K. (2000) Determination of marker constituents in *Radix Glycyrrhizae* and *Radix Notoginseng* by near infrared spectroscopy. *Fresenius J. Anal. Chem.* **367**, 491–496.

Chuang, W.C., Wu, H.K., Sheu, S.J., Chiou, S.H., Chang, H.C. and Chen, Y.P. (1995) A comparative study on commercial samples of Ginseng Radix. *Planta Med.* **61**, 459–465.

Cui, X.M., Lo, C.K., Yip, K.L., Dong, T.T.X. and Tsim, K.W.K. (2003) Authentication of *Panax notoginseng* by 5S-rRNA spacer domain and random amplified polymorphic DNA (RAPD) analysis. *Planta Med.* **69**, 582–584.

Di, X., Shellie, R.A., Marriott, P.J. and Huie, C.W. (2004) Application of headspace solid-phase microextraction (HS-SPME) and comprehensive two-dimensional gas chromatography (GC × GC) for the chemical profiling of volatile oils in complex herbal mixtures. *J. Sep. Sci.* **27**, 451–458.

Dong, T.T.X., Cui, X.M., Song, Z.H., Zhao, K.J., Ji, Z.N., Lo, C.K. and Tsim, K.W. (2003) Chemical assessment of roots of *Panax notoginseng* in China: regional and seasonal variations in its active constituents. *J. Agric. Food Chem.* **51**, 4617–4623.

Fukuda, N., Tanaka, H. and Shoyama, Y. (2000) Applications of ELISA, western blotting and immunoaffinity concentration for survey of ginsenosides in crude drugs of *Panax* species and traditional Chinese herbal medicines. *Analyst* **125**, 1425–1429.

Gao, W., Lin, S., Chen, Y., Chen, A., Li, Y., Chen, X. and Hu, Z. (2005) Non-aqueous capillary electrophoresis for rapid and sensitive determination of fangchinoline and tetrandrine in radix *Stephaniae tetrandrae* and its medicinal preparations. *J. Sep. Sci.* **28**, 639–646.

Gorenstein, M.V. (2004) Method and devices for chromatographic pattern analysis employing chromatographic variability characterisation. US Patent 1999, No. 5,969,228 (http://www.uspto.gov/), accessed 2nd July 2004.

Guo, J., Zong, Y., Yao, G. and Li, J. (1996) *Zhong Hua Ben Cao Jin Xuan Ben*, Vol. 1. Shanghai Science and Technology Publishers, Shanghai (in Chinese).

Gu, M., Zhang, S., Su, Z., Chen, Y. and Ouyang, F. (2004) Fingerprinting of *Salvia miltiorrhiza* Bunge by non-aqueous capillary electrophoresis compared with high-speed counter-current chromatography. *J. Chromatogr. A* **1057**, 133–140.

Harkey, M.R., Henderson, G.L., Gershwin, M.E., Stern, J.S. and Hackman, R.M. (2001) Variability in commercial ginseng products: an analysis of 25 preparations. *Am. J. Clin. Nutr.* **73**, 1101–1106.

Hu, P., Liang, Q.L., Luo, G.A., Zhao, Z.Z. and Jiang, Z.H. (2005a) Multi-component HPLC fingerprinting of Radix Salviae Miltiorrhizae and its LC-MS-MS identification. *Chem. Pharm. Bull.* **53**, 677–683.

Hu, P., Luo, G.A., Zhao, Z. and Jiang, Z.H. (2005b) Quality assessment of Radix Salviae Miltiorrhizae. *Chem. Pharm. Bull.* **53**, 481–486.

Jiang, Y.Q., Wang, Q., Ma, S.P. and Dang, X.D. (2000) Quantitative determination of saponins in the root of *Panax pseudo-ginseng* var. *notoginseng* by HPLC-ELSD and UV spectrophotometry. *Chin. Tradit. Herbal Drugs* **31**, 737–739.

Kim, H.S., Lee, E.H., Ko, S.R., Choi, K.J., Park, J.H. and Im, D.S. (2004) Effects of ginsenosides Rg3 and Rh2 on the proliferation of prostrate cancer cells. *Arch. Pharm. Res.* **27**, 429–435.

Kim, W.Y., Kim, J.M., Han, S.B., Lee, S.K., Kim, N.D., Park, M.K., Kim, C.K. and Park, J.H. (2000) Steaming of ginseng at high temperature enhances biological activity. *J. Nat. Prod.* **63**, 1702–1704.

Kite, G.C., Howes, M.J., Leon, C.J. and Simmonds, M.S. (2003) Liquid chromatography/mass spectrometry of malonyl-ginsenosides in the authentication of ginseng. *Rapid Commun. Mass Spectrom.* **17**, 238–244.

Koh, H.L., Lau, A.J. and Chan, E.C.Y. (2005a) Hydrophilic interaction liquid chromatography with tandem mass spectrometry for the determination of underivatized dencichine (β-N-oxalyl-L-α,β-diaminopropionic acid) in *Panax* medicinal plant species. *Rapid Commun. Mass Spectrom.* **19**, 1237–1244.

Koh, H.L., Wang, H., Zhou, S., Chan, E. and Woo, S.O. (2005b) Detection of aristolochic acid I, tetrandrine and fangchinoline in medicinal plants by high performance liquid chromatography and liquid chromatography/mass spectrometry. *J. Pharm. Biomed. Anal.*, in press.

Kuo, Y.H., Ikegami, F. and Lambein, F. (2003) Neuroactive and other free amino acids in seed and young plants of *Panax ginseng*. *Phytochemistry* **62**, 1087–1091.

Lau, A.J., Seo, B.H., Woo, S.O. and Koh, H.L. (2004) High-performance liquid chromatographic method with quantitative comparisons of whole chromatograms of raw and steamed *Panax notoginseng*. *J. Chromatogr. A* **1057**, 141–149.

Lau, A.J., Woo, S.O. and Koh, H.L. (2003) Analysis of saponins in raw and steamed *Panax notoginseng* using high performance liquid chromatography with diode array detection. *J. Chromatogr. A* **1011**, 77–87.

Li, L., Zhang, J.L., Sheng, Y.X., Guo, D.A., Wang, Q. and Guo, H.Z. (2005) Simultaneous quantification of six major active saponins of *Panax notoginseng* by high-performance liquid chromatography-UV method. *J. Pharm. Biomed. Anal.* **38**, 45–51.

Li, W.K. and Fitzloff, J.F. (2001) A validated method for quantitative determination of saponins in notoginseng (*Panax notoginseng*) using high-performance liquid chromatography with evaporative light-scattering detection. *J. Pharm. Pharmacol.* **53**, 1637–1643.

Liang, Y.Z., Xie, P. and Chan, K. (2004) Quality control of herbal medicines. *J. Chromatogr. B* **812**, 53–70.

Long, Y.C., Ye, Y.H. and Xing, Q.Y. (1996) Studies on the neuroexcitotoxin β-N-oxalyl-L-α,β-diaminopropionic acid and its isomer α-N-oxalyl-L-α,β-diaminopropionic acid from the root of *Panax* species. *Int. J. Peptide Res.* **47**, 42–46.

Lu, G.H., Chan, K., Leung, K., Chan, C.L., Zhao, Z.Z. and Jiang, Z.H. (2005a) Assay of free ferulic acid and total ferulic acid for quality assessment of *Angelica sinensis*. *J. Chromatogr. A* **1068**, 209–219.

Lu, G.H., Chan, K., Liang, Y.Z., Leung, K., Chan, C.L., Jiang, Z.H. and Zhao, Z.Z. (2005b) Development of high-performance liquid chromatographic fingerprints for distinguishing Chinese Angelica from related umbelliferae herbs. *J. Chromatogr. A* **1073**, 383–392.

Mahady, G.B., Fong, H.H.S. and Farnsworth, N.R. (2001) *Botanical Dietary Supplements: Quality, Safety and Efficacy.* Swets and Zeitlinger, Netherlands.

Ngan, F., Shaw, P., But, P. and Wang, J. (1999) Molecular authentication of *Panax* species. *Phytochemistry* **50**, 787–791.

Quereshi, M.Y., Pilbeam, D.J., Evans, C.S. and Bell, E.A. (1977) The neurolathyrogen, α-amino-β-oxalylaminopropionic acid in legume seeds. *Phytochemistry* **16**, 477–479.

Rao, S.L.N., Adiga, P.R. and Sarma, P.S. (1964) The isolation and characterisation of β-N-oxalyl-L-α,β-diaminopropionic acid: a neurotoxin from the seeds of *Lathyrus sativus*. *Biochemistry* **47**, 432–436.

Sha, D.X. and Zhang, M.L. (2005) Determination of notoginsenoside R1, ginsenoside Rg1 and Rb1 in *Radix Notoginseng* and its preparation by HPLC-ELSD. *China J. Chin. Mater. Med.* **30**, 112–115.

Shaw, P.C. and But, P.P.H. (1995) Authentication of *Panax* species and their adulterants by random-primed polymerase chain reaction. *Planta Med.* **61**, 466–469.

Shellie, R.A., Marriott, P.J. and Huie, C.W. (2003) Comprehensive two-dimensional gas chromatography (GC × GC) and GC × GC-quadrupole MS analysis of Asian and American ginseng. *J. Sep. Sci.* **26**, 1185–1192.

Shim, Y.H., Park, C.D., Kim, D.H., Cho, J.H., Cho, M.H. and Kim, H.J. (2005) Identification of *Panax* species in the herbal medicine preparations using gradient PCR method. *Biol. Pharm. Bull.* **28**, 671–676.

Tang, W. and Eisenbrand, G. (1992) *Chinese Drugs of Plant Origin — Chemistry, Pharmacology and Use in Traditional and Modern Medicine.* Springer-Verlag, New York, pp. 745–751.

The European Agency for the Evaluation of Medicinal Products (2000) Committee for Proprietary Medicinal Products, Note for guidance on specifications: test procedures and acceptance criterion for herbal drugs, herbal drug preparations, and herbal medicinal and herbal medicinal products.

The State Pharmacopoeia Commission of PR China (2000) *Pharmacopoeia of the People's Republic of China*, Vol. 1. Chemical Industry Press, Beijing.

US FDA (2004) Centre for Drug Evaluation and Research, Guidance for Industry, Botanical Drug Products, draft guidance.

Wang, M., Fan, Y.G. and Gao, W.F. (2000) Quantitative determination of notoginsenoside R1 and ginsenoside Rg1, Rb1 content in total notoginsenosides of *Panax notoginseng* and Xuesaitong injection by HPLC gradient elution method. *Chin. J. Pharm. Anal.* **20**, 410–413.

Wang, Y. and Bi, K.S. (2003) Fingerprint construction of *Panax notoginseng. China J. Chin. Mater. Med.* **28**, 316–320.

Wang, Z.G. and Ren, J. (2002) Current status and future direction of Chinese herbal medicine. *Trends Pharmacol. Sci.* **23**, 347–348.

World Health Organization (2003) *Media Center: Traditional Medicine.* Fact Sheet, Issue No. 134.

Xiao, S.Y., Luo, G.A., Wang, Y.M., Yang, X.D. and Liang, Q.L. (2004) Identification of *Panax notoginseng* and its preparations by LC/MS. *Acta Pharm. Sin.* **39**, 127–131.

Xie, P.S. and Wong, E. (2005) Direction of TCM modernisation and quality control mode. In: *Annals of Traditional Chinese Medicine: Chinese Medicine — Modern Practice*, Vol. 1. (eds.) Leung, P.C. and Xue, C.C.L. World Scientific Publishing, Singapore, pp. 99–105.

Yamaguchi, H., Kasai, R., Matsuura, H., Tanaka, O. and Fuwa, T. (1988) High-performance liquid chromatographic analysis of acidic saponins of ginseng and related plants. *Chem. Pharm. Bull.* **36**, 3468–3473.

Yang, C.R., Cui, Z.H. and Wu, M.Z. (1985) Isolation and identification of saponins from raw and processed *Panax notoginseng. Zhong Yao Tong Bao* **10**, 33–34, 23 (in Chinese).

Zhai, W.M., Yuan, Y.S., Zhou, Y.X. and Wei, L.X. (2001) HPLC fingerprints identification of *Panax ginseng* C. A. Mey., *P. quinquefolin* L. and *P. notoginseng* (Burk. F. H. Chen). *China J. Chin. Mater. Med.* **26**, 481–482.

Zhang, G.D., Cui, J.F. and Liu, H.Y. (1990) HPTLC fluorometric determination of dencichine, a haemostatic component of *Panax notoginseng. Chin. J. Pharm. Anal.* **10**, 209–212.

Zhang, J.L., Cui, M., He, Y., Yu, H.L. and Guo, D.A. (2005) Chemical fingerprint and metabolic fingerprint analysis of Danshen injection by HPLC-UV and HPLC-MS methods. *J. Pharm. Biomed. Anal.* **36**, 1029–1035.

Zhao, G.Q. and Wang, X.X. (1986) Haemostatic constituent of Sanchi (*Panax notoginseng*)-Dencichin. *Chin. Tradit. Herbal Drugs* **17**, 34–35, 20.

Zhao, K.J., Dong, T.T., Tu, P.F., Song, Z.H., Lo, C.K. and Tsim, K.W. (2003) Molecular genetic and chemical assessment of radix Angelica (Danggui) in China. *J. Agric. Food Chem.* **51**, 2576–2583.

Zhao, Y., Chen, B. and Yao, S. (2005) Simultaneous determination of abietane-type diterpenes, flavonolignans and phenolic compounds in compound preparations of *Silybum marianum* and *Salvia miltiorrhiza* by HPLC-DAD-ESI-MS. *J. Pharm. Biomed. Anal.* **38**, 564–570.

Zhou, Y.X., Yuan, Y.S., Gao, X., Wei, L.X. and Du, S.S. (2001) Studies on the fingerprint of *Radix notoginseng* and its preparation. *China J. Chin. Mater. Med.* **26**, 122–123.

Zhu, S., Zou, K., Fushimi, H., Cai, S. and Komatsu, K. (2004a) Comparative study on triterpene saponins of ginseng drugs. *Planta Med.* **70**, 666–677.

Zhu, S., Fushimi, H., Cai, S. and Komatsu, K. (2004b) Species identification from Ginseng drugs by multiplex amplification refractory mutation system. *Planta Med.* **70**, 189–192.

Zhu, Y.P. (1998) *Chinese Material Medica.* Harwood Medicine Association, Australia.

Zou, P., Hong, Y. and Koh, H.L. (2005) Chemical fingerprinting of *Isatis indigotica* root by RP-HPLC and hierarchical clustering analysis. *J. Pharm. Biomed. Anal.* **38**, 514–520.

Chapter 7

DNA Profiling for Quality Control of Medical Herbs, Utilities and Issues

Yan Hong & Baolin Guo

Abstract

While gaining popularity worldwide, botanical products are facing the challenge of product quality and safety. Authentication and quality control of medical herbs have become critical issues. Since DNA composition for a living organism remains consistent throughout development and is not affected by various environmental conditions, DNA profiling can specifically identify a herb species or cultivar, to ensure its quality if there is linkage of its genetic identity with either chemical constituents or bioactivities and to ensure the genetic uniformity of herb materials. Among the many techniques, Amplified Fragment Length Polymorphism (AFLP) and Simple Sequence Repeat (SSR or microsatellite) are gaining popularity due to their high level of polymorphism, reliability and robustness. DNA sequencing of rDNAs, internal transcribed spacers (ITS) and chloroplast genes have also been used. While DNA profiling has been used successfully in differentiating authenticated herbs from other related species and adulterants, in finding intra-specific variation and even genetic diversity in a single farm, there has been comparatively less work done on correlating genetic identity with chemical constituents or bioactivities. In view of the fact that no single authentication procedure can be applied to every medical herb, we suggest a holistic approach by combining use of DNA profiling together with chemical profiling and/or biological activity testing for authentication of medical herbs. For the wider adoption and acceptance of DNA profiling, there is a need for international collaboration in gaining access to authenticated specimens, working out standard operating procedures (SOPs) for DNA profiling, sharing DNA profile information and building mechanisms to deposit and gain access to DNAs.

Keywords: Herbs; Genetic Profiling; Authentication; Quality Control; DNA Fingerprinting; Amplified Fragment Length Polymorphism; Simple Sequence Repeat; Microsatellite.

7.1 The Need for Authentication and Quality Control of Medical Herbs

Botanical products are gaining popularity worldwide. In 2001, US$4.2 billion was spent on herbs and other botanicals in the United States, accounting for over half of the total nutraceuticals consumer sales (NBJ, 2002). The market for Chinese Herbal Medicine has been projected to be US$400 billion by 2010 (Wang and Ren, 2002) worldwide. Beyond the use as food and supplement, botanic products have been given more serious consideration as complementary and alternative medicine. In June 2004, the US FDA issued the "*Guidance for Industry Botanical Drug Products*" (http://www.fda.gov/cder/guidance/index.htm). Taking certain unique characteristics of botanical drug product into consideration, this guidance allows sponsor of a botanical drug not to identify the active constituents. Instead, "FDA may rely on a combination of tests and controls to ensure the identity, purity, quality, strength, potency, and consistency of botanical drugs. These tests and controls include (1) multiple tests for drug substance and drug product (e.g., spectroscopic and/or chromatographic fingerprints, chemical assay of characteristic markers, and biological assay), (2) raw material and process controls (e.g., strict quality controls for the botanical raw materials and adequate in-process controls), and (3) process validation (especially for the drug substance)."

Despite the increasing sales, consumers eagerly embracing botanical products and opening opportunity for botanical drug products, the botanical products are facing the challenge of product quality and safety (Cardellina, 2002). Several accidents that involved botanical products became the targets of negative media attention.

In one case, two women were hospitalised with symptoms suggestive of digoxin poisoning. Analysis of serum samples confirmed the presence of significant blood levels of digoxin. The source of digoxin was finally traced to the herb *Digitalis lanata* that was accidentally mixed with plantain, a component of a herbal combination that they both took

(Slifman *et al.*, 1998). In the second instance, a number of participants in a clinical study of a weight loss Chinese herbal product developed serious nephrotoxicity, to the extent that some required kidney replacement (Vanherweghem *et al.*, 1996). Continuous monitoring of the study population revealed a higher number of kidney tumours (Nortier *et al.*, 2000). It was determined that this incident was caused by inappropriate substitution of the expected *Stephania tetrandra* by an aristolochic acid containing *Arastolochia fangchi*, probably because of the confusion arising of the similar Chinese names (*Han Fang Ji* versus *Guang Fang Ji*). The above two widely covered incidents highlighted the situation that harvested or wildcrafted botanicals could be intentionally or unwittingly mixed with other plant species, which could result in diluted physiological effect or have dire consequences. Reliable authentication procedures for plant materials are becoming critical for the protection of public health, for sustainable development of the industry and in integrating folk medicine into mainstream medicine. However, there are many hurdles to overcome.

7.2 Hurdles to Authentication and Quality Control of Medical Herbs

7.2.1 *The lack of clear botanic identity of some traditional medical herbs*

The lack of clear botanic identity for herbs is a general phenomenon to many schools of traditional medicine, even for the best-recorded traditional Chinese medicine. Chinese materia medica has had its scope expanded from a handful of drugs recorded around 1000 BC to over 12,800 today. Among the many herbal books by different authors at different times, there were often conflicting records on the identity of herbs under the same common names. People in different geographic regions might have used different plant sources under the same common name. One example is the medical herb *Guan Zhong*. As many as 31 different herbals have been used in different parts of China, all under the same generic name (Li *et al.*, 1996). Different plant species under the same common name may have different medical efficacies, illustrated by the report that common name *Fang Chi* includes more than ten plant species from the family *Aristolochiaceae* and the family *Menispermaceae*, but only one species (*Feng Fangchi*, *Stephania tetrandra* S. Moore) contains the muscle relaxing alkaloid tetrandrine (Li *et al.*, 1996). However, in order to ensure continuation and to accommodate such traditional usage, even the new *Chinese Pharmacopoeia* (2005) still allows some interchangeable use of herbals under the similar generic names like 金钱草 (*Lysimachia christinae* from Primulaceae) and 广金钱草 (*Desmodium styracifolium* from Leguminosae). Different species are also allowed to be used under one generic name. The herb Epimedii (淫羊藿, Yin Yang Huo) can be any one from the five plant species *Epimedium sagittatum*, *Epimedium brevicornum*, *Epimedium koreanum*, *Epimedium pubescens* or *Epimedium wushanense*. This practice is acceptable in the context of traditional medicine, but it creates possible confusion due to the lack of scientific research on "total equality" and "uniformity". It also adds to the difficulty in correct identification and specific use of a particular plant species.

7.2.2 *The arguable use of the term "Dao Di Herbs" or "Authenticated Herbs"*

Chinese traditional medicine emphasises the use of "*Dao Di* Herbs" or "Authenticated Herbs", referring literally to those particular plant species, subspecies or cultivars grown in a particular area and harvested and/or processed in a certain way. Such a term from traditional herbal book has been adapted and widely used as indication of quality. "*Dao Di*" becomes the equivalence of high quality. Other similar terms like "geoherb", "genuineness" and "trueborn" have also been used. However, there is the lack of systematic study on qualities and criteria of "*Dao Di* Herbs". With no clear and well-accepted definition, the term "*Dao Di* Herbs" has been liberally adapted to refer either one or more of the following situations:

(a) the herb and its production area were mentioned in one of the old herbal books;
(b) the area with the most trading volume for a herb;

(c) the current main production area for a herb; or
(d) the areas with the tradition of collection and use of a widely available herb.

There is, understandably, loose linkage between "*Dao Di* Herbs" and clinical efficacy. Actually, there have been many reports on superior qualities of herbs that were not classified as "*Dao Di* Herbs".

7.2.3 *Problem in not having clear active components*

For those herbs with known active components, authentication and quality control can be conducted by evaluating content and activity of these active components. However, active principles of many medical herbs remain unknown. A practical solution was adapted by checking marker compounds that were usually the major or specific compounds. Use of marker compounds can be misleading since they might not have direct linkage to bioactivities. Such practice may also lead to the possibility of adulteration with the specified marker compounds. On the other hand, there are many herbs with no criteria of quality control at all. Even the newest *Chinese Pharmacopoeia* (2005) only gives criteria of quality control for less than half of the herbs listed.

7.2.4 *Lack of clear bioactivity target for authentication and quality control*

Many herbs have been traditionally used for multiple purposes, presumably due to multiple bioactivities conferred by various chemical constituents. Take *Sanqi* (*P. notoginseng*) as an example; it has been recorded for use in promoting blood circulation, removal of blood stasis, induction of blood clotting, relief of swelling and alleviation of pain. It was even reported by recent research with oestrogen activity and activity to sensitise an experimental tumour to ionising radiation. Many of these bioactivities have been attributed to different saponins (Hong *et al.*, 2005). If only one bioactivity or component is used for authentication and quality control, other components and bioactivities are not taken into consideration then.

Table 7.1. Summary of DNA profiling techniques for herbal authentication and quality control.

Techniques	Development cost	Throughput	Operating cost	Polymorphisms	Reliability	Comments
RAPD	Low	High	Low	Low	Low	Easy to start but difficult to get reliable results
RFLP	Medium	Low	High	Low	High	Obsolete due to low resolution and high cost
AFLP	Low	High	Medium	High	High	Highly polymorphic, easier to start but difficult to database
Simple Sequence Repeat (SSR) or microsatellite	High	High	Medium	High	High	Highly polymorphic but expensive to develop; used for intra-specific analysis or closely related species

Table 7.1. *(Continued)*

Techniques	Development cost	Throughput	Operating cost	Polymorphisms	Reliability	Comments
SCAR	High	Low	Low	Low	High	Suitable for differentiation of targeted herbs
Sequencing: • rDNA • ITS • chloroplast genes and intervening sequences	Medium/High	Low/Medium	Medium	Low/Medium	High	Good for differentiating plants from different families and genera, not polymorphic enough for intervening sequences

Abbreviations: RAPD: Random Amplified Polymorphic DNA, RFLP: Restriction Fragment Length Polymorphism, SCAR: Sequence Characterised Amplified Region, AFLP: Amplified Fragment Length Polymorphism, SSR: Simple Sequence Repeat (or microsatellite), rDNA: ribosomal DNAs, ITS: Internal-Transcribed Spacer.

7.2.5 *Other safety issues*

The safety of botanical products are also affected by adulteration with Western drugs, presence of toxic heavy metals, intrinsic toxicity, contamination, etc. (Koh and Woo, 2000).

7.3 Introduction to DNA Profiling

Deoxyribonucleic acid (DNA) is the fundamental building components of all living cells. The specific arrangement of DNA base pair sequences guides the production of proteins and enzymes, which in turn will direct the synthesis of wide range of phytochemicals. DNA profiling including PCR-based techniques and DNA sequencing can reveal differences in genomic DNAs of living organisms including plants, and their results are generally independent of environment and developmental stages. Such techniques can distinguish plants from different families, genera and even closely related cultivars. The different techniques vary in setting up cost, throughput, operation cost and reliability (see Table 7.1 for a summary). The two most popular and robust techniques are Amplified Fragment Length Polymorphism (AFLP) and Simple Sequence Repeat (SSR or microsatellite). DNA sequencing is also widely used in differentiating herbs.

7.4 Amplified Fragment Length Polymorphism (AFLP)

AFLP is technique developed by Vos *et al.* (1995) through which selected restriction fragments from the digestion of total plant DNA are amplified by the polymerase chain reaction. It has a higher multiplex ratio, defined as the number of information points analysed per experiment, than other types of techniques. It has proven to be an extremely effective tool for distinguishing closely related genotypes. This technique has been used to analyse genetic diversity in hop (*Humulus lupulus* L.) cultivars (Hartl and Seefelder, 1998). Fluorescent AFLP profiling gave accurate and objective estimation of genetic relationship of the *Dendrobium* hybrids tested (Xiang *et al.*, 2003); each cultivar had a distinct genetic profile that was uniform in different parts of tested plants, stable among individuals in vegetatively propagated populations throughout different growth periods. The advantages of AFLP, especially fluorescent AFLP are:

- it does not require prior sequence or identification of target regions; and
- it is a robust and very reliable technique and easy to automate.

Chinese medical herbs under common names *Radix quinquefolii* (American Ginseng or *Xiyangshen*), *Radix Astragali* (*Huangqi*), *Radix Notoginseng* (*Tianqi*), *Coxtex Cinnamomum* (*Guipi*), *Radix Isatidis* (*Banlangen*), *Radix Codonopsis* (*Dangshen*) and *Radix Rehmannia* (*Shengdi*) were collected from three independent herbal shops in Singapore and their DNAs were isolated and subjected to fluorescent AFLP analysis (Yuan and Hong, 2003). While samples for *Radix quinquefolii* and *Radix Astragali* were genetically homogenous across three shops, genetic heterogeneity was found for other herbs (SI < 0.7). For example, four samples of *Radix Codonopsis* were of three distinct patterns (SI < 0.6). This result highlighted the situation that genetic distinct Chinese medical herbs are labelled and marketed under same common names in international markets. This work also showcased AFLP as a robust technique that was insensitive to DNA degradation due to light processing and storage.

To check amenability to AFLP analysis of dried herbs sold in the market, the same lab conducted a screening of 118 herbs representing most Chinese medicinal herbs available in Singapore. Their DNAs were isolated with the same modified CTAB protocol and quality verified. Eighteen commercially available primer pairs were tested for AFLP analysis of those herbs with good quality DNA. Based on the criteria of intensity and distribution of fragments, at least two good primer combinations were selected for 45 herbs (unpublished data). This result suggests that specific AFLP protocol can be easily developed for many medical herbs. An example is given in Fig. 7.1 to showcase AFLP profiles for two subspecies of *Epimedium myrianthum*. With a high throughput DNA sequence analyser like Applied Biosystem 3730xl, as many as 1500 samples can be analysed in a day.

Since AFLP involves the digestion of restriction enzymes, ligation and two rounds of PCR, it is a relatively expensive, time consuming and technically challenging technique. A robust and high throughput set-up

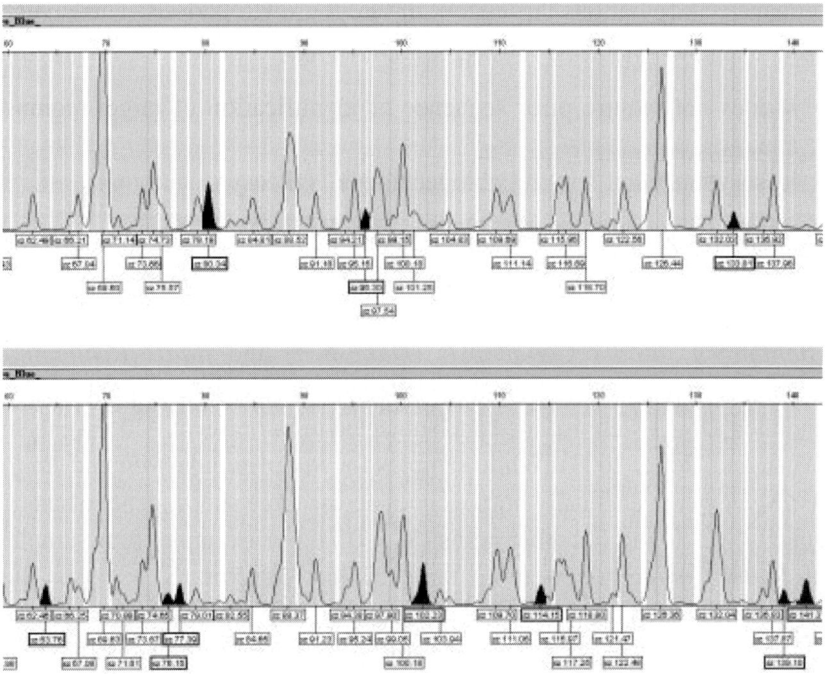

Fig. 7.1. Part of AFLP electrophoregram for two sub-species of *E. myrianthum*. Each fragment is labelled by size. Differential peaks are labelled in black.

requires using fluorescent-labelled primers and expensive DNA sequencing machine. Moreover, AFLP data are difficult to database and compare. These limitations make it difficult to be widely adopted for authentication of medical herbs. To address the difficulty of databasing and comparing AFLP profiles, a scheme was reported to represent an AFLP DNA profile with a nucleotide sequence-like format to facilitate databasing and exchange of data (Hajdukiewicz *et al.*, 1994). In such a format, the information line contains the minimal but necessary details to interpret a DNA fingerprint profile. They include technique used, information on restriction enzymes, primer combination, biological source for DNA materials, sizing information and annotation. The nucleotide sequence-like bodylines contain information on size and relative intensity of DNA bands by a string of defined alphabets or symbols. Algorithms for normalising raw data, binning of fragments and comparing AFLP DNA fingerprint profiles were also described. A software package was developed based on the scheme and proposed algorithms. Such software can be helpful in databasing AFLP fingerprint profiles for medicinal herbs. It allows easy keeping of experiment data and comparison across different laboratories.

7.5 Simple Sequence Repeats (SSRs) or Microsatellites

Simple sequence repeats (SSRs) or microsatellites are short (mostly 24 bp) tandem repeats of DNA sequences. It is hypothesised that the variation or polymorphism of SSRs are a result of polymerase slippage during DNA replication or unequal crossing-over (Levinson and Gutman, 1987). SSRs are not only very common but also hypervariable among the types of tandem repetitive DNA in the genomes of eukaryotes. SSR markers are becoming the preferred molecular markers in crop breeding because of their properties of genetic co-dominance, high reproducibility and multiallelic variation. They are beginning to find applications in herbal identification and quality control. SSR markers have been successfully developed and used for *Cannabis sativa* (Kojoma *et al.*, 2002), *P. ginseng* and *P. quinquefolius* (Hon *et al.*, 2003). Being highly polymorphic, SSR markers even detected genetic variations among samples form different *P. quinquefolius* farms.

However, it takes time and effort to identify suitable polymorphic SSR markers for a particular plant species. Annealing temperature can also change banding patterns when all other PCR conditions are held constant. SSR markers are generally useful for intra-specific analysis or closely related species.

7.6 Other DNA Profiling Techniques

Other techniques like RAPD and RFLP pale in the features of polymorphism, reliability and throughput and are less used nowadays.

7.7 DNA Sequencing

For species identification and identification at genera and family level, sequencing of more conservative regions like ribosomal DNAs (rDNA),

Table 7.2. A collection of recent reports on DNA profiling of medical herbs.

Herbs	Techniques	Highlights of finding	Reference
Hop	Fluorescent AFLP	Some of the hop cultivars could be discriminated	Hartl and Seefelder (1998)
Radix Astragali, *Radix Notoginseng*, *Radix Quinquefolii*, *Coxtex Cinnamomum*, *Radix Isatidis*, *Radix Codonopsis*, and *Radix Rehmannia*	Fluorescent AFLP	Genetic heterogeneity of some of the commonly used herbs was found in the Singapore market; optimised DNA extraction protocol gave DNAs of enough quality for AFLP analysis	Yuan and Hong (2003)
Panax notoginseng	Fluorescent AFLP; ITS 2	Genetic diversity and variation of saponin contents among individual roots from the same farm	Hong *et al.* (2005)
Panax ginseng and *Panax quinquefolius*	AFLP and directed amplification of minisatellite region DNA (DAMD)	*P. ginseng* samples were homogeneous, whereas samples of *P. quinquefolius* from different sources were much more heterogeneous	Ha *et al.* (2002)
Panax ginseng and *Panax quinquefolius*	SSR coupled with microchip electrophoresis	Two microsatellite loci (CT 12, CA 33) could tell American ginseng from Oriental ginseng. Cultivated and wild American ginseng could also be distinguished	Qin *et al.* (2005)
Panax ginseng and *Panax quinquefolius*	SSR	Nine SSR loci with 11–26 alleles per locus could differentiate *Panax ginseng* from *Panax quinquefolius*; different allelic patterns among *P. quinquefolius* samples from some farms	Hon *et al.* (2003)

Table 7.2. (*Continued*)

Herbs	Techniques	Highlights of finding	Reference
Cannabis sativa	SSR	Cannabis samples of different chemo types could be differentiated	Kojoma *et al.* (2002)
Dendrobium species for medical use	Sequencing ITS 2	Medical *Dendrobium* species were shown to be significantly different from one another and from non-orchids and Pholidota (an adulterant of Shihu)	Lau *et al.* (2001)
Panax vietnamensis and other *Panax* species	Sequencing of 18S rDNA and chloroplast matK gene	*P. vietnamensis* was sympatric with other *Panax* species and had a close relationship with *P. japonicus* var. Major and *P. pseudo-ginseng* subsp. Himalaicus	Komatsu *et al.* (2001)
Curcuma wenyujin, *Curcuma phaeocaulis*, and *Curcuma kwangsiensis*	Sequencing ITS	Diversity in DNA sequences among various species was found	Xia *et al.* (2005)
Ephedra species	Sequencing of rDNA, ITS regions and chloroplast intergenic spacer between trnL and trnF	ITS and trnL/trnF differentiated the Ephedra species; intra-specific variation of the nucleotide sequence in *E. przewalskii* was found in different habitats in Xinjiang; Ephedrine alkaloids were absent in *E. regeliana* and *E. przewalskii*.	Long *et al.* (2004 and 2005)

internal transcribed spacer sequence (ITS) of rRNA genes and chloroplast genes like chloroplast tRNA genes have been employed. For example, combined analysis of ITS and chloroplast *trnL/trnF* sequence differentiated the eight *Ephedra* species (Long *et al.*, 2004). Analysis of 18S rRNA genes and *mat*K gene proved that *Panax vietnamensis* was sympatric with other *Panax* species (Komatsu *et al.*, 2001). Comparing DNA sequences in the same genetic regions is very reliable. In general, one nuclear and one chloroplast region are used for this comparison. The key to this approach is to choose a region with the conserved outer portions to allow use of same PCR primers to amplify the same genetic regions for different plants. For this reason, ITS regions located between the more conserved ribosomal 18S rDNA and 5.8S rRNA (ITS 1), between 5.8S rDNA and 28S rDNA (ITS 2) are the popular choices. In chloroplast DNA, rbcL gene and tRNA genes or non-coding intervening sequences are used. Another advantage of the DNA sequencing approach is the ease of PCR cloning rDNAs and chloroplast DNAs because of their multiple copies in the cell.

Since systematists have also used these same genetic regions, there has been a wealth of sequence information in the public databases for a large number of plants. It takes little effort to put together a comprehensive collection of chosen genetic regions for authentication of medical herbs (Table 7.2).

The limitation of the sequence-based approach is the requirement of conserved regions among samples for PCR amplification with the same primers. The other problem is the lack of diversity. Chloroplast DNAs can have difficulty differentiating some species apart. According to a recent analysis of *P. notoginseng* roots from a single farm, ITS was much less polymorphic than AFLP and hence was not suitable for intra-specific analysis. The sequence-based approach is generally not used to detect variation below species level.

7.8 New Developments

It is noted that new technology is diffusing into authentication of medical herbs. In a most recent report (Carles *et al.*, 2005), an oligo-microarray system was developed to detect toxic medical herbs by their specific 5S

DNA fragments. These herbs include *Aconitum carmichaeli*, *A. kusnezoffi*, *Alocasia macrorrhiza*, *Croton tiglium*, *Datura inoxia*, *D. metel*, *D. tatula*, *Dysosma pleiantha*, *Dy. versipellis*, *Euphorbia kansui*, *Hyoscyamus niger*, *Pinellia cordato*, *P. pedatisecta*, *A. ternata*, *Rhododendron molle*, *Strychnos nux-vomica*, *Typhonium divaricatum and T. giganteum*. Such an approach can be similarly used for other medical herbs. With high density of specific probes to different herbs on gene chips, it will even be possible to tell exact composition of herbs in a powdered mixture in the near future.

It can be concluded that genetic profiling can clearly identify adulterants, differentiate herbals of different families, genera, species and even sub-species or cultivars. Genetic identify of a medical herbal can be unambiguously used as proof of genetic uniformity. This will be very useful for proving consistency in plantation and harvest of herbals of the same genetic identity.

7.9 Link of DNA Profile with Chemical Constituents and Bioactivities

DNA profiling will be more useful if a linkage is created between a genetic profile (or a marker) and content of bioactive components and even bioactivities. There are, however, few reports in this area. This is a difficult task because of the uncertainty of relative contribution of genetic factor and environmental conditions. It is possible for those species/varieties with strong genetic contribution or with relative uniform growth environment. It is reported that sequences in ITS region and chloroplast trnL/trnF could differentiate *Ephedra* species with Ephedrine alkaloids from those without (Long *et al.*, 2005). Such linkage could be very useful in authentication and quality control of chemical constituents. In another report (Hong *et al.*, 2005), both genetic diversity and variation in saponin contents were found among individual *P. notoginseng* roots. However, there was no strict correlation between genetic diversity with the variation in saponin contents. The authors suggested that most genetic changes might have occurred at non-coding sequences, changes in coding regions could be silent and those mutated proteins might not have contributed to saponin biosynthesis. Linkage of a particular genetic profile or markers to a desirable saponin content would only possible with both genetic and chemical analysis of a much bigger population followed by statistical analysis.

7.10 Limitation of Utility of DNA Fingerprinting

While DNA profiling is very efficient in ensuring genetic authenticity or uniformity of herbal materials, it cannot ensure chemical composition, less of clinical efficacy. Linkage of DNA profile or marker to chemical composition/bioactivity might be possible for some herbs but it will take effort to establish any strong cause-effect linkage.

DNA profiling also requires the presence of DNAs. Even the most tolerant and sensitive techniques like AFLP and SSR have minimum requirements for DNA quality. It is not applicable to materials free of DNA or with highly degraded DNA. We found that steamed *Tianqi* (*P. notoginseng*) and steamed *Radix Rehmannia* (*Shou di*) were not amenable to AFLP analysis due to absence of DNA or highly degraded DNA (unpublished data). This makes DNA profiling not applicable for in line process monitoring.

Another issue is the difficulty of comparing DNA profiling results. Any DNA profile, either a DNA sequence or a banding pattern from a PCR-based technique, is specific to a sample, the particular technique chosen (with multiple variable parameters) and the set up (both manpower and equipment). Fair comparison is only possible with a clear identification/description of samples analysed and the necessary technical details on DNA isolation protocol and primer information, etc.

Other limiting factors include the cost for equipment, reagent and necessary skill for cloning, DNA sequencing and especially AFLP and SSR analysis.

7.11 The Future of DNA Profiling-Credibility and International Collaboration

7.11.1 *Building credibility of DNA profiling*

It is foreseeable that DNA profiling will be further developed and widely used in research. The challenge is to enable DNA profiling to be adopted by regulatory agencies and the herbal industry in regulation and manufacturing of herbal products. For academic research, many DNA profiling techniques can be used as long as they can differentiate targeted herbs. For regulation and quality control in manufacturing, tracebility, credibility, repetitiveness, ease to adopt and cost are all important considerations. There is also the need of linkage between DNA profile and chemical components and bioactivities. A tight relationship of DNA profile with efficacy or biological activity will make it easier for it to be recognised and adopted. Such linkage takes time and effort to work out. Reliable results are only possible after comparative analysis of large population of samples with both DNA profiling and chemical profiling/bioactivity profiling. Factors like variation within a sampled population, variation among populations collected from different areas should all be taken into consideration.

For any research with the intention to develop DNA profiling system and protocols for regulation and quality control for manufacturing, the following principles should always be adhered to:

(1) Voucher plant(s) will be deposited in a recognised herbarium (such as the Singapore Herbarium).
(2) A standard operation procedure (SOP) should be followed for each test. Date and operator name together with other relevant technical details should be clearly recorded.
(3) Each sample will be tested at least twice. In case of controversy, another researcher should conduct more tests.
(4) For each test, a positive and a negative control should always be included. This is important especially for PCR-based techniques since false negative does not necessary indicate the absence of targeted sequence. Poor quality and too little quantity of DNA and some variation of protocol could all result in negative results. For AFLP, it is important to have a positive band across all samples before registering negative bands smaller than this common band. For SSR system, a positive PCR fragment for all tested samples should be incorporated into the system. Experiment results should be disregarded in case of false positive or false negative results.
(5) All DNA samples will be maintained during the whole project period for possible verification and cross-examination.

(6) For a sample number too big to be handled in one test, some common samples should be included in each subsequent test. Results of different tests are deemed comparable only when the common samples gave the same results in different tests.

7.11.2 *International collaboration*

For the ultimate protection of the consumers, authentication should occur throughout the various processing stages, from the raw materials to the finished products. These many stages can happen in different countries. International collaboration is therefore necessary for effective authentication and quality control of medical herbs in the following areas:

(1) Deposit and allow access to voucher specimen

Voucher specimens are a cornerstone to the whole authentication procedure. They serve as reference material and prove chain of custody. Researchers and manufacturers should be encouraged to deposit sample specimen of herbs that have been properly examined and authenticated to a recognised international herbarium, such as the Singapore Herbarium. Such specimen should be made available either physically or as high quality digital photos for examination by others. Such specimen should also include macro- and microscopic examination date.

(2) Deposit and exchange of DNA samples

Together with specimen, DNA samples should also be deposited. DNAs should be made available to others for verify published results, to compare different protocols and further technical development.

(3) Standard protocols for DNA profiling of herbs of certain species

There should be an international effort in working out standard protocols that can be widely adopted. It would be easier for sequencing-based approach. Recommendation should be given as to what nuclear and chloroplast genes are recommended with list of primers. More development and more technical details are necessary to standardise SSR or AFLP protocols. Important information like amplification primers, amplification conditions, equipment and parameters for analysis are all important for others to interpret and repeat experiments. It is not an easy task but possible as exemplified by the widely used 13 SSR loci endorsed by the FBI Laboratory's Combined DNA Index System (CODIS) for human typing.

(4) Sharing of chemical profiling and DNA fingerprinting information

This is also an important part of international coordinated effort. Chemical profiling results and DNA profiles should be deposited and shared, which are clearly beneficial to the authentication procedure. There is the need for a common platform to present and database such information. The proposed scheme for AFLP data (Hong and Chuah, 2003) can be a possible choice for sharing and databasing AFLP profiles.

7.12 Summary

In summary, authentication and quality control of herbal materials have become the key issues to modernisation of traditional medicine and wider acceptance of herbal products. They are also critical to any research project on herbal medicine to ensure credible research results. Due to the chemical complexity controlled by a particular genetic make-up and environmental conditions, a holistic and integrated approach should be adapted. Such an approach should start from certification of medical herbs by herbalists follow by DNA profiling, chemical fingerprinting and biological activity testing. More efforts are needed to link DNA profile to chemical components and bioactivities. On the other hand, a comprehensive database containing voucher specimens, macro- and microscopic data, standardised recommended protocols for every herbal species, chemical profiling data and DNA profile information will be very helpful to authenticate medical herbs and to provide consumers with safe products. This requires international collaboration. Scientists and regulatory agencies in the big herbal source countries and consuming countries will be important in this endeavor. International organisations like the newly formed Consortium for Globalisation of Chinese Medicine can also play active and important roles.

References

Cardellina, J.H. (2002) Second challenges and opportunities confronting the botanical dietary supplement industry. *J. Nat. Prod.* **65**, 1073–1084.

Carles, M., Cheung, M.K.L., Moganti, S., Dong, T.T.X., Tsim, K.W., Ip, N.Y. and Sucher, N.J. (2005) A DNA microarray for the authentication of toxic traditional Chinese medicinal plants. *Planta Med.* **71**, 580–584.

Ha, W.Y., Shaw, P.C., Liu, J., Yau, F.C.F. and Wang, J. (2002) Authentication of *Panax ginseng* and *Panax quinquefolius* using amplified fragment length polymorphism (AFLP) and directed amplification of minisatellite region DNA (DAMD). *J. Agric. Food Chem.* **50**, 1871–1875.

Hajdukiewicz, P., Svab, Z. and Maliga, P. (1994) The small, versatile pPZP family of Agrobacterium binary vectors for plant transformation. *Plant Mol. Biol.* **25**, 989–994.

Hartl, L. and Seefelder, S. (1998) Diversity of selected hop cultivars detected by fluorescent AFLPs. *Theor. Appl. Genet.* **96**, 112–116.

Hon, C.C., Chow, Y.C., Zeng, F.Y. and Leung, F.C. (2003) Genetic authentication of ginseng and other traditional Chinese medicine. *Acta. Pharmacol. Sin.* **24**, 841–846.

Hong, D.Y.Q., Lau, A.J., Yeo, C.L., Liu, X.K., Yang, C.R., Koh, H.L. and Hong, Y. (2005) Genetic diversity and variation of saponin contents in *Panax notoginseng* roots from a single farm. *J. Agric. Food. Chem.* (DOI: 10.1021/jf051248g).

Hong, Y. and Chuah, A. (2003) A format for databasing and comparison of AFLP fingerprint profiles. *BMC Bioinform.* **4**, 7.

Koh, H.L. and Woo, S.O. (2000) Chinese proprietary medicine in Singapore: regulatory control of toxic heavy metals and undeclared drugs. *Drug Saf.* **23**, 351–362.

Kojoma, M., Iida, O., Makino, Y., Sekita, S. and Satake, M. (2002) DNA fingerprinting of *Cannabis sativa* using inter-simple sequence repeat (ISSR) amplification. *Planta Med.* **68**, 60–63.

Komatsu, K., Zhu, S., Fushimi, H., Qui, T.K., Cai, S.Q. and Kadota, S. (2001) Phylogenetic analysis based on 18S rRNA gene and matK gene sequences of *Panax vietnamensis* and five related species. *Planta Med.* **67**, 461–465.

Lau, D.T.W., Shaw, P.C., Wang, J. and But, P.P.H. (2001) Authentication of medicinal Dendrobium species by the internal transcribed spacer of ribosomal DNA. *Planta Med.* **67**, 456–460.

Levinson, G. and Gutman, G.A. (1987) Slipped-strand mispairing: a major mechanism for DNA sequence evolution. *Mol. Biol. Evol.* **4**, 203–221.

Li, J.S., Jia, M.R. and Wan, D.G. (eds.) (1996) *Chinese Medicine Pharmacognosy*. Shanghai Science and Technology Press (in Chinese).

Long, C., Kakiuchi, N., Takahashi, A., Komatsu, K., Cai, S. and Mikage, M. (2004) Phylogenetic analysis of the DNA sequence of the non-coding region of nuclear ribosomal DNA and chloroplast of Ephedra plants in China. *Planta Med.* **70**, 1080–1084.

Long, C.F., Kakiuchi, N., Zhong, G.Y. and Mikage, M. (2005) Survey on resources of Ephedra plants in Xinjiang. *Biol. Pharm. Bull.* **28**, 285–288.

NBJ (2002) NBJ's annual industry overview VII. *Nutrit. Bus. J.*

Nortier, J.L., Martinez, M.C., Schmeiser, H.H., Arlt, V.M., Bieler, C.A., Petein, M., Depierreux, M.F., De Pauw, L., Abramowicz, D., Vereerstraeten, P. and Vanherweghem, J.L. (2000) Urothelial carcinoma associated with the use of a Chinese herb (*Aristolochia fangchi*). *N. Engl. J. Med.* **342**, 1686–1692.

Qin, J.H., Leung, F.C., Fung, Y.S., Zhu, D.R. and Lin, B.C. (2005) Rapid authentication of ginseng species using microchip electrophoresis with laser-induced fluorescence detection. *Anal. Bioanal. Chem.* **381**, 812–819.

Slifman, N.R., Obermeyer, W.R., Aloi, B.K., Musser, S.M., Correll, W.A., Jr., Cichowicz, S.M., Betz, J.M. and Love, L.A. (1998) Contamination of botanical dietary supplements by *Digitalis lanata*. *N. Engl. J. Med.* **339**, 806–811.

The State Pharmacopoeia Commission (eds.) (2005) *Pharmacopoeia of the People's Republic of China*. Chemical Industry Press.

Vanherweghem, J.L., Abramowicz, D., Tielemans, C. and Depierreux, M. (1996) Effects of steroids on the progression of renal failure in chronic interstitial renal fibrosis: a pilot study in Chinese herbs nephropathy. *Am. J. Kidney Dis.* **27**, 209–215.

Vos, P., Hogers, R., Bleeker, M., Reijans, M., van de Lee, T., Hornes, M., Frijters, A., Pot, J., Peleman, J., Kuiper, M. *et al.* (1995) AFLP: a new technique for DNA fingerprinting. *Nucleic Acids Res.* **23**, 4407–4414.

Wang, Z.G. and Ren, J. (2002) Current status and future direction of Chinese herbal medicine. *Trends Pharmacol. Sci.* **23**, 347–348.

Xia, Q., Zhao, K.J., Huang, Z.G., Zhang, P., Dong, T.T.X., Li, S.P. and Tsim, K.W.K. (2005) Molecular genetic and chemical assessment of *Rhizoma curcumae* in China. *J. Agric. Food Chem.* **53**, 6019–6026.

Xiang, N., Lam-Chan, L.T. and Hong, Y. (2003) Genetic analysis of tropical orchid hybrids (Dendrobium) with fluorescence amplified fragment-length polymorphism (AFLP). *J. Am. Soc. Hort. Sci.* **128**, 731–735.

Yuan, M. and Hong, Y. (2003) Heterogeneity of Chinese medical herbs in Singapore assessed by fluorescence AFLP analysis. *Am. J. Chin. Med.* **31**, 773–779.

Chapter 8

Modern FT-IR Spectroscopy and Quality Control of Traditional Chinese Medicines

Suqin Sun

Abstract

A protocol based on Fourier transform infra-red spectroscopy, two-dimensional correlation IR spectroscopy and computer-aided analysis technology has been established for the quality control of traditional Chinese medicine (TCM) commodities. This method does not need the extraction and separation that follow the integrated principle of TCM, and has obtained many amazing achievements during the years.

Keywords: Fourier Transform Infra-Red Spectroscopy; Two-Dimensional Correlation IR Spectroscopy; Computer-Aided Technique; Quality Control; Traditional Chinese Medicines.

8.1 Introduction

At present, there is an overwhelmingly preferred procedure in the study of traditional Chinese medicines (TCM), which is based on the hypothesis that one should strive to find out "the most effective active component" as the "index component" in the complicated TCM raw herbs or pharmaceutics. To obtain the chemical structure of the "index component", researchers have made great efforts in the extraction and separation of the complicated TCM matrix. This idea is feasible for the pure chemical medicines because the system has a stable molecular structure and fixed chemical compositions. However, as far as TCM is concerned, it comprises thousands of different compositions and attains its curative effect only through the interactions of many ingredients, therefore, under the guidance of the traditional Chinese therapeutics, it is assumed any kind of active composition cannot reflect the overall curative effect of the medicine used by a TCM doctor.

For this reason, the integrative analyses will inevitably play an important role in TCM research. In our research, a protocol based on Fourier transform infra-red (FTIR) spectroscopy and two-dimensional correlation infrared (2D-IR) spectroscopy has been established for the macroscopic quality control of TCM commodities.

In the pharmacopoeia of many different countries, IR spectroscopy is a common technique used for medicine analysis. However, it is only applicable for identification of chemical medicines. For a TCM sample, a complicated matrix, its IR spectrum only provides total information based on the constituents present in the system, embodying highly overlapped IR bands and with fewer features than that of pure compound. In this case, some problems arise, for example, how to explain the spectrum? How to identify and resolve similar spectra? How to differentiate the overlapped peaks in the spectrum? These questions have blocked the application of IR technique on matrix analysis to a great extent! In the 1980s, some reports about IR identification of TCM have emerged, which were based on research of three different TCM extracts. It has not obtained remarkable development because it still needed separation. In 1990s, our group has advanced a non-destructive technique for TCM infra-red analysis. Without separation, the samples can be identified directly via FTIR spectroscopy. Furthermore, we have introduced two-dimensional correlation IR spectroscopy and some computer-aided technique into our analysis, which can provide detailed information complementary to conventional IR spectroscopy. These serial achievements prove convincingly that the modern IR spectroscopy, allied with traditional Chinese pharmacology, mathematics, and analytical chemistry, and complementing each other, will undoubtedly play an important role in the macroscopic quality control of the traditional Chinese medicines.

For over eight years, we have utilised this "macro-fingerprint IR identification method" together with the computer-aided technique to do macroscopic quality control of different TCM commodities successfully.

From raw materials, processed medicines to Chinese patent medicines, this technique has already covered all kinds of TCM commodities. In this article, the special features and advantages of "macroscopic fingerprint" spectroscopy, as well as its function and position in traditional Chinese medicine modernisation, standardisation, and internationalisation are expounded in the following aspects.

8.2 Classification and Identification of TCM Raw Materials

Based on their major chemical compositions, TCM herbs can be divided into several types, such as those abundant in volatile oil, lipid, protein, alkaloid, flavonoids, glucide, starch, etc. Each type has its own subject chemical composition, and each composition has its own characteristic functional groups. Thus the TCM herbs can be distinguished and classified via those IR characteristic absorptions exactly. In addition, the TCM herbs within the same class may have various kinds of chemical compositions and different content. Also, the peak locations and intensities of the characteristic functional groups are different. These distinctions can be identified through corresponding characteristic peaks of IR spectra exactly. For example, 280 kinds of TCM have been classified and distinguished in literature (Sun *et al.*, 2003a). The hemp seeds, magnolia vine fruits, crotons and peach kernels, which mainly contain fatty oils, may have peaks within the range of 2930–2850 cm^{-1} and 722 cm^{-1} belonged to the CH_3 and CH_2 functional groups, and the characteristic peaks of fat are located around 1745 cm^{-1}, 1240 cm^{-1} and 1162 cm^{-1} (Fig. 8.1).

8.2.1 *Identification of different kinds of materials with conventional IR spectrum*

Danggui and *Chuanxiong* are two kinds of medicines that are difficult to identify by HPLC, however, in their conventional IR spectrum, they have obvious features (Fig. 8.2). Compared with the IR spectrum of pure sucrose, we can find the shape of the *Danggui* spectrum to be very similar with that of sucrose, therefore, we think it contains a lot of sucrose.

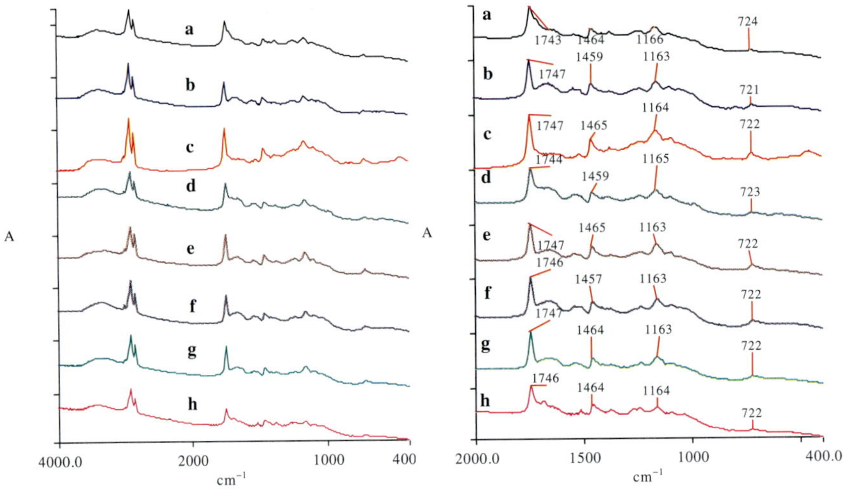

Fig. 8.1. FTIR spectra of medicinal herbs, which mainly contain lipids. (a) Crotons, (b) white mustard seeds, (c) climbing fern, (d) *fructus cannabis*, (e) radish seeds, (f) pumpkin seeds, (g) peach kernels, and (h) magnolia vine fruit.

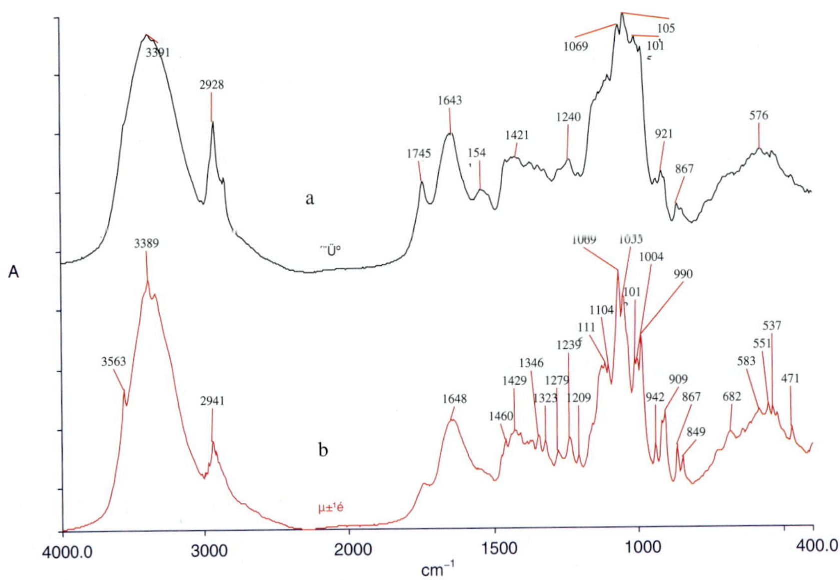

Fig. 8.2. IR spectra of (a) *Chuanxiong* and (b) *Danggui*.

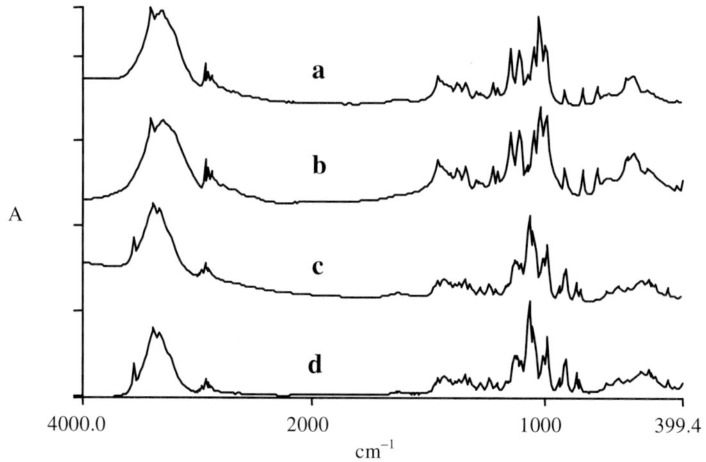

Fig. 8.3. FTIR spectra of ginseng teabags and the excipients. (a) Teabag sample 1, (b) glucose, (c) teabag sample 6, and (d) saccharose.

8.2.2 *Evaluation of TCM and dietary supplements with conventional IR spectrum*

Seven kinds of ginseng teabags, which are used as dietary supplements, were determined directly by IR spectrum. It can be seen from Fig. 8.3 that according to IR characteristic spectra, commercial ginseng teabags can be divided into two classes. One is made by pure ginseng powder, another by the extract of ginseng plus glucose and saccharose as excipients. The relative intensities of characteristic peaks of saccharose or glucose can be utilised to approximate their qualities. This conclusion has already been further proved by HPLC (Sun *et al.*, 2002b).

Thirty-six kinds of ganoderma products were identified by FTIR. Great differences were shown in the IR spectra of ganoderma, spore powder and mycelium (Fig. 8.4). The IR spectra differ a lot in the peak positions and relative intensities. This is due to the various producing areas selected by different manufacturers, the different excipients, and the excipient contents added into the products. Results show that 36 kinds of ganoderma products can be classified and distinguished according to the IR characteristic spectra (Sun *et al.*, 2001a).

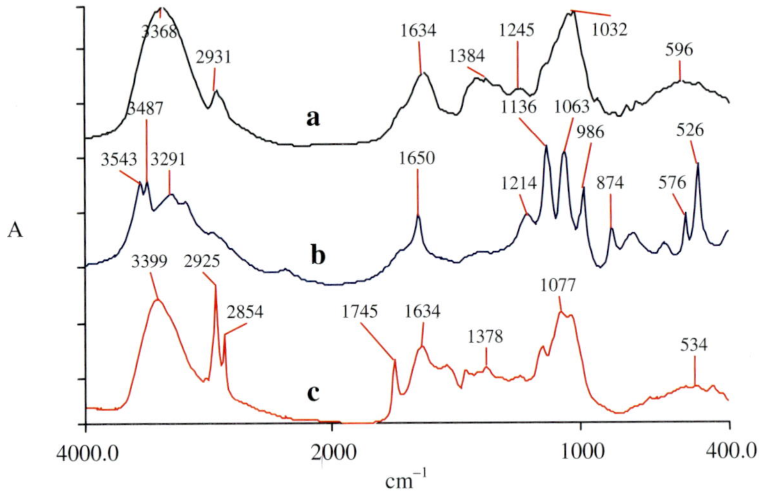

Fig. 8.4. FTIR spectra of different *ganoderma lucidum* products. (a) Chinese crude *ganoderma lucidum*, (b) *lucidum mycelium*, and (c) lucidum spore.

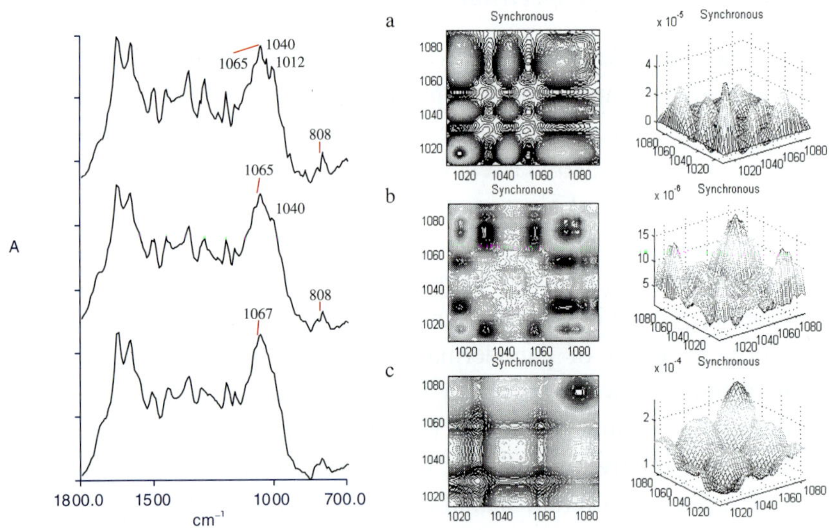

Fig. 8.5. Conventional and 2D IR spectra of sophora flowers at different processing stages. (a) Raw Sophora, (b) roasted Sophora, and (c) charred Sophora.

8.2.3 *Identification of different processed TCM by conventional and 2D IR spectroscopy*

The functions of non-processed and processed-at-different stages TCM materials are greatly different, so controlling the processing procedure and identifying samples at different procedures are highly important in guaranteeing the curative effect. Figure 8.5 shows the spectra of Sophora flowers at different processing stages. We can identify them by conventional IR spectra according to the numbers of shoulder peaks in the area around 1065 cm^{-1}, which are due to the vibrations of C–O bond linking to different kinds of hydrogen bonds. Along with the increase in heating time, the shoulder peaks at 1012 cm^{-1} and 1040 cm^{-1} begin to disappear. In their 2D correlation IR spectra, the features of samples in different processed stages are much more distinct.

8.2.4 *Computer-aided analysis on the spectra information of the same medicines*

The same kinds of traditional Chinese medicine are extremely similar to each other, and are thus very difficult to identify. However, because of the differences in geographic origins, climate, planting methods, gathering time, producing area, wild and artificial culture, whether they are planted in sunny slope or northern slope of mountains etc., they do show differences in practical applications. With the aid of the computer, using many kinds of software treating the IR spectra, those medicines can be discerned directly too.

Rhizoma Cimicifuga (*Shengma*) samples from 15 different origins are determined by FTIR combined with comparison software. The correlation coefficient is gained by different genus of *Shengma* compared with the standard *Shengma* (*C. dahurica*, *Xing'an Shengma*). The results show that the spectra of these samples rely on the difference of the chemical components and the contents of related components. The differences of spectra among samples belonging to different families were distinct, and this is also true for different species within the same genus. For two samples of the same species from different producing areas, or with same

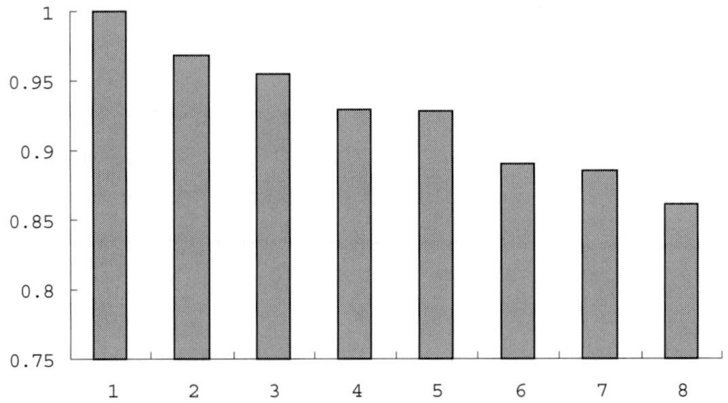

Fig. 8.6. The correlation coefficient of various *Shengma* (*C. dahurica* as standard). (1) *C. dahurica*, (2) *C. heracleifolia*, (3) *C. foetida*, (4) *C. simplex*, (5) *C. yunnanensis*, (6) *C. nanchuanensis*, (7) *C. brachycarpa*, and (8) *C. acerina*.

producing area but different collection dates, the spectra differences are not obvious (Fig. 8.6). This approach provides a quick and accurate determination method of raw drugs without extraction and separation (Wang *et al.*, 2001).

Software is used to compare the IR spectra of TCM injections one by one. Results show that the correlation coefficient of different kinds of injections is less than 0.8; if the main compositions of injections are similar to each other, the coefficient will be greater than 0.8. The correlation coefficient of the same kind of products from different manufacturers is over 0.9, and for those from the same manufacturers, the value would exceed 0.95 (Zuo *et al.*, 2001).

FTIR spectroscopy combined with pattern recognition is used to classify and identify the skullcaps (*Huangqin*). Sixty-nine samples from 15 producing areas are classified, of which 59 samples are wild and 10 samples are cultivated. According to the macroscopic fingerprint characteristic, using Principle Component Regression (PCR) method, the *Huangqin* samples can be divided into six areas, one of which is cultivated *Huangqin*. This classification result is consistent with the quality evaluation results of traditional and modern theory. It is related with the geography and climate conditions. So this can be regarded as the gist in

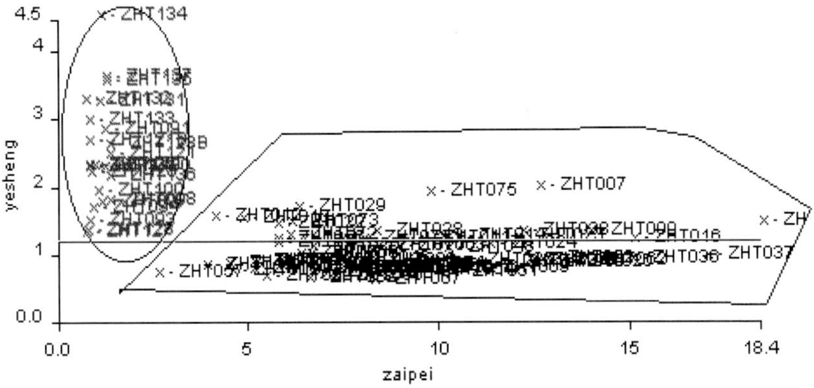

Fig. 8.7. The clustering result of wild (grey) and cultivated (black) *Chishao.*

the quality control of *Huangqin* objectively (Sun *et al.*, 2001b). Three artificial neural network (ANN) models: non-linear-linear, linear-linear and non-linear-non-linear, are set up to identify three classes of skullcaps (cultivated, wild *Scutellaria baicalense* Georgi and *Scutellaria viscidula* Bge). Among them, 43 samples are gathered as training set and 34 as test set, and both sets are trained by ANN separately. From the recognition results, the most reliable model is the non-linear-linear model of ANN, with the hidden layer as 3. Its recognition rate is up to 97% (Xu and Sun, 2002).

Based on the IR spectra of *Paeonia lactiflora* Pall, 90 samples from 18 geographical origins are classified into six groups with principal component analysis (Fig. 8.7). This result is in agreement with their geographical origins; 45 geographical origins are predicted with radial basis function, and it is demonstrated to be a powerful ANN method in discrimination. The accuracy rate is 97.8% (Xu *et al.*, 2003; Dong and Sun, 2002).

The authenticity of *tuber dioscoreae* (Chinese yam) can be discerned by various softwares based on IR spectra. Using the comparison software, if the correlation coefficient between the sample and standard exceeds 0.98, it can be regarded as genuine (Sun *et al.*, 2002a). While using the pattern recognition software along with the instrument, soft independent modeling of class analogy (SIMCA), the discern rate of the genuine one is up to 70% with the credibility exceeding 60% (Sun *et al.*, 2003a). Also, while carrying principal components analysis (PCA), the discern rate can be up to 90.9% (Xu *et al.*, 2002b).

In addition, based on the pattern recognition concept, a new array co-efficient correlation software is designed, namely multi-band compassion software. Comparison with the routine single-band programme, the new one shows good features in identification, flexibility and anti-interference. More than 300 kinds of herbs have been chosen for analysis, and the results show that the efficiency and differentiation accuracies of new software are superior to the routine one, moreover, the recognition capability has also been improved greatly (Xu *et al.*, 2002a and c).

8.2.5 *IR fingerprint characteristic of TCM formula granules*

TCM formula granules and their auxiliary materials are studied via FTIR. It can be seen from the spectra that the formula granules from different pharmaceutical factories have great disparities in the contents and sorts of auxiliary materials. The spectra can be assigned directly when the formula granules have lower contents of auxiliary materials, whereas when the contents are higher, differential spectra technology can be used to improve the resolution. Thus the TCM formula granules can be identified one by one (Zhou *et al.*, 2003). Then via the macroscopic fingerprint spectra of formula granules made from herbs or animals, the following points can be gained. First, the granules can be classified easily and quickly. Second, according to the similarity with the original medicines, the quality of granules can be analysed conveniently. Third, it is possible to study the effects of TCM preparation procedures on the chemical composition of medicines. Fourth, the method can be used to distinguish the products from different manufacturers. The result is shown in Fig. 8.8. Fifth, the method can be employed to carry out quality control on different batches from the same manufacturers (Fig. 8.9). Sixth, the method can also be used to monitor and analyse the ingredients and amount of the auxiliary materials added into the granules. Overall, effective, simple and convenient quality control has been realised in the manufacture of formula granules (Huang *et al.*, 2003).

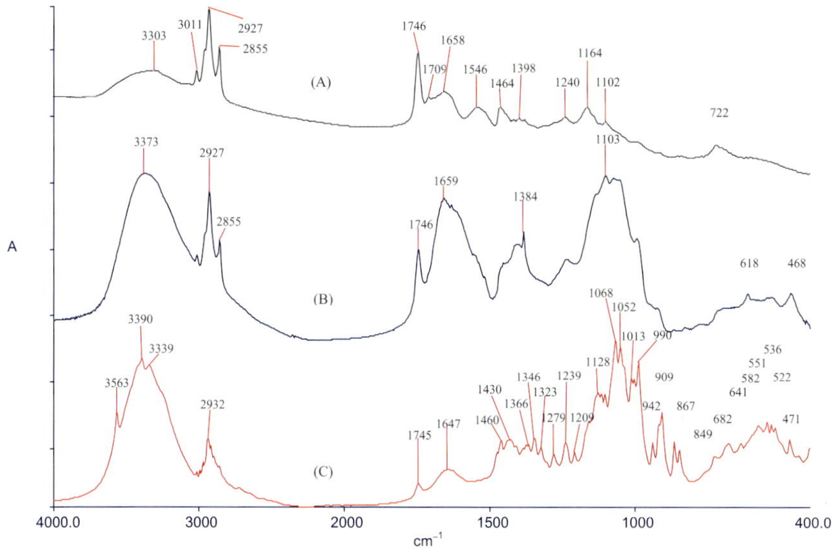

Fig. 8.8. Formula granules of *fructus cannabis* from different manufacturers. (A) Reference medicine, (B) product of manufacturer A, and (C) product of manufacturer B.

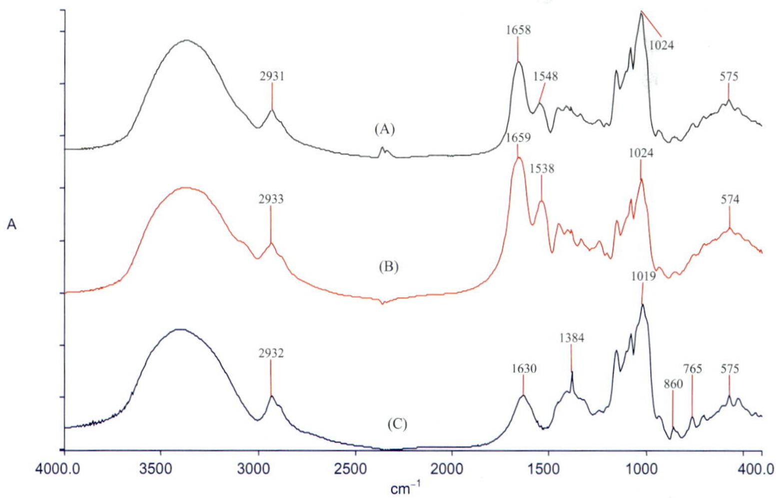

Fig. 8.9. FTIR spectra of deer horn formula granules with different batches.

8.2.6 *IR fingerprint characteristic of TCM injections*

In the case of injections where samples contain a large amount of water, Attenuated Total Reflection (ATR) accessory can be used. More than 20 kinds of injections from different manufacturers and batches, including "*Qingkailing*", "compound *danshen*", "*Hekui*" and "*Huangqi*" etc., are determined. The results show that first, various kinds of TCM injections possess the characteristic spectra, which can be used for distinguishing. Second, the similarities of the injections reflect several components, such as carbohydrates, proteins, starch, lipid, etc. are the carrier and basic materials of effective compositions in TCM. However, they can be identified via the various ratios of these components. Third, every injection has its own characteristic functional groups. For example, based on the relative intensity of C–O stretching of glucoside around 1000–1100 cm^{-1}, aromatic ring skeleton stretching at 1560–1640 cm^{-1} of alkaloid, and carbonyl stretching around 1600–1760 cm^{-1} of terpene or flavonoids, etc. TCM injections can be identified (Zuo *et al.*, 2001).

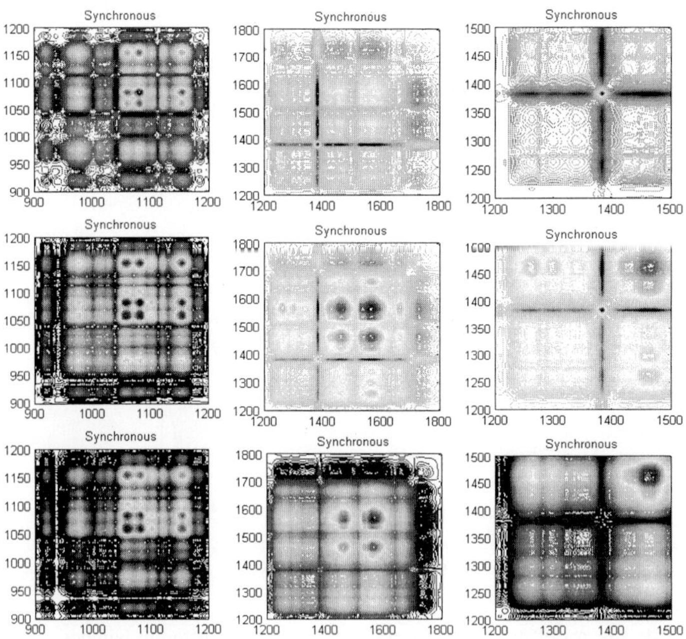

Fig. 8.10. 2D correlation IR spectra of *Danshen* injections with different batches.

For the same TCM injections from different manufacturers and batches, the main components in them are highly similar; their conventional IR spectra embody many similarities. In this case, we apply 2D correlation IR spectroscopy, which can enhance the spectral resolution to a great extent, to analyse them. Figure 8.10 shows 2D correlation IR spectra of *Danshen* injections with different batches. They have obvious features in the peak positions and intensities at different ranges.

8.2.7 *2D correlation IR analyses and the stability verification of TCM*

The thermal stability of the materials can be monitored by FTIR combined with a temperature controller. The deterioration of TCM injection is a gradual changing process. Generally it is very difficulty to identify the presence of deterioration by routine analytical methods if the compulsive

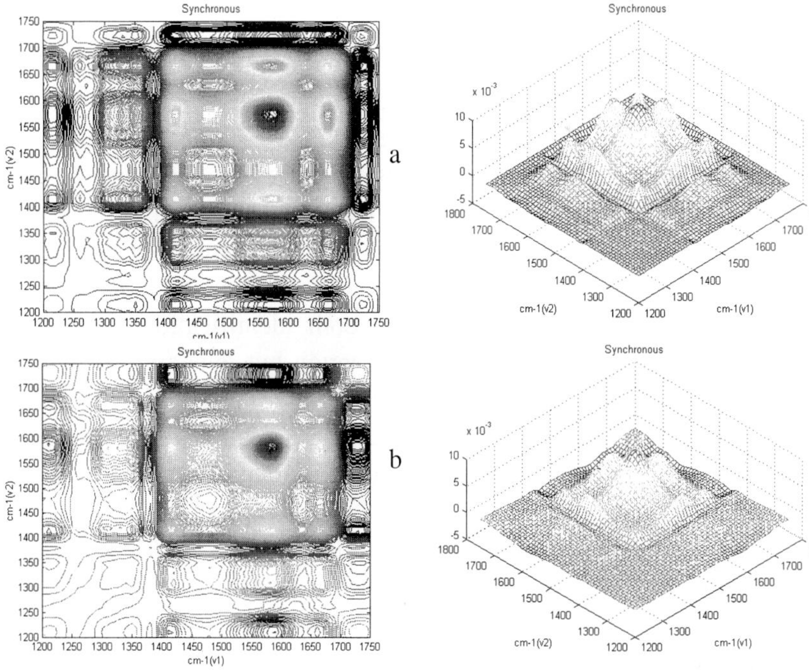

Fig. 8.11. 2D-IR spectra of (a) original and (b) deteriorative *Qingkailing* injection.

ageing time is not long enough or if the temperature range is not wide enough. However, we may use 2D-IR correlation analysis to trace this change. Now, the "*Qingkailing*" injections can be monitored in real time, and further analysed using 2D-IR correlation analysis technique. Figure 8.11 shows the original and deteriorative samples' contour and fishnet 2D-IR spectra deduced under the thermal perturbation. The relative intensities of auto-peaks and cross-peaks are greatly different for these two samples. According to our research, we condude that the deterioration of the injection in air at room temperature is due to the oxidation of flavone and even the changes in conformation and structure of the flavones compounds in "*Qingkailing*" injection. These changes may be related to the conjugate carbonyl and hetero-aromatic rings. Thus, the 2D correlation analysis provides a powerful method for the deterioration mechanism and quality control of the traditional Chinese medicine injection (Zuo *et al.*, 2003).

8.3 Conclusion

In short, the IR spectrum can be used as routine techniques to identify the TCM. Utilising macroscopic fingerprint spectra, not only the raw herbs, but also TCM patent medicines, namely formula granules and injections, can be identified directly. Both quality analysis and quantity analysis can be carried out. The TCM herbs can be classified and even identified by the producing areas. Not only can we discriminate the counterfelt samples, but we can also evaluate the qualities of the TCM samples. This method can be used in both identification and quality control. Moreover, not only static information but dynamic information can be gained as well. This is a non-destructive, fast, accurate, simple and cheap method without sample separation. We call this kind of method macroscopic fingerprint spectroscopy. It has unique merits that cannot be substituted by other methods and means.

This IR macro-fingerprint identification method is a fast, authentic, comprehensive and macroscopic technique for TCM quality control. Also, the method, a non-destructive technique, follows the integrative principle of TCM and does not destroy original natural instinct and compatibility of TCM. The only procedure required before IR analysis is the grinding of the herbal medicine, and thus the whole process for IR research takes only three minutes since no extraction and separation is necessary. According to the IR "fingerprint" characteristic of TCM, we can identify them directly. Furthermore, the IR spectrometer is easy to handle and promote. Most importantly, there is no need to design the contrast medicines; some generally acknowledged and stable TCM commodities can be chosen to generate standard spectra for the macroscopic quality control. With these remarkable features, the technique is worthy to be promoted and applied in macroscopic quality control of TCM commodities.

Besides this technique, we have established a multi-step IR database system based on IR spectra of hundreds of different kinds of TCM commodities, which comprises of a general database, a sorted database, as well as a comparative database. Different kinds of TCM in large amounts were gathered equally, including those belonging to different species, raw drags of true and false. Under the survey conditions of the relative standard, the standard atlas of different traditional Chinese medicines was obtained, and the database was set up according to the TCM characteristics.

When spectrum search is done using the general database, one can judge what medicine the sample is. The sorted database can identify the main type of components involved in the medicine. For the same kind of materials, to know their different geographic origins and growing environments, one can search the comparative database. Depending on the requirements, different databases can be selected for spectrum search. Not only can this database guarantee a good control of the quality of the traditional Chinese medicine, it can also be regarded as the fast appraisal system of the traditional Chinese medicine with good from bad and true from false. The set-up of the database and its application will strengthen traditional Chinese medicine in its production and market development. This will promote the standardisation, and thus the internationalisation of traditional Chinese medicine.

References

Dong, B. and Sun, S.-Q. (2002) *Spectrosc. Spect. Anal.* **22**(2), 232.

Huang, H., Li, J., Qin, Z., Zhou, Q. and Sun, S.-Q. (2003) *Chin. J. Anal. Chem.* **31**(7), 828.

Sun, S.-Q., Du, D.-G., Leung, H.-W. and Yeung, H.-W. (2001a) *Chin. J. Anal. Chem.* **29**(3), 309.

Sun, S.-Q., Huang, H., Xu, Y.-Q. and Cai, S.-Q. (2001b) *Anal. Sci.* **17**(Suppl.), a451.

Sun, S.-Q., Tang, J.-M., Yuan, Z.-M. and Bai, Y. (2003a) *Spectrosc. Spect. Anal.* **23**(2), 258.

Sun, S.-Q., Yuan, Z.-M. and Bai, Y. (2002a) *Comp. Appl. Chem.* **19**(1), 77.

Sun, S.-Q., Zhou, Q., Leung, H.-W. and Yeung, H.-W. (2002b) *Spectrosc. Spect. Anal.* **22**(4), 600.

Sun, S.-Q., Zhou, Q. and Qin, Z. (2003b) *Atlas of Two-Dimensional Correlation Infra-Red Spectroscopy for Traditional Chinese Medicine Identification.* Chemistry Industry Press, Beijing.

Wang, Z., Sun, S.-Q., Li, X.-B. and Zhou, Q. (2001) *Spectrosc. Spect. Anal.* **20**(3), 311.

Xu, Y.-Q., Huang, H. and Sun, S.-Q. (2003) *Chin. J. Anal. Chem.* **31**(1), 5.

Xu, Y.-Q. and Sun, S.-Q. (2002) *Spectrosc. Spect. Anal.* **22**(6), 945.

Xu, Y.-Q., Sun, S.-Q. and Xu, J.-W. (2002a) *Chin. J. Spectro. Lab.* **19**(5), 606.

Xu, Y.-Q., Sun, S.-Q., Yuan, Z.-M. and Bai, Y. (2002b) *Chin. J. Anal. Chem.* **30**(10), 1231.

Xu, Y.-Q., Zhu, J., Qin, Z. and Sun, S.-Q. (2002c) *Comp. Appl. Chem.* **19**(3), 223.

Zhou, Q., Jing, Li, Sun, S.-Q. and Leung, H.-W. (2003) *Chin. J. Anal. Chem.* **31**(3), 292.

Zuo, L., Sun, S.-Q. and Tang, J.-M. (2001) *Anal. Sci.* **17**(Suppl.), a447.

Zuo, L., Sun, S.-Q., Zhou, Q., Tao, J.-X. and Noda, I. (2003) *J. Pharm. Biomed.* **30**(5), 1491.

Chapter 9

GLP Requirements and Herbal Medicines

King-Fai Cheng, Mavis Y.-H. Lee & Kwok-Pui Fung

Abstract

Good Laboratory Practice (GLP) is becoming more and more important in the research and development of Traditional Chinese Medicine (TCM) and its globalisation. If a TCM product is to be registered as Over-the-Counter (OTC) drug and enter international markets, the safety and efficacy studies conducted according to GLP requirements is necessary. The article introduces the content of GLP requirements and the recent development of GLP in China. The safety and efficacy assessment for TCM or herbal medicines under GLP are also covered. This paper also briefly describes the areas that should be covered by GLP regulation and the areas that do not need to follow GLP requirements.

Keywords: Good Laboratory Practice (GLP); Traditional Chinese Medicine (TCM); Herbal Medicine; Safety and Efficacy; Quality Control.

9.1 Introduction

Laboratory tests are essential for drug development. They provide the screening requirements to rule out toxicity, the conformation for quality, the bioassay for adverse effects and drug interaction, and other specific steps towards chemical analysis and development.

Good Laboratory Practice (GLP) is a quality system concerned with the organisational process and the conditions under which non-clinical quality and safety studies for drugs, food additives, agrichemicals, chemicals and cosmetics are planned, performed, monitored, recorded, archived and reported in the laboratory. The ultimate purpose of GLP regulation is intended to assure that non-clinical laboratory study data are of high quality, integrity and reliability.

The results of pre-clinical laboratory studies determine whether a new preparation is appropriate to undergo clinical studies or if it has to undergo further development. To maintain a high quality pre-clinical study, the whole study processes must meet all requirements of GLP. Since the USA issued its first GLP guideline in 1978 (Liu *et al.*, 2000; Liang and Huang, 2000), it has since been adopted by many other countries. Since then, many countries had launched their own GLP Guidelines (Harston *et al.*, 1994). China has also issued its GLP Guideline in 1993 (Li, 1999). China certified seven GLP-compliant facilities in January 2005, and as of the early of July 2005, the total number of GLP-compliant facilities has reached 11. Starting 1 September 2003, all data submitted for new drug's safety evaluation must come from GLP-complied labs, according to SFDA.

9.2 Background of GLP

In the 1970s, fraud practices were quite common in the research of agri-chemicals and drugs in the world. This aroused much caused public concern in the USA (Liang and Huang, 2000; FDA, 1997). In order to stop such dangerous practice in health care product research, the US Food and Drug Administration (FDA) issued a regulation, which was based on the US Public Health Service Act (PHSA), to guide the non-clinical laboratory studies. The drug manufacturers must demonstrate the efficacy and safety of the drugs in the laboratory before they could be tested on humans (Tian, 2001). The current GLP guideline was developed from the US Regulation. During the ten years of GLP implementation, FDA inspected their research institutes located domestically and abroad a total of 690 times. The results of any study should be repeatable, wherever the study was conducted, at any time and by any operators. The investigations did indicate that if a research were conducted according to GLP, the results obtained in different organisations and at different ountries and regions, should be comparable (Turnheim, 1993).

9.3 GLP in the World

As the basic principles and requirements of GLP in different countries are quite similar, testing data may be exchanged freely internationally. In fact, the US FDA has reached an agreement with the United Kingdom, the Federal Republic of Germany, France, Switzerland, Italy, Japan, Sweden and Netherlands for a mutual acceptance of laboratory data. Cross acceptance of data eliminates duplications of laboratory procedures (Turnheim, 1993; OECD; UK Department of Health, 1992; Taiwan Health Administration, 2000).

In 1989, a round table meeting was held in the USA for GLP evaluation. During the meeting, all participants coming from relevant countries agreed on the absolute value of GLP for the safety assessment of healthcare product. The GLP guidelines therefore were internationally endorsed.

9.4 GLP in China

In 1991, the Chinese government started to draft its first GLP guideline. Two years later (December 1993), the first issue of "*Good Practice of Non-clinical Drug Research (Trial)*" was announced by the Ministry of Science cooperating with relevant departments in former State Medicine Bureau (State Sciences and Technology Committee Life Sciences Centre; Du and Ye, 2001), which would be effective since January 1st, 1994.

From the data given for the pre-clinical safety assessment for new drug application in China, it was obvious that more requirements were put in place to completely satisfy the GLP requirements. In the past, practice in China might not be ideal because:

(1) Incomplete legal system;
(2) Lacking management methods and legal warranty;
(3) Lack of academic leaders and management talents;
(4) Insufficient training;
(5) No certificate, weak management;
(6) Inadequate specific requirements, no supervising inspection;
(7) Severe insufficient investment; or
(8) Few laboratories meets the international standard in real science.

Hence, China is now speeding up her efforts to implement GLP so as to facilitate the entry of new domestic drugs into the international market (Huang, 2002).

In the quest for the modernisation of TCM in the 21st century, the Chinese government has set the following national goals for the period of 1996–2005 (State Administration of TCM of PRC):

- Develop 30 highly effective TCM formulas and to push ten into the international market.
- Establish and improve research standards and development systems with the compliant standards: GAP and GMP for TCM cultivation and quality control; GLP for TCM experiments in pharmacology bio-assays and safety evaluations; and GCP for clinical trials.
- Establish ten standardised TCM production bases for herbal raw material and five modern high-tech production bases.
- Foster five internally recognised TCM-based industrial groups.

In order to stimulate the new drug research and development, a State New Drug Research and a Committee for Developmental Harmonisation was set up. The committee was leaded by the State Sciences and Technology Committee and was composed of 18 State Bureaus. A "National Medicinal and Pharmaceutical Innovation Project", the so-called "*<1035> Project*" was established (Du and Ye, 2001; Wang, 1999). The project included:

The establishment of six new Drug Screening Centres and Key Laboratories. They are:

(1) Shanghai Institute of Pharmacology of the Chinese Academy of Sciences;
(2) Institute of Pharmacology of the Chinese Academy of Medical Sciences;
(3) College of Pharmacy of Beijing Medical University;
(4) Institute of Bio-medical and Pharmaceutical Technology of the Chinese Academy of Medical Sciences;
(5) Fujian Institute of Microbiology; and
(6) New TCM Screening Key Laboratory at the Chinese University of Pharmacy and Xin Hua Pharmaceutical Co.

The establishment of three new Drug Safety Assessment Centres (GLP):

(1) Institute of Toxicology and Pharmacology at The Military Academy of Medical Sciences;
(2) Shanghai Pharmaceutical Research Institute; and
(3) Chinese Pharmaceutical and Biological Product Testing and Inspection Centre.

The establishment of three GLP Key Laboratories:

(1) Guangzhou Pharmaceutical Research Institute;
(2) Zhejiang Academy of Medical Sciences; and
(3) Union of Shenyang Pharmacological University and Shenyang Chemical Industry Research Institute.

Up to August 2005, 11 laboratories have been certified by SFDA as GLP compliant laboratories (Table 9.1).

The establishment of ten clinical research centres with GCP standards are to be located at:

(1) Zhongshan Hospital of Shanghai Medical University;
(2) Huashan Hospital of Shanghai Medical University;
(3) Beijing Medical University;
(4) Beijing Union Hospital;
(5) Beijing Fuwai Hospital;
(6) Beijing Tumour Hospital;
(7) Affiliated Tumour Hospital of Sun Yet-Sen University of Medical Sciences;
(8) Guangdong Province Traditional Chinese Medicine Hospital;
(9) Affiliated Xiyuan Hospital of Chinese Academy of Traditional Chinese Medicine; and
(10) Harbin Medical University.

During the process of setting up the GLP laboratories, the following problems were observed:

(1) Innovative new drugs appeared insufficient.

From 1985 to 1995, only 26 Class 1 new drugs were approved by the Ministry of Health (MOH) of China. If a drug was only developed

Table 9.1. GLP-compliant facilities.

No.	Name	Test items
1.	National Institute for the Control of Pharmaceutical and Biological Products (NICPBP) (National Centre for Safety Evaluation of Drug) (NCSED)	1. Single and repeated dose toxicity testing (rodent and non-rodent) 2. Reproduction toxicity testing 3. Genotoxicity testing 4. Carcinogenicity testing 5. Local toxicity testing 6. Immunogenicity testing 7. Safety pharmacotesting 8. Toxicokinetics testing
2.	Shanghai Institute of Pharmaceutical Industry (SIPI) National (Shanghai) Centre for New Drug Safety Evaluation and Research	1. Single and repeated dose toxicity testing (rodent and non-rodent) 2. Reproduction toxicity testing 3. Genotoxicity testing 4. Carcinogenicity testing 5. Local toxicity testing 6. Immunogenicity testing 7. Safety pharmacotesting 8. Toxicokinetics testing
3.	Jiangsu Provincial Institute of Materia Medica (Jiangsu Province Drug Safety Evaluation Centre)	1. Single and repeated dose toxicity testing (rodent and non-rodent) 2. Reproduction toxicity testing 3. Genotoxicity testing 4. Carcinogenicity testing 5. Local toxicity testing 6. Immunogenicity testing 7. Safety pharmacotesting
4.	Shengyang Safe Appraisal Centre of the Shengyang Research Institute of Chemical Industry (Shengyang New Drug Safety Evaluation and Research Centre)	1. Single and repeated dose toxicity testing (rodent and non-rodent) 2. Reproduction toxicity testing 3. Genotoxicity testing 4. Carcinogenicity testing 5. Local toxicity testing 6. Immunogenicity testing 7. Safety pharmacotesting 8. Toxicokinetics testing

Table 9.1. (*Continued*)

No.	Name	Test items
5.	Sichuan Nature Herb Institute (Safety Evaluation Centre)	1. Single dose toxicity testing (rodent and non-rodent) 2. Repeated dose toxicity testing (rodent and non-rodent) 3. Reproduction toxicity testing 4. Genotoxicity testing 5. Local toxicity testing 6. Safety pharmacotesting
6.	Shanghai Institute of Materia Medica, Chinese Academy of Sciences (Drug Safety Evaluation and Research Centre)	1. Single dose toxicity testing (rodent and non-rodent) 2. Repeated dose toxicity testing (rodent and non-rodent) 3. Reproduction toxicity testing 4. Genotoxicity testing (Ames, micronuclei, chromosome aberration) 5. Carcinogenicity testing 6. Local toxicity testing 7. Immunogenicity testing
7.	Guangzhou Pharmaceutical Industry Research Institute (Key Laboratory of New Drug Safety Evaluation and Research)	1. Single dose toxicity testing (rodent and non-rodent) 2. Repeated dose toxicity testing (rodent and non-rodent) 3. Local toxicity testing 4. Immunogenicity testing 5. Safety pharmacotesting 8. Safety pharmacotesting 9. Toxicokinetics testing
8.	Zhenjiang Academy of Medical Sciences (Key Laboratory of New Drug Safety Evaluation and Research)	1. Single dose toxicity testing (rodent and non-rodent) 2. Repeated dose toxicity testing (rodent and non-rodent) 3. Reproduction toxicity testing 4. Genotoxicity testing 5. Local toxicity testing 6. Immunogenicity testing 7. Safety pharmacotesting

Table 9.1. (*Continued*)

No.	Name	Test items
9.	National (Chengdu) TCM Safety Evaluation Centre	1. Single dose toxicity testing (rodent and non-rodent) 2. Repeated dose toxicity testing (rodent and non-rodent) 3. Reproduction toxicity testing 4. Genotoxicity testing (Ames, micronuclei, chromosome aberration) 5. Carcinogenicity testing 6. Local toxicity testing 7. Immunogenicity testing 8. Safety pharmacotesting 9. Toxicokinetics testing
10.	Jilin Nature Pharmaceutical Co. Ltd.	1. Single dose toxicity testing (rodent and non-rodent) 2. Repeated dose toxicity testing (rodent and non-rodent) 3. Reproduction toxicity testing 4. Genotoxicity testing (Ames, micronuclei, chromosome aberration) 5. Carcinogenicity testing 6. Local toxicity testing 7. Immunogenicity testing 8. Safety pharmacotesting
11.	Beijing Union Pharmaceutical Factory Institute of Materia Medica, Chinese Academy of Medica Sciences and Peking Union Medical College	1. Single dose toxicity testing (rodent and non-rodent) 2. Repeated dose toxicity testing (rodent and non-rodent) 3. Reproduction toxicity testing 4. Genotoxicity testing (Ames, micronuclei, chromosome aberration) 5. Carcinogenicity testing 6. Local toxicity testing 7. Immunogenicity testing 8. Safety pharmacotesting

for the domestic market and the data was only aimed to meet the basic requirements of "New Drug Assessment Regulation", the sponsors used to arrange pre-clinical studies at a non-GLP lab in order to cut costs. They did not select the State GLP Safety Assessment Centres. In fact, the GLP laboratories approved by the State did not always command privileges in drug development. Only a few sponsors were willing to register their drugs overseas using the test data collected domestically because they worried about the acceptability of such data. Hence, sponsors preferred to seek collaboration with overseas companies or out-source overseas GLP laboratories to undertake the pre-clinical tests.

Among the 783 items of Western medicine produced in 1990, 97.4% of them were generic drugs. Only 20 drugs belonged to the innovative group which included one anti-malaria drug, Southenwood Methyl Ether (蒿甲醚) and one heavy metal eliminating drug, Sodium Dimeraptosccinate (DMS). These two drugs had been approved by the US FDA. From the above data we could see that the R&D ability for the development of innovative new drugs in China was still far from being satisfactory.

(2) Research funds were deficient.

In developed countries, the successful development of a new drug usually costs 200–300 million USD. In China, the R&D cost for a Class 1 New Drug has been only 2–3 million RMB, which is only 1% or 2% of the sales turnover. Compared with the 10–15% of sales turnover in affluent countries, the differences are quite large.

9.5 Safety and Efficacy Assessment of Herbal Medicines and GLP Requirements

Today, many herbal remedies are being used prophylactically to maintain or enhance good health or prevent certain conditions from occurring. The World Health Organization (WHO) estimates that four billion people — 80% of the world population — use herbal medicine for some aspects of primary healthcare (Farnsworth *et al.*, 1985).

Written records about medicinal plants dated back at least 5000 years to the Sumerians (Swerdlow, 2000). Since the early 19th century, attempts have been made to understand the actions and properties of TCM through scientific research.

In 1984, the People's Republic of China implemented the Drug Administration Law, which said that traditional herbal preparations were generally considered "old drugs" and, except for new uses, were exempt from testing for efficacy or side-effects. The Chinese Ministry of Public Health would oversee the administration of new herbal products (Gilhooley, 1989). In China, there are about 6000 pharmaceuticals manufacturers, among them 2000 are Traditional Chinese Medicinal Products manufacturers. However, so far only four GLP laboratories are approved by State Food and Drug Administration (SFDA). These are the Shanghai State New Drug Safety Control Centre, the National Institute for the Control Pharmaceutical and Biological Product, the Shenyang Research Institute of Chemical Industry, and the Jiangsu Institute of Pharmaceutical Research. If these 2000 TCM manufacturers want to sell their TCM products on the international markets, they have to test the safety and efficacy of their products according to GLP requirements. These four GLP laboratories cannot meet the tremendous demand. For example, the simple acute toxicity test requires at least three months if conducted in a GLP laboratory.

Reform of China's TCM sector began in 1996 under the principles of standardisation, modernisation and internationalisation. The Chinese government started phasing in a set of regulations, known as the five Ps:

- Good Agricultural Practice (GAP);
- Good Manufacturing Practice (GMP);
- Good Laboratory Practice (GLP);
- Good Clinical Practice (GCP); and
- Good Selling Practice (GSP).

Herbs are natural products and thus do not have a consistent, standardised composition. Herbs contain numerous chemical constituents (up to several hundred in some cases). Different parts of the plant (e.g. roots, leaves) contain a different profile of constituents. Furthermore, the content and concentration of the constituents can be influenced by climate, growing conditions, time of harvesting and post-harvesting treatment. If a TCM medication can be proofed for its safety and efficacy as well as its batch-to-batch and manufacture-to-manufacture consistency, it is possible to be registered as an OTC drug in the US or Europe markets. GLP is one of the most important requirements in drug development, which is usually required in drug safety and efficacy study. Implementation of GLP requirements will increase the costs by about 20% (Fleischhauer, 1984); the cost is used for quality control, documentation (e.g. SOPs) and archiving and analysis of reagents and test samples. For example, in the US, the cost of Ames test (a test for determining if a chemical is a mutagen) conducted by a GLP laboratory is around 4500–6000 USD; if conduced according to non-GLP standard at same laboratory, the cost is only 800–1600 USD (Fu, 2002). So some GLP laboratories of international pharmaceutical companies have two systems: GLP standard research and non-GLP standard research. Only research intended for registration are performed according to GLP requirements (Fu, 2002). From the general recognised principles of GLP, safety evaluations usually include single dose toxicity test, repeated dose toxicity test, foetal development toxicity test, reproductive toxicity test, mutagenicity test and carcinogenicity test (Harston *et al.*, 1994).

A number of barriers must be overcome before China's TCM industry can claim the place on the world stage it feels it deserves. Official statistics show that some 96% of TCM manufacturers in China are small- or medium-sized enterprises, with less than 10% of them holding GMP accreditation.

Opinions about the safety, efficacy, and appropriateness of medicinal herbs vary widely among medical and health professionals in countries where herbal remedies are used. Some countries' professionals accept historical, empirical evidence as the only necessary criterion for herbal medicine's efficacy. Others would ban all herbal remedies as dangerous or of questionable value.

9.6 Main Contents and Requirements of GLP

GLP regulations usually cover the following types of studies:

- non-clinical studies;
- safety studies, and
- studies in support of an application for a research or marketing permit.

In administrative practices, GLP should include:

- facility organisation;
- facilities;
- equipment maintenance;
- personnel and training;
- animal care;
- record keeping;
- reporting; and
- quality assurance.

However, GLP regulations do not cover scientific practices, such as:

- protocol design;
- testing methods;
- types of equipment;
- personnel qualification;
- animal selection; or
- data interpretation.

The following are the main contents of GLP regulations:

(1) Personnel (Wang, 2001a)

According to GLP guidelines, the study team should include a Study Director, a Principal Investigator, Study and Quality Assurance Personnel.

The Study Director should be a toxicologist with many years of experience. He is the focal point of study control and has the responsibility for the overall conduct of the study and for its final report.

The Principal Investigator should have the ability to ensure that the delegated phases of the study are conducted in accordance with the applicable principles of GLP.

All personnel involved in the conduct of the study must be knowledgeable in the principles of GLP, which are applicable to their involvement in the study. The Quality Assurance Personnel are independent of the study and assure test facility management of compliance with these principles of GLP.

(2) Test facility (Wang, 2001b)

The basic facilities for a GLP lab should include animal raising and housing apparatus, equipment for testing various functional parameters, storage facilities for study supplies and test medication preparation equipment, as well as washing and disinfecting apparatus. Among them, animal housing and relative equipment are critical for a GLP lab because they are the core of safety assessment. In addition to controlling the timing of the tests, advanced and automatic apparatus ensure that the test results are accurate, objective and reliable.

(3) Standard Operating Procedures (Li, 2003)

Standard Operating Procedures (SOPs) mean documented procedures, which describe how to perform tests or activities normally not specified in detail in study plans or test guidelines. SOPs are very important for GLP implementation because it makes the test result accurate, comparative, authentic and repeatable. In order to avoid the deviation of the test result such as "fault positive" or "fault negative", each step of operating procedure of a safety assessment study must follow the unified guideline that is SOP, including:

- the requirements for receipt, identification, labelling, handling and storage of the test medication;
- the requirements for experimental animals of reservation, acceptance, weighing, health examination, antiscolic, animal selection criteria, animal raising procedures, nutritional standard, drinking water hygienic standard, animal room clearing and disinfecting standards and dead animal treatment procedures;
- various calculating formulas for test medication preparation and administration;
- apparatus maintenance, cleaning and calibration;

- the requirements for testing observation record procedures, data treatment, storage and archive;
- the requirement for specimens in sampling, handling and treating;
- procedures of lab supplies purchasing, storage and getting for use;
- the requirement for the moving route of staff, study material and animals; and
- the requirements for experimental data collection, summary of results, calculations and determinations of statistical significance and final report writing.

(4) Management (Kang, 2003)

Apart from equipping with advanced facilities/equipment, the establishment of a rigorous control system is also important. The system should include:

- the project research management;
- animal raising and environmental monitoring;
- reagents and apparatus management;
- specimen of test medications and biological material handling;
- SOPs management; and
- archive management for all test data including study plans, raw data, final reports.

The heart of GLP regulation implementation is reflected in its Quality Assurance Program. The main responsibility of Quality Assurance Program are to:

- prepare the study schedule;
- inspect the study plans;
- conduct the inspections during the study in progress, which include study-based inspections, facility-based inspections and process-based inspections;
- prepare quality Assurance documents;
- inspect the study results and the reports;
- inspect the qualification of study personnel;
- inspect the documents for submission; and
- inspect the study plans and SOPs being followed.

9.7 GLP Laboratory Establishment

(1) Hardware

The general GLP requirements for test facilities are making sure the data and the results obtained should be reliable and the quality management system should be maintained and monitored according to GLP standards (Wang, 2001b). The following aspects are essential:

- animal housing facility;
- apparatus for various parameters testing;
- sufficient storage and supply facilities;
- test medications handling, washing and disinfecting facilities; and
- archive facility.

To build up a GLP laboratory that meet all international requirements would require an area of 3000–4000 square metres and cost about 30–40 million RMB (Yuan and Lu, 1999). The construction of Shanghai New Drugs Safety Evaluation Centre has been completed and investment of 50 million RMB was estimated (Ye, 1997).

(2) Software

Construction of hardware of a GLP laboratory is relative simple, but construction and following the software according to GLP requirements is not easy (Guo *et al.*, 2003). The overall principles of GLP is assure that data obtained are a true reflection of the results obtained during the study and can therefore be relied upon when making risk/safety assessments (UK GLP MA). In order to achieve the goal, the following aspects should be carried out:

- preparation of the study personnel training programme
- formulation of a series Standard Operating Procedures; and
- formulation a set of rigorous Quality Assurance Program.

9.8 Pharmaceutical Industry in China

In general, China does not yet have strong drug development capabilities, and most of its drug development facilities do not meet the global standards. As a result, China does not have a robust pipeline for innovative drugs. Up to now, most domestic manufacturers in China concentrate on copying existing drugs rather than developing original one. Between 1985 and 1996, only 82 drug approvals were Chinese patented drugs, and most of these were raw materials or herbal medicine products (Espicom Business Intelligence, 2005). So far China has had only two drugs, arteannin and sodium di-mercaptosuccinate, approved internationally (Wang, 2002).

In 1998, China streamlined its centralised regulatory processes for all medical products sold or manufactured in China. The State Food and Drug Administration (SFDA) was organised to formulate and implement relevant regulations in the same year. The SFDA is now more restrictive and moving closer to the way the US FDA and the European Agency for Evaluation of Medicinal Products (EMEA) operate.

Historically China has not been an attractive pharmaceutical market. Its domestic pharmaceutical market is still small scale — less than 2% of the worldwide market. On a per capita basis, the average Chinese is spending approximately US$60 a year on healthcare with 45–58% of that going toward drugs. However this situation has been rapidly changing. Because there are several advantages have made China pharmaceutical market more and more important in the world:

- High growth potential with aging population and improved personal income
- Growing trend of global out-sourcing to Asia due to low costs in R&D and manufacturing
- Large researcher talent pool with technology and industry knowledge and skills
- Strong central and local government support, with favourable tax policies and grants

So we can expect that the Chinese Pharmaceutical Industry will play an increasingly important role in the world.

9.9 Conclusion

All herbal products including TCM when supplied, as medications, should be regulated for safety, quality and for appropriate evidence of efficacy.

The purpose of Good Laboratory Practice is to promote the quality of drug research and development. In the future, TCM products should be strictly studied to prove safety and efficacy, according to GLP requirements. The quality of test data under the GLP regulations is the basis for the mutual acceptance of data among different countries. If individual countries can rely on test data developed independently with confidence, duplicated testings can be avoided, thereby saving time and resources.

References

Department of Health, The United Kingdom (1992) Good laboratory practice, The United Kingdom compliance programme. London, The United Kingdom.

Du, G.-Y. and Ye, Z.-G. (2001) Necessity of making SOPs for traditional Chinese medicine research. *China J. Chin. Mat. Med.* **16**(6), 430–432.

Espicom Business Intelligence (2005) *World Pharmaceutical Market Outlook — BRIC Market for Pharmaceuticals*, January.

Farnsworth, N.R., Akerele, O., Bingel, A.S., Soejarta, D.D. and Eno, Z. (1985) Medicinal plants in therapy. *Bull. World Health Organ.* **63**(6), 965, 981.

Fleischhauer, H. (1984) The cost of GLP compliance. *Pharm. Tech.*, 26 January.

Fu, L.-J. (2002) Suggestions and opinion for the construction of GLP Laboratory in China. *Chin. Pharm. Affairs* **16**(2), 89–91.

Gilhooley, M. (1989) Pharmaceutical drug regulation in China. *Food Drug Cosmetic Law J.* **44**, 21–39.

Good Laboratory Practice for Non-clinical Laboratory Studies (Third Version). Taiwan Health Administration, June 2000.

Guo, J.-Q, Zhang, H., Chai, H.-L. *et al.* (2003) The existing problems of actualizing GLP in China is the software construction. *Sci. Manage.* **18**(6), 46–47, 63.

Harston, S.J., Pharm, B. and Sc, M. (1994) Implementation of good laboratory practices by European pharmaceutical companies. *Drug Inf. J.* **28**, 1055.

Huang, Z.-Y. (2002) Pre-clinical safety study of traditional Chinese medicine and GLP. *J. Chin. Med. Mat.* **25**(1), 52–53.

Inspection: The United Kingdom Good Laboratory Practice Monitoring Authority (UK GLP MA).

Kang, Y. (2003) Implementation of GLP in quality control for new drug research. *Chin. J. Pharm.* **34**(12), 633–635.

Li, P.-Z. (1999) *Quality Control for Non-clinical Safety Study Guideline Training Book.* pp. 5.

Li, P.-Z. (2003) Standard Operating Procedures (SOPs) for GLP laboratory. *Chin. J. New Drug* **12**(5), 321–323.

Liang, Z. and Huang, Y.-S. (2000) Safety assessment of agricultural chemicals and GLP. *Agric. Chem.* **39**(12), 45–46.

Liu, L., Hu, T.-J. and Zhang, X.-L. (2000) Implementation of GLP in European countries. *Chin. Pharm. Affairs* **14**(4), 275–277.

OECD. Good laboratory practice in the testing of chemicals: Final report of the group of experts on good laboratory practice.

Pharmaceuticals Non-clinical Study Guidelines issued by State Sciences and Technology Committee Life Sciences Centre.

State Administration of Traditional Chinese Medicine of People's Republic of China (http://www.satcm.gov.cn).

Swerdlow, J. (2000) Nature's medicine. Plants that heal. In: *Natural Geographic Society*.

Tian, S.-L. (2001) Importance of GLP for the quality of drug non-clinical safety study. *Chin. J. New Drug* **10**(12), 952–954.

Turnheim, D. (1993) Benefits of good laboratory practice as a tool to improve testing. *Hum. Exp. Toxicol.* **12**(6), 528–532.

United States Food and Drug Administration (1997) Good laboratory practice for non-clinical laboratory studies. Part 58. In: *Title of the US Code of Federal Regulations*.

Wang, K.-M. (1999) The problems and considerations of construction and implementation of GLP in China. *Chin. Pharm. Affairs* **13**(6), 384–387.

Wang, K.-M. (2001a) Organisation and personal for GLP implementation. *Chin. Pharm. Affairs* **15**(3), 174–178.

Wang, K.-M. (2001b) Implementation of GLP and laboratory facilities management. *Chin. Pharm. Affairs* **15**(5), 311–315.

Wang, J. (2002) The internal and external environment facing the domestic pharmaceutical industry, July (http://www.tdctrade.com/report/indprof/indprof_20703.htm).

Ye, Z.-G. (1997) GLP Introduction. *Foreign Med. J. TCM Branch* **19**(3), 38–40.

Yuan, P.-J. and Lu, G.-C. (1999) Non-clinical GLP study and new drug development. *Chin. New Drug J.* **8**(5), 289–293.

Chapter 10

The Recognition and Challenge of Drug Metabolism and Pharmacokinetics in Modernisation Research in Traditional Chinese Medicine

Changxiao Liu

Abstract

Traditional Chinese medicine (TCM) has an ancient history and a unique system that includes theory, methodology, prescription formulation and drugs. It has been widely used clinically for thousands of years in China. Therefore, TCM plays an important role in health care in China. This paper will briefly introduce about the present state of pharmacokinetics and drug metabolism research in TCM. This article includes five parts: (1) advances on pharmacokinetic studies of major active compounds from TCM; (2) characteristics on pharmacokinetic studies by combination of diagnosis (*Zheng*); and recipe (*Fangji*) and pharmacokinetics of TCM; (3) effects of traditional Chinese herbal medicine on cytochrome P450 enzymes; (4) key issues in the modernisation of TCM, which are the *lack of standardisation of TCM products and the lack of scientifically accepted clinical efficacy and safety data*. Thus, valid data from well-designed studies pertaining to these two areas are needed to modernise of TCM. The pharmacokinetics of TCM, including quantitatively describing the kinetic changes of absorption, distribution, metabolism and elimination/excretion of TCM, involving many theories and technologies, is a marginalised subject that focuses on pharmacology, chemistry of TCM, analytical chemistry, mathematics in one entity; and (5) challenges and opportunities in pharmacokinetic research of TCM. In fact, *Fanji* is different from chemical drug as it is a mixture of many clear and unclear single chemical entities. It integrates the theory, therapeutics and pharmacy of

TCM. It has often used as tool to study the physiology, pathophysiology and action mechanism of TCM. So, it has important significance in exploring the mechanism of TCM and the scientific connotation, accelerating the improvement of new medicine and quality control and the globalisation of TCM. It needs mutual collaboration and the efforts of different experts in multiple subjects. Pharmacokinetic studies can be very helpful towards the modernisation of TCM.

Keywords: Traditional Chinese Medicine; Modern Research; Traditional Theory; Pharmacokinetics; Metabolism; Metabonomics; Cytochromes P450; Drug Interaction.

10.1 Introduction

Traditional Chinese medicine (TCM) has an ancient history and a unique system that includes theory, methodology, prescription formulation and drugs. Therefore, TCM plays an important role in the health care in China. This article includes four parts: (1) advances on pharmacokinetic studies of major active compounds from TCM; (2) characteristics on pharmacokinetics studies by combination of diagnosis and treatment (*Zheng*, 证), recipe (*fangji*, 方剂) and pharmacokinetics of TCM; (3) the effects of traditional Chinese herbal medicine on cytochrome P450 enzymes; and (4) the challenge and opportunity in pharmacokinetics research of TCM. It will briefly introduce the present state of pharmacokinetics and drug metabolism research of TCM. It has important significance in exploring the mechanism of TCM and the scientific connotation, accelerating the improvement of new medicine and quality control and the globalisation of TCM.

10.2 Advances on Pharmacokinetic Studies of Major Active Compounds from TCM

Studies on metabolism and pharmacokinetics of TCM were reported as early as the 1960s in China (Chen *et al.*, 1963; Song and He, 1964). From then on, especially from 1980, the range and quality of metabolic and pharmacokinetic studies have made considerable progress. Chinese researchers are only recently paying increasing attention to the study on metabolic chemistry of active constituents of TCM; previously, they have mainly focused on pharmacokinetics. The studies on metabolic chemistry of active constituents of TCM before 1990 were reviewed (Gu *et al.*, 1993). Dr. Yang summarised recent advances in this field (Yang *et al.*, 2001).

10.2.1 *Metabolism and pharmacokinetics of active compounds from TCM*

Modern bioanalytical methods (such as HPLC, TLC, GC, MS, LC-MS, etc.) are applied to study the pharmacokinetics of single active compounds or active fractions of TCM. In the past 25 years (1980–2004), more than 1000 research papers were published in academic journals. The obtained pharmacokinetic parameters played important roles in the basic research and clinical application of TCM. Here, this chapter would only cover some information on metabolism of TCM.

10.2.1.1 Alkaloids

Tetramethylpyrazine (TMPZ) is isolated from the rhizomes of *Ligusticum wallichii* Franch. It has the effects of dilating blood vessel, increasing blood discharge of coronary and cerebral circulation, inhibiting blood platelet from aggregating, etc. The metabolites of TMPZ in rabbits administrated by *IP* were separated by HPLC and solvent extraction. TMPZ and its metabolites, 2-hydroxymethyl-3,5,6-trimethylpyrazine (TMPZ D1) and 3,5,6-trimethylpyrazine-2-carboxylic acid (TMPZ D2), were determined in serum (Chen and Dong, 1996). The possible metabolic pathways of TMPZ are oxidisation of the four methyl groups to hydroxymethyl and carboxyl group to form TMPZ D1 and TMPZ D2. TMPZ and its three metabolites existed in rat urine after administration of TMPZ by intra-gastric perfusion. The possible structures of three metabolites were identified (Jiang *et al.*, 1993). The metabolism and transformation of TMPZ in human are similar to those in rats (Ye *et al.*, 1996). Its major metabolite is 3,5,6-trimethylpyrazine carboxylic acid in human urine.

Clausenamide (CL) was isolated from the water extract of leaves of *Clausena lansium* (Lour.) Skeels. The metabolic transformation of (−)-CL was studied *in vitro* with phenobarbital-induced rat liver microsomal incubate containing the NADPH-generating system. The major metabolites were isolated and purified by silica gel column chromatography, preparative TLC and HPLC, and their structures were determined as 6-OH CL and 5-OH CL by HNMR and MS (Yao and Wang, 1998). The metabolic transformation of (−)-CL and 6-hydroxyl-clausenamide was studied in rats administered by intravenous (*IV*) injection (Zhu *et al.*, 2000). The major metabolite of (−)-CL is 6-hydroxyl-clausenamide, which is consistent with the study in rat liver microsomes. The distribution, transformation and elimination of (−)-CL in rat plasma are all relatively rapid. The elimination of 6-hydroxyl-clausenamide is slower than that of (−)-CL.

Hainanensine (HA) was isolated from the bark of *Cephalotaxus hainanensis* Li. Its derivative HH07A is a new anti-cancer drug synthesised from HA as leading compound. The studies *in vitro* indicated that it has better anti-cancer effect. The metabolic transformation of HH07A was studied both *in vitro* and *in vivo*. The metabolic transformation of HH07A was studied *in vitro* with phenobarbital-induced rat liver microsomal incubate containing the NADPH-generating system. The study stated that two metabolites of HH07A existed in the system, and one metabolite structure was determined (Zhang *et al.*, 1997). After oral administration, the metabolism of HH07A in the rat was investigated by GC-MS. HH07A and its four metabolites were determined in the rat urine, and existed mainly as glycosides of glucquronic acid (Zhang and Zhou, 1998).

10.2.1.2 Lignins

Schisandrin (SC) isolated from the seeds of *Schisandra chinensis* (Turcz.) Baill. has good effect of centre tranquilisation. It was widely distributed in various tissues and organs, metabolised and excreted rapidly. There was a small amount of the original drug in urine. The metabolic transformation of SC was studied *in vitro* by rat liver microsomes (Cui and Wang, 1992). The major metabolites were identified as 7,8-dihydroxy-schizandrin, 7,8-dihydroxy-2-demethyl SC and 7,8-dihydroxy- 3-demethyl

SC. The three metabolites were also determined in rat bile and urine after administration of SC. It has demonstrated that 7,8-dihydroxy-schizandrin has the same tranquilisation effect as SC.

10.2.1.3 Lactones

n-butyl phthalide (NBP) is isolated from the seeds of *Apium graveolens* L. It has an anti-convulsant action and is able to protect animals from seizures induced by sodium glutamate, spasm induced by acetylcholine and tremorine spasm as well as electroshock. It also has brain protective action and improves ischaemic brain energy metabolism. After oral administration of NBP to rats, urine was collected, hydrolysed with β-glucuronidase, extracted and concentrated for TMS derivatisation, and then analysed by GC-MS. NBP and its four oxidative metabolites were determined in 0–24 h, and 24–48 h rat urine, and the metabolites mainly existed as the derivatives of γ–OH and β–OH of NBP (Peng and Zhou, 1996).

10.2.1.4 Phenols

Gastrodin and gastrodigenin are the main active principles of *Gastrodia elata* Bl, and have tranquilisation and anti-convulsion effects. The bio-distribution and metabolism of ^{3}H-gastrodigenin and ^{3}H-gastrodin after intravenous injection were studied by the detection of their radioactivity in mice tissues (You *et al.*, 1994). The results demonstrated that gastrodin could penetrate through the blood-brain barrier into the brain, and it was rapidly decomposed into the gastrodigenin in brain, liver and blood. Then, gastrodigenin was preserved in the brain and mediated its pharmacological inhibitive effects on the central nervous system. Most of the gastrodigenin and gastrodin were excreted by the kidney. Gastrodin might exist in the enterohepatic circulation, but Liu *et al.* proposed that gastrodin might not exist in the enterohepatic circulation in rats (Lu *et al.*, 1985).

10.2.1.5 Quinones

Cryptotanshinone (CT) was isolated from the roots of *Salvia miltiorrhiza* Bunge and *S. Przewaquskii* Maxim. The experiments *in vitro* demonstrated that it has strong bacteriostasis against pathogenic bacteria such as *Staphylococcus pyogenes var. aureus* and its drug-resistant bacterium, *Streptococcus bacteroide ramosus*. Clinical observations stated that total ketones mainly containing CT have good curative effects on human infectious disease. The pharmacokinetics and excretion of CT and its metabolite tanshinone II A(TS) in pigs were studied (Xue, 1999). The concentrations of CT and TS in porcine plasma, urine and bile were determined. After *IV* administration of CT, four constituents were isolated from porcine urine. Plasma concentrations of CT and TS, after *IV*, *PO* and *IM* administration of CT, were low, and eliminated rapidly especially after *PO* and *IM*. The absorption in pigs after *PO* administration of CT was low or it was rapidly transformed. Some of CT was first transformed to TS, and TS was further transformed to hydroxyl-metabolite, combined with endogenous substance to increase polarity and then was beneficial to excretion.

10.2.1.6 Flavones and isoflavones

Icariin is a compound of the main flavones in *Epimedium koreaum* Nakai. After oral administration of icariin to rats, the major metabolites in gastric, small intestinal, urine and bile were determined (Qiu *et al.*, 1999). Two metabolites, icariside II and icaritin in both small intestine and urine, and two metabolites, icaritin-3-*O*-*a*-*L*-rhamnopyranosyl-7-*O*-*β*-*D*-glucopyranuronoside and icariside II in bile, were identified. The major metabolic pathway of icariin administered orally in rats was proposed. Icariin is metabolised prior to absorption and exists mainly as its metabolites *in vivo*. The result is different from the report in which flavonoids is decomposed to a glycone and then is absorbed in intestinal. It is possible that it was not the enzyme or microbe that decomposed icariside II or whose effect was weak.

Puerarin and daidzin are the major components in the roots of *Pueraria labata* (Willd.) Ohwi or *P. thomsonii* Benth. After oral administration of puerarin to rats, the urine contained puerarin and four major metabolites, daidzein 4′,7-di-*O*-sulfate, daidzein 7-*O*-*β*-*D*-glucuronide, daidzein 4′-*O*-sulfate, daidzein. Total cumulative amounts of the puerarin and four metabolites excreted in the urine at 48 h following the oral administration of puerarin were approximately 3.6% of the doses administered. The bile contained puerarin and two major metabolites, which were identified as puerarin 4′-*O*-sulfate and puerarin 7-*O*-*β*-*D*-glucuronide on the basis of chemical and spectroscopic data. These experimental data suggest that *C*-glycoside pueraron could be partially hydrolysed to aglycone in the body, but mainly excreted in the urine as puerarin (Zhang and Yang, 1996).

10.2.1.7 Glycosides

Sennoside C is an active ingredient in *Cassia augustifolia* (leaves of *Cassia angustifolia* Vahl or *Cassia tacutifolia* Delile) and Dahuang (root and rhizome of *Rheum palmatum* L., *R. tanguticum* Maxim. Ex Balf. or *R. officinale* Baill.). Its final active metabolites in rats are aloe-emodin anthrone and rheinanthrone. They have purgative action in coordination to mice and rats (Xue, 1993). Sennosides were transformed to an extremely purgative ingredient rheinanthrone, barbaloin was metabolised to aloe-emodin anthrone by the hydrolysis under the action of enteric bacteria (He *et al.*, 1990a).

Swertiamarin (SW), a seco-iridoid glycosides, is from *Swertia pseudochinensis* Hara. The metabolites, erythrocentaurin, $C_{10}H_{20}O_2$ and $C_{10}H_{20}O_4$, were obtained from the culture solution of SW and *Lactobacillus plantarum*. SW is metabolised by 24 isolated intestinal strains. The major metabolites are erythrocentaurin and $C_{10}H_{20}O_2$. The hydrolysates, gentiopicral and a small amount of $C_{10}H_{20}O_2$, were produced by *β*-glucosidase (He *et al.*, 1990b).

Ginseng saponins are the main active constituents in radix ginseng (the root of *Panax ginseng* C.A. Meyer). Ginsenoside Rb1 (G-Rb1) and Rg1 (G-Rg1) were metabolised to varied metabolites in intestines after *PO* administration. G-Rb1 was decomposed easily *in vitro* by rat and human intestinal bacteria, and consequently four metabolites (Rd, Rg3/F2, Rh2/C-K and 20(s)-protopanaxadion [PPD]) were observed on TLC with prolongation of incubation time. The mode of metabolism of G-Rb1 by rat and human intestinal bacteria was Rb1 → Rd → F → C-K(compound K) and the final metabolite was PPD in the faeces of rats and human; after *IG* administration of G-Rb1, Rb1 and its metabolites

Rd and Rg3/F2 were observed in faeces (Chen *et al.*, 1999), and G-Rb1 and its metabolites Rd and F2 were observed in serum after *IG* administration of Rb1 to rats (Ye, 1990). Two metabolites, Rh1 and F1, were detected in the urine and serum of rats by ESI-MS and HPLC. Glycyrrhizin (GL), an active ingredient of liquorice, is widely used in medicine, especially in treating hepatitis. Part of GL, after oral administration, was hydrolysed to the aglycone, 18-β-glycyrrhetic acid (GA), which was then partially transformed by human intestinal flora to 3-*epi*-18-β-glycyrrhetic acid and 3-dehydro-18-β-glycyrrhetic acid (Jin and Xia, 1994).

10.2.2 *Studies on complex preparation of TCM*

The study on metabolism of complex preparation of TCM is void on the whole, while there are relatively more abroad such as a series of studies on pharmacological properties of a preparation reported by Yoshihiro *et al.* Qualitative analysis of components in rat plasma after oral administration of "Kanzobusito" (KB) was carried out by HPLC. Two major compounds were detected, and identified as cinnamic acid and 6*E*,12*E*-tetradecadiene-8,10-diyne-1,3-diol. The former could be the compound originally existing in KB and absorbed from the gastrointestinal tracts, or the metabolite from cinnamic aldehyde; the latter could be metabolite of 6*E*,12*E*-tetradecadiene-8,10-diyne-1,3-diol diacetate, contained in Chinese atractylodes, or the compound originally existing in KB and absorbed from the gastrointestinal tracts (Ye, 1990).

10.2.2.1 The *in vitro* study

The incubation of drug along with the gastrointestinal contents or faeces is a praising method to study metabolism of drug in gastrointestinal tracts. Many active constituents of TCM are metabolised by the action of intestinal flora, especially the hydrolysis of drug with glycoside bond by hydrolytic enzymes of glycoside in intestinal flora is a character of drug metabolism by intestinal bacteria. Cultivating human or animal's faeces as a suspension containing intestinal bacteria and drug under anaerobic condition, and detecting its original constituent and its metabolites are an effective method to study drug metabolism by the action of intestinal bacteria. It is also a good method treating gastrointestinal contents along with drug by heating, such as the study on metabolisms of ginsenoside Rb1 (Chen *et al.*, 1999). Metabolism in animal liver microsomes is used to study drug metabolism in liver. Rat is the classical animal used in drug metabolic studies, such as investigation of SC metabolism (Cui and Wang, 1992).

10.2.2.2 The *in vivo* study

After administration, drug metabolism in gastrointestinal can be investigated by killing animals to obtain each partial gastrointestinal contents to be analysed. To study drug metabolism and propose the pathway of metabolism in gastrointestinal, it can also be used in determining metabolite structures and detecting metabolites contents via time in urine, faeces and bile. Sometimes the sweat and the gas exhaled were analysed. Labelling ^{14}C or ^{3}H is a good method to investigate the absorption, distribution, metabolism and excretion of a drug. The method was used in the study of the metabolism of gastrodin (You *et al.*, 1994; Lu *et al.*, 1985). Metabolism *in vitro* can rapidly solve some complex problems in drug metabolism, and can also easily control metabolic conditions such as the kinds of intestinal bacteria. As its metabolic system is relative pure, isolating and extracting metabolite from the system can be easily done. The result could be obtained in a relative short period of time. This method is especially suitable for studying the metabolism of TCM. If direct metabolic study *in vivo* has some difficulties, metabolism *in vitro* can be first studied to determine the metabolite structures, and then a method can be found for detecting metabolite according to metabolite property in order to investigate drug metabolic situation and the pathway of metabolism *in vivo*, such as the studies on metabolisms of SC (Cui and Wang, 1992). Metabolism *in vitro* might be different from that *in vivo*. To evaluate drug metabolism correctly, metabolism *in vivo* should be further studied on the basis of metabolism *in vitro*.

10.2.2.3 Detection method study

The process of detecting metabolite includes: collecting and treating properly assay mixtures, solvent extracting or preparing sample by column chromatography or TLC, purifying by preparative HPLC, sometimes, and then identifying the metabolite structure by UV, IR, MS and NMR, confirming further by comparison with the spectral and chromatographic behavior of the authentic or synthesised compound, or detecting the treated solution by GC/MS to determine its structure, and further confirming its structure by MS or GC/MS of its derivatives. The RP-HPLC-DAD method, which easily finds the peak of metabolite in extensive range, is suitable for detection of drug and its metabolites. As the metabolite polarity is usually increased, the retention time of metabolite is less than the retention time of original drug during HPLC analysis. Electrospray ionisation mass spectrometry (ESI-MS) is a useful tool for detecting metabolite and its structure. More information could be obtained from MS^n.

10.3 Characteristics on Pharmacokinetics Studies by Combination of Diagnosis and Treatment (*Zheng*, 证), Recipe (*fangji*, 方剂) and Pharmacokinetics of TCM

Since 1985, one of the significant changes in the field of TCM and pharmacology is the combination of TCM "*zheng*" (证), recipe (*fangji*, 方剂) (TCM terminology, object of diagnosis and treatment of TCM), recipe (*fangji*) and pharmacokinetics. The above-mentioned idea and its research job have changed gradually from no to yes. The academic idea of modern research of traditional Chinese medicine (TCM) has changed in combination of the pharmacokinetics and *Zheng* or recipe (Huang *et al.*, 1994 and 2004; Huang, 1999).

10.3.1 *The change in determining chemical component derived from TCM recipe in vivo from NO to YES*

The determination of chemical components derived from TCM recipe *in vivo* had not been reported before 1985. It is mainly the result of the idea that it is impossible or difficult to determine chemical components entering into circulation for an oral TCM recipe. The positive viewpoint considered that the chemical components content and number is too low, complex and unclear.

The pharmacokinetic interaction of glycyrrhetic acid (GA) and other component when oral administration of *Radix Glycyrrhizae* alone or combination of *Radix Paeoniae* Alba was first reported in 1985. So far, over 100 first published papers in the literature supported the above element 1. However, it is only the first step in elucidating the *in vivo* pharmacodynamic substance base of TCM recipe.

It is interesting for several scholars to advance a similar idea about the above positive viewpoint. In 1992, Simon indicated that it is necessary to determine chemical component fate *in vivo* following oral administration of herbal extracts. In 1987, Hiroko Iwama *et al.* developed a new pharmacological testing method, in which two *in vitro* experimental systems were compared in evaluating the pharmacological effects of Shosaikoto, a Japanese and Chinese traditional herbal medicinal mixture, on the mitogenic activity of lipopolysaccharide (LPS) using murine splenic cell culture. The first system involved the addition of serum obtained from mice treated orally with Shosaikoto to the medium. And Shinichi Tashiro termed the method "serum pharmacology" in 1991. In 1991, Chen Keji appealed to the specialist to study pharmacokinetics of TCM recipe and we advance a hypothesis defining the absorption, distribution, metabolism and elimination of traditional Chinese recipe-derived component in blood of healthy subject and patient, and estimate its correctness.

The above hypothesis is divided into *Zheng* and recipe pharmacokinetics. The former indicates that the pharmacokinetic differences between the different *Zheng* have statistical significance and the latter means that the circulatory pharmacokinetics among recipe-derived chemical components are influenced markedly following oral administration of recipe (which is a mixture of more than two herbs). The above two pharmacokinetic characteristics are related to the therapeutic, toxic responses and theory of TCM. Besides the definition described in the above method, we summarised the main elements as follows: (1) recipe-derived components *in vivo* are possibly detected; (2) their number are relatively restricted; (3) they could represent the therapeutic effect of the parent recipe; (4) their concentration and pharmacokinetics could be affected by the combination of herbs in recipe; (5) effects of new bioactive components related with those of their parent recipe; and (6) the *Zheng* state could affect their pharmacokinetics significantly. All the ideas of *Zheng* and recipe pharmacokinetics exhibited the characteristics of combining TCM theory and pharmacokinetics (Huang, 1999).

10.3.2 *The numerable change of recipe-derived chemical components absorbed into circulatory from INFINITE to FINITE*

The orthodox academic circles thought that recipe-derived chemical components *in vivo* and their pharmacokinetics are not detectable and suitable for study because they are too complicated, trace in quantity or unable to represent curative effect of their parent recipes. However, the recipe pharmacokinetics theory says that these numbers are relatively restricted because: (1) most chemical component contents in herbs are too low to be detected when they are distributed throughout the entire circulatory system; (2) only a few recipe-derived high content chemical components in herbs are determined; (3) not all are dissolved into decoction when boiled and not all are absorbed into the circulatory system from the gastrointestinal tract. However, only less than ten chemical components are found from our obtained literature and only nine chemical components in serum were determined, five of them were identified as tetramethylpyrazime, ferulic acid, danshensu, protocatechuic aldehyde and paeoniflorin after oral administration of Coronary Heart No. II, which consists of five herbs. Huang *et al.* developed a novel method called a water bath, in which the above five chemical components in serum following oral Coronary Heart No. II are first extracted and then determined (Huang, 1999).

10.3.3 *The change in academic viewpoint about the relationship between recipe-derived chemical component entered into circulatory and their recipe-induced therapeutic effects: from NO to YES*

The pessimistic opinion is that recipe chemical components are too complicated to represent their parent's recipe effects. Our above-mentioned hypothesis postulates that it is necessary for recipe therapeutic effect to relate with the chemical components that have entered into the circulatory system. Our recently published paper reported the double peak of the serum tetramethylpyrazime concentration-time curve, the second peak of which was related to the acute haemodynamic effect induced by intravenous injection of *Ligusticum wachilli* Hort recipe. Similarly, three evidences published in the journal supported the above-mentioned hypothesis (Huang, 1999).

10.3.4 *The study on Zheng essences according to the pharmacokinetic theory and method*

Many experimental data indicated that the disease state affects the pharmacokinetic parameters significantly. Similarly, the hypothesis of *Zheng* pharmacokinetics studies the effect of *Zheng* state on pharmacokinetics. The related orthodox idea only studied the effect of recipe on body. Since 1994, our research showed that the reserpine-induced rat model (it is often used as spleen deficiency model of TCM) and coronary artery stenosis model, which is used as blood stasis model of TCM influence absorption, distribution, metabolism and elimination of drug. The action mechanism of TCM recipe is still unclear. The key problem is that we do not know the effect(s) of the components that enters the body's circulatory system. However, this problem is gradually solved according to pharmacokinetic theory and methodology.

10.4 The Effects of Traditional Chinese Herbal Medicine on Cytochrome P450 Enzymes

Studying enzyme induction and inhibition is an important part in understanding drug-drug interaction. Herbal medicines are widely consumed by patients in different clinical settings all over the world. Interest in the use of herbal products has grown dramatically in the Western world. Recent estimates suggest an overall prevalence for herbal preparation use of 13% to 63% among cancer patients, thus there is an increasing need for understanding possible adverse drug interactions in medical oncology. Herbs with the potential to significantly modulate the activity of drug-metabolising enzymes (notably cytochrome p450 isozymes) and/or the drug transporter P-glycoprotein include garlic (*Allium sativum*), ginkgo (*Ginkgo biloba*), echinacea (*Echinacea purpurea*), ginseng (*Panax ginseng*), *Hypericum perforatum*, and *Piper methysticum*. All of these products participate in potential pharmacokinetic interactions with anti-cancer drugs. It is suggested that health care professionals and consumers should be aware of the potential for adverse interactions with these herbs, question their patients on their use of them, especially among patients whose disease is not responding to treatments as expected, and urge patients to avoid herbs that could confound their cancer care (Sparreboom *et al.*, 2004). Seven herbal components ginsenosides Rb1, Rb2, Rc, and Rd (from *Ginseng quercetin*) ginkgolides A and B (from *Ginkgo biloba*), were investigated for their inhibitory effects on hepatic CYP2C9 and CYP3A4 catalytic activities in human liver microsomes. Tolbutamide 4-methylhydroxylation and testosterone 6-beta-hydroxylation were used as index reactions of CYP2C9 or CYP3A4 catalytic activities, respectively. The metabolites of both reactions were measured by high-performance liquid chromatography and used as indicators of whether enzymes were inhibited or unaffected by these agents. Herbal components were studied at various concentrations (0.1, 1, 10, 100, 200 μmol/L). The herbal compounds investigated were capable of inhibiting CYP2C9 and CYP3A4 catalytic activities, but the potencies differed. Quercetin showed marked inhibitory effects on both tolbutamide 4-methylhydroxylation and testosterone 6-beta-hydroxylation, with IC_{50} values of 35 and 38 μmol/L, respectively. Ginsenoside Rd also had significant inhibitory potency on both CYP2C9- and CYP3A4-mediated index reactions with IC_{50} values of 105 and 62 μmol/L, respectively. Ginsenosides Rb1, Rb2, and Rc had limited inhibitory activities on both enzyme reaction systems, whereas the effects of ginkgolides A and B appeared negligible. It is concluded that the components of ginseng and *ginkgo biloba* screened are capable of inhibiting CYP2C9- and CYP3A4-mediated metabolic reactions. It suggests that quercetin and ginsenoside Rd have the potential to interact with conventional medicines that are metabolised by CYP2C9 and CYP3A4 (He and Edeki, 2004).

A Chinese herbal medicine formulation sho-saiko-to which is a mixture of seven herbal components (Bupleurum root, Pinellia tuber, Scutellaria root, Jujube fruit, Ginseng root, Glycyrrhiza root and Ginger rhizome), is widely administered to patients with chronic hepatitis in Japan. We assessed the effects of sho-saiko-to on the activity of cytochrome P450 (CYP) 1A2, CYP3A and xanthine oxidase (XO) in 26 healthy subjects, evaluating their CYP1A2 and XO baseline activity by the respective urinary metabolic ratios of an 8-h urine sample after an oral 150 mg dose of caffeine and of CYP3A by a urinary excretion ratio of 6-beta-hydroxycortisol (6-beta-HC) to free cortisol (FC). Thereafter, the subjects received a twice daily 2.5 g dose of this formulation for five days. The mean activity of CYP1A2 decreased by 16% on both days 1 and 5 compared with the baseline ($p = 0.001$). The mean activity of XO also significantly decreased by 25% on day 1 and 20% on day 5 ($p < 0.0001$) compared with the baseline value. The activity of CYP3A tended to be lower on day 5 than the baseline ($p = 0.146$). It is concluded that this drug reduces CYP1A2 and XO activity in man (Saruwatari *et al.*, 2003).

10.5 *Panax Ginseng* and Siberian Ginseng Extracts and Ginsenosides Effects on CYPs Activities

Ginseng extracts and Ginsenosides effects on CYPs activities were studied by many researchers (Yu *et al.*, 2004, He and Edeki, 2004; Anderson *et al.*, 2003; Raucy, 2003; Park *et al.*, 2002; Chang *et al.*, 2002; Henderson *et al.*, 1999). Treatment of rats with a single oral dose (10–30 mg kg^{-1}) of a crude *Panax ginseng* extract of unknown ginsenoside content has been reported to modestly increase hepatic microsomal cytochrome P450-mediated aminopyrine *N*-demethylation activity. In the present study, we compared the effect of *Panax ginseng* and *Panax quinquefolius* extracts on rat hepatic CYP2B1, CYP3A23, and CYP1A2 gene expression. Adult male Sprague–Dawley rats (250–275 g) were administered by oral gavage or *IP* with *Panax ginseng* extract (4% w/w total ginsenosides; 30 or 100 mg $kg^{-1}d^{-1}$ for one or four days), *Panax quinquefolius* extract (10% w/w total ginsenosides; 100 or 400 mg $kg^{-1}d^{-1}$ for 21 consecutive days), or an equivalent volume (2 mL kg^{-1}) of the vehicle (0.9% NaCl or 0.3% carboxymethylcellulose) and terminated one day after the last dose. *Panax ginseng* and *Panax quinquefolius* extracts did not affect body weight gain, absolute or relative liver weight, hepatic CYP2B1,

CYP3A23, or CYP1A2 mRNA expression, or microsomal CYP2B-mediated 7-benzyloxy-resorufin O-dealkylation (BROD) or CYP1A-mediated 7-ethoxyresorufin O-dealkylation (EROD) activity. In contrast, results from positive control experiments indicated that phenobarbital increased CYP2B1 mRNA and BROD activity, dexamethasone increased CYP3A23 mRNA, and beta-naphtho-flavone increased CYP1A2 mRNA and EROD activity levels. Treatment of primary cultures of rat hepatocytes with either of the ginseng extracts (0.1–1000 μg mL^{-1} for two days) also did not affect CYP2B1 or CYP3A23 mRNA expression. Overall, our data indicated that *Panax ginseng* and *Panax quinquefolius* extracts do not increase rat hepatic CYP2B1, CYP3A23, or CYP1A2 gene expression (Yu *et al.*, 2004).

In a study, seven herbal components ginsenosides Rb1, Rb2, Rc, and Rd (from *Ginseng quercetin*) ginkgolides A and B (from *Ginkgo biloba*) were investigated for their inhibitory effects on hepatic CYP2C9 and CYP3A4 catalytic activities in human liver microsomes. Tolbutamide 4-methylhydroxylation and testosterone 6β-hydroxylation were used as index reactions of CYP2C9 or CYP3A4 catalytic activities, respectively. The metabolites of both reactions were measured by high-performance liquid chromatography and used as indicators of whether enzymes were inhibited or unaffected by these agents. Herbal components were studied at various concentrations (0.1, 1, 10, 100, 200 μmol L^{-1}). The herbal compounds investigated were capable of inhibiting CYP2C9 and CYP3A4 catalytic activities, but the potencies differed. *Quercetin* showed marked inhibitory effects on both tolbutamide 4-methyl-hydroxylation and testosterone 6β-hydroxylation with IC_{50} values of 35 and 38 μmol L^{-1}, respectively. Ginsenoside Rd also had significant inhibitory potency on both CYP2C9- and CYP3A4-mediated index reactions with IC_{50} values of 105 and 62 μmol L^{-1}, respectively. Ginsenosides Rb1, Rb2, and Rc had limited inhibitory activities on both enzyme reaction systems, whereas the effects of ginkgolides A and B appeared negligible. It is concluded that the components of ginseng and *Ginkgo biloba* screened are capable of inhibiting CYP2C9- and CYP3A4-mediated metabolic reactions. Our findings suggest that quercetin and ginsenoside Rd have the potential to interact with conventional medicines that are metabolised by CYP2C9 and CYP3A4 *in vivo* (He and Edeki, 2004).

Studies *in vitro* using human liver microsomes were performed to determine the effect of soy extract on probe substrates of CYP and UDP glucuronosyltransferase (UGT). Unhydrolysed soy extract produced very little inhibition of CYP1A2, CYP2A6, and CYP2D6 and a trend of activation of CYP3A4. Hydrolysed soy extract showed inhibition of all of the CYPs tested, particularly CYP2C9 and CYP3A4. UGT2B15 was the only UGT significantly inhibited. Ginseng has been shown to activate CYP3A4 *in vitro*; there is a lack of an *in vitro* correlation with the *in vivo* effects (Anderson *et al.*, 2003).

A reporter gene assay using the human pregnane X receptor (hPXR) and promoter regions of CYP3A4 transiently transfected into HepG2 cells, exhibited inductive properties by the aforementioned therapeutics that were similar to those observed in hepatocytes. Several flavonoids including quercetin, resveratrol, and curcumin were also examined for their ability to induce CYP3A4 in human hepatocytes. Only quercetin produced accumulation of CYP3A4 mRNA (230 ± 73% of control). When examined in a reporter gene assay, this flavonoid exhibited negligible increases in luciferase activity suggesting that quercetin induced CYP3A4 by mechanisms that may not involve PXR. We also examined the effects of herbals on CYP3A4 expression in human hepatocytes. Grapeseed extract, ginseng, silymarin, and kava-kava produced 270 ± 73%, 155 ± 83%, 100 ± 10%, and 386 ± 185% of control CYP3A4 mRNA, respectively. Of these botanicals only kava-kava produced enhanced luciferase activity (11.6 ± 2.1% fold above DMSO treated cells). Such results indicate that kava-kava required PXR to mediate CYP3A4 induction. Collectively, results demonstrated that several botanicals induce CYP3A4, suggesting the potential for drug-herbal interactions (Raucy, 2003).

Park *et al.* have studied the effects of ginsenoside Rb1 (GRb1) on the change in lipid contents in rat liver. When GRb1 was administered intraperitoneally to rats, liver microsomal cytochrome P-450 content and NADPH-cytochrome P-450 reductase activity were lower than those in control rats. The contents of triglyceride (TG) and cholesterol were decreased, but those of total phospholipid, phosphatidylcholine, and phosphatidylethanolamine were increased in the GRb1-treated group compared with controls. These results indicate that GRb1 might be involved in lipid metabolism by regulating the activity of microsomal cytochrome P-450 monooxygenase. Although liver TG levels were reduced by GRb1, the levels of TG and beta-lipoprotein in serum from the GRb1-treated group did not change as compared with those in controls. Thus we suggest that the decrease in liver TG levels with GRb1-treatment is not associated with the secretion of TG-rich very low-density lipoprotein. Furthermore, the level of cAMP was also significantly increased in the GRb1-treated group as compared with that in controls. Additionally, the cAMP level was more markedly increased as compared with that in the GRb1-treated or control groups when GRb was exogenously added to the reaction system for measuring cAMP production in homogenates from the control group liver. Accordingly, these results demonstrate that GRb1 might lower TG levels via cAMP-production in the liver, and GRb1 might be an interesting candidate to search for a modulator of cAMP-mediated effects, especially within the liver steatosis system (Park *et al.*, 2002).

Ginseng extract has been reported to decrease the incidence of 7,12-dimethylbenz[a]anthracene (DMBA)-initiated tumourigenesis in mice. A potential mechanism for this effect by ginseng is inhibition of DMBA-bioactivating cytochrome P450 enzymes. In the present *in vitro* study, we examined the effect of a standardised *Panax ginseng* extract (G115), a standardised *Panax quinquefolius* extract (NAGE), and individual ginsenosides (Rb1, Rb2, Rc, Rd, Re, Rf, and Rg1) on CYP1 catalytic activities, as assessed by 7-ethoxyresorufin *O*-dealkylation. G115 and NAGE decreased human recombinant CYP1A1, CYP1A2, and CYP1B1 activities in a concentration-dependent manner. Except for the competitive inhibition of CYP1A1 by G115, the mode of inhibition was the mixed-type. A striking find was that NAGE was 45-fold more potent than G115 in inhibiting CYP1A2. Compared with G115, NAGE also preferentially inhibited 7-ethoxyresorufin *O*-dealkylation activity in human liver microsomes. Rb1, Rb2, Rc, Rd, Re, Rf, and Rg1, either individually or as a mixture and at the levels reflecting those found in an inhibitory concentration (100 μg mL^{-1}) of NAGE or G115, but did not influence CYP1 activities. However, at a higher ginsenoside concentration (50 μg mL^{-1}), Rb1, Rb2, Rc, Rd, and Rf inhibited these activities. Overall, our *in vitro* findings indicate that standardised NAGE and G115 extracts, which were not treated with calf serum or subjected to acid hydrolysis, inhibited CYP1 catalytic activity in an enzyme-selective and extract-specific manner, but the effects were not due to Rb1, Rb2, Rc, Rd, Re, Rf, or Rg1 (Chang *et al.*, 2002).

Because little is known about the interactions between herbal products and standard medications, the effects of seven ginsenosides and two eleutherosides (active components of the ginseng root) on the catalytic activity of c-DNA expressed cytochrome P450 isoforms were studied in *in vitro* experiments. Increasing concentrations of ginsenosides Rb1, Rb2, Rc, Rd, Re, Rf, and Rg1 and eleutherosides B and E were incubated with a panel of recombinant human CYP isoforms (CYP1A2, CYP2C9, CYP2C19, CYP2D6 and CYP3A4) and their effects on the conversion of specific surrogate substrates measured fluorometrically in a 96-well plate format. For each test substance, the IC_{50} (the concentration required to inhibit the metabolism of the surrogate substrates by 50%) was estimated and this value compared with that obtained for positive control inhibitory drugs furafylline, sulfaphenazole, tryanylcypromine, quinidine, and ketoconizole. Of the components tested, three ginsenosides (Rd, Rc, and Rf) modified the activity of the recombinant enzymes. Ginsenoside Rd produced weak inhibitory activity against the surrogate substrates for CYP3A4 and CYP2D6 and even weaker inhibitory activity against the surrogate substrates for CYP2C19 and CYP2C9. The IC_{50} values of 58 and 74 μmol for the two substrates for CYP3A4 are orders of magnitude higher than that for the potent inhibitor ketoconazole used as a positive control. Ginsenoside Rc produced an increase in the activity of CYP2C9 (70% at 200 μmol) and ginsenoside Rf produced an increase in the activity of CYP3A4 (54% at 200 μmol). The biological significance of this is unclear at this time. Enzyme "activation", the process by which direct addition of one compound to an enzyme enhances the rate of reaction of the substrate, has been observed in a number of cases with P450 enzymes; however, a matrix effect caused by the test compound fluorescing at the same wavelength as the metabolite of the marker substrate cannot be ruled out. These studies suggest that the ginsenosides and eleutherosides tested are not likely to inhibit the metabolism of co-administered medications in which the primary route of elimination is via cytochrome P450; the potential of ginsenosides to enhance the catalysis of certain substrates requires further investigation (Henderson *et al.*, 1999).

Siberian ginseng ([SG]; *Eleutherococcus senticosus*) is a commonly used herbal preparation. The objective of this study was to assess in normal volunteers (n = 12) the influence of a standardised SG extract on the activity of cytochrome P450 CYP2D6 and 3A4. Probe substrates dextromethorphan (CYP2D6 activity) and alprazolam (CYP3A4 activity) were administered orally at baseline and again following treatment with SG (1 × 485 mg twice daily) for 14 days. Urinary concentrations of dextromethorphan and dextorphan were quantified, and dextromethorphan metabolic ratios (DMRs) were determined at baseline and after SG treatment. Likewise, plasma samples were collected (0–60 h) for alprazolam pharmacokinetics at baseline and after SG treatment to assess effects on CYP3A4 activity. Validated high performance liquid chromatography methods were used to quantify all compounds and relevant metabolites. There were no statistically significant differences between pre- and post-SG treatment DMRs indicating a lack of effect on CYP2D6. For alprazolam there also were no significant differences in the pharmacokinetic parameters determined by non-compartmental modelling (C(max), T(max), area under the curve, half-life of elimination), indicating that SG does not significantly induce or inhibit CYP3A4. The results indicate that standardised extracts of SG at generally recommended doses for over-the-counter use are unlikely to alter the disposition of co-administered medications primarily dependent on the CYP2D6 or CYP3A4 pathways for elimination (Donovan *et al.*, 2003).

10.6 Interaction of Drugs and Chinese Herbs

The inhibitory effects of *Angelica dahurica* root extract on rat liver microsomal cytochrome P450 and drug-drug interactions were studied. The 2α- and 16α-hydroxylase activity of testosterone were most strongly inhibited, with 17.2% and 28–5% of their activity remaining, respectively, after oral administration of *A. dahurica* extract at a 1 g kg^{-1}) dose. 6β-hydroxylase activity was also inhibited, with 70% of its activity remaining, under the same conditions. In addition, treatment with the extract inhibited the metabolism of tolbutamide, nifedipine and bufuralol. These results showed that the extract inhibited the various isoforms of cytochrome P450 such as CYP2C, CYP3A and CYP2D1. The *A. dahurica* extract delayed elimination of tolbutamide after intravenous administration at a 10 mg kg^{-1} dose to rats. Thus, the extract altered the liver intrinsic clearance. It had little effect, however, on the pharmacokinetic parameters of diazepam after intravenous administration at 10 mg kg^{-1}. Since diazepam showed high clearance, it underwent hepatic blood flow rate-limited metabolism. Therefore, the change of intrinsic clearance had little effect on hepatic clearance. However, the C_{max} value after oral administration of diazepam with extract treatment was four times that with non-treatment. It was suggested that the first-pass effect was changed markedly by the extract. High-dose (1 g kg^{-1}), but not low dose (0.3 g kg^{-1}), administration of *A. dahurica* extract increased significantly the duration of rotarod disruption following intravenous administration of diazepam at 5 mg kg^{-1}. It was concluded that administration of *A. dahurica* extract has the potential to interfere with the metabolism, by liver cytochrome P450, of other drugs (Ishihara *et al.*, 2000).

10.7 Challenges and Opportunities in Pharmacokinetics Research of TCM

The pharmacokinetics of TCM, including quantitatively describing the kinetic changes of absorption, distribution, metabolism and elimination/excretion of the medicine, and involving many theories and technologies, is a marginalised subject that focuses on the pharmacology, chemistry of TCM, analytical chemistry, and mathematics in one entity. It needs the mutual collaboration and efforts of different experts in various subjects. Pharmacokinetic studies can be very helpful towards the modernisation of TCM. Not only can such studies provide useful data to support efficacy and safety of TCM, but such studies can potentially contribute to *in vivo* standardisation of TCM. There are three aspects in which pharmacokinetic studies can be utilised in contributing towards the modernisations of TCM pharmacokinetic studies: (1) can clarify the oral absorption of TCM; (2) can determine activity of different components as well as herb-herb and herb-drug interaction; and (3) together with well-developed analytical techniques, can potentially provide a method for *in vivo* standardisation of TCM (Chow *et al.*, 2004). Challenges in pharmacokinetics research of TCM include: (1) the correlation between fundamental theory and traditional medicine; (2) the difficulty in research methods, the characteristic of minute amount research objects and the controllability of quality; and (3) the application of advanced technology in the world requires a relatively higher standard in the pharmacokinetics research the challenge coming from foreign countries.

Metabonomics is a new "-omics" science in post-gene time. Metabonomics can be directly understood as the physiological and biochemical situation by its "metabolome profile" as a whole. Therefore it can provide a lot of information that differed from those that came out of other "-omics". Metabonomics has been used to evaluate test animal models and to evaluate xenobiotics, each producing a distinctive series of metabolic perturbations that are characteristic of the type of action mechanism, target organ of toxicity and tissue damage (Lindon *et al.*, 2003; Liu *et al.*, 2004; Liu 2004a and b). It is hopeful that metabonomics would play a necessary role in research and development of new drugs from TCM. Applying metabonomics involves metabolic databases for the discovery of new biomarkers, in screening of new drugs, in drug safety testing and action mechanism research.

The development of genomics, proteomics, toxicogenomics and metabonomics can influence several areas of drug discovery and development. The opportunities presented by this development, the application of these tools and the progress of these new genomic approaches will herald a new revolution in drug discovery development and impact on modern research of TCM. Metabonomics can be applied at any stage in drug discovery and development processes when used in one or more of the following settings: (1) predictive biomarkers for drug-related effects in animal models; (2) understanding of the biochemical mechanisms of action to target-organ or to target-organ pathologies in animal to man; (3) developing biomarkers for toxicities in non-clinical development; and (4) predictive biomarkers for drug-related effects in man during Phase II and Phase III clinical trials.

There is a need to modernise TCM to gain greater acceptance by medical and regulatory agencies internationally so that the benefits from TCM can be realised. The key issues in the modernisation of TCM are: (1) lack of standardisation of TCM products; and (2) lack of scientifically accepted clinical efficacy and safety data. Thus, valid data from well-designed studies pertaining to these two areas are needed to modernise TCM (Chow *et al.*, 2004). We believe that the pharmacokinetics of TCM is critical in the modernisation of TCM leading to international acceptance, just like the "Western" drugs. We urge that pharmacokinetic studies be carried out for all TCM products for human use.

References

Anderson, G.D., Rosito, G., Mohustsy, M.A. and Elmer, G.W. (2003) Drug interaction potential of soy extract and Panax ginseng. *J. Clin. Pharmacol.* **43**(6), 643–648.

Chang, T.K., Chen, J. and Benetton, S.A. (2002) *In vitro* effect of standardised ginseng extracts and individual ginsenosides on the catalytic activity of human CYP1A1, CYP1A2, and CYP1B1. *Drug Metab. Dispos.* **30**(4), 378–384.

Chen, C.H., Kao, S.M., Du, X.F. and Yu, W.H. (1963) Studies on Chinese rhubarb IV. Absorption, distribution and excretion of anthraquinone derivatives. *Acta Pharm. Sin.* **10**, 525–530.

Chen, X. and Dong, S.N. (1996) Studies on the metabolites of tetramethylpyrazine in rabbits. *Acta Pharm. Sin.* **31**(8), 617–621.

Chen, X., Zhou, Q.L. and Wang, B.X. (1999) The metabolism of ginsenoside Rb1 by intestinal bacteria. *Acta Pharm. Sin.* **34**(6), 410–414.

Chow, M.S.S., Yin, O.Q.P., Zuo, Z. and Lau, C.B.S. (2004) Application of pharmacokinetics in the modernisation of traditional Chinese medicine key issues and challenges. *Asian J. Drug Metab. Pharmacokinet.* **3**(2), 89–92.

Cui, Y.Y. and Wang, M.Z. (1992) Metabolic transformation of schizandrin. *Acta Pharm. Sin.* **27**(1), 57–63.

Donovan, J.L., DeVane, C.L., Chavin, K.D., Taylor, R.M. and Markowitz, J.S. (2003) Siberian ginseng (*Eleutheroccus senticosus*) effects on CYP2D6 and CYP3A4 activity in normal volunteers. *Drug Metab. Dispos.* **31**(5), 519–522.

Fan, H.R., He, F., Li, Q.S., Huang, Y.R., Wei, G.L., Xiao, S.H. and Liu, C.X. (2004) Study on influence of ginsenoside Re on cytochrome P450 isoforms by cocktail approach using probe drugs, caffeine, chlorzoxazone, omeprazole and dapsone in rats. *Asian J. Drug Metab. Pharmacokinet.* **4**(3), 177–186.

Gu, L.H., Chen, Y.J. and Liu, L. (1993) Advances on metabolic chemistry of traditional Chinese drugs. *J. Shenyang College Pharm.* **10**(3), 225–230, 234.

He, N. and Edeki, T. (2004) The inhibitory effects of herbal components on CYP2C9 and CYP3A4 catalytic activities in human liver microsomes. *Am. J. Ther.* **11**(3), 206–212.

He, Y.Z., Wang, Q. and Du, G.Y. (1990a) The metabolism of TCD by intestinal bacteria. *Tradit. Chin. Med. Foreign Med. Sci.* **12**(6), 44.

He, Y.Z., Wang, Q. and Cai, Z.D. (1990b) The metabolism of TCD by intestinal bacteria. *Tradit. Chin. Med. Foreign Med. Sci.* **12**(1), 56.

Henderson, G.L., Harkey, M.R., Gershwin, M.E., Hackman, R.M., Stern, J.S. and Stresser, D.M. (1999) Effects of ginseng components on c-DNA-expressed cytochrome P450 enzyme catalytic activity. *Life Sci.* **65**(15), PL209–214.

Huang, X. (1999) Significance of recipe/serum components and target components. *J. Fourth Mil. Med. U.* **20**(4), 277–280.

Huang, X., Run, P., Zhang, L. and Wen, A.D. (2004) The combination of traditional Chinese medicine and pharmacokinetics L the change in academic idea and its research. *Asian J. Drug Metab. Pharmacokinet.* **4**(1), 27–28.

Huang, X., Zhang, Y.M. and Xia, T. (1994) On "zheng"-knetics. *Pharmacol. Clin. Res. Tradit. Chin. Med.* **14**(6), 43–46.

Ishihara, K., Kushida, H., Yuzurihara, M., Wakui, Y., Yanagisawa, T., Kamei, H., Ohmori, S. and Kitada, M. (2000) Interaction of drugs and Chinese herbs: pharmacokinetic changes of tolbutamide and diazepam caused by extract of *Angelica dahurica*. *J. Pharm. Pharmacol.* **52**(8), 1023–1029.

Jiang, J., Jiang, G.F., Ye, Y.P. and Wang, S.Z. (1993) The metabolism of TMPz *in vivo*. *Acta Acad. Med. Sin.* **15**(2), 79–82.

Jin, J.J. and Xia, D.Q. (1994) The advances on pharmacokinetics of glycyrrhizin. *Tradit. Chin. Med.* **16**(1), 13.

Lindon, J.C., Holmes, E. and Nicholson, J.K. (2003) So what's the deal with metabonomics? *Anal. Chem.* **75**(17), 384A–391A.

Liu, C.-X. (2004a) Application of metabonomics in drug discovery and development. In: *Post-Gene-Time: Drug Discovery* (ed.) He, F.C. Military Medical Science Press, Beijing, pp. 17–20.

Liu, C.-X. (2004b) Significance of metabonomics in modern research of Chinese traditional and herbal drugs. *Chin. Tradit. Herb. Drug* **35**(6), 601–605.

Liu, C.X., Li, C., Lin, D.H. and Song, N.N. (2004) Significance of metabonomics in drug discovery and development. *Asian J. Drug Metab. Pharmacokinet.* **4**(2), 87–96.

Lu, G.W., Zou, Y.J. and Mo, Q.Z. (1985) Kinetic aspects of absorption, distribution, metabolism and excretion of ^{3}H-gastrodin in rats. *Acta Pharm. Sin.* **20**, 167–172.

Nguyen, T.D., Villard, P.H., Barlatier, A., Elsisi, A.E., Jouve, E., Duc, N.M., Sauze, C., Durand, A. and Lacarelle, B. (2000) *Panax vietnamensis* protects mice against carbon tetrachloride-induced hepatotoxicity without any modification of CYP2E1 gene expression. *Planta Med.* **66**(8), 714–719.

Park, K.H., Shin, H.J., Song, Y.B., Hyun, H.C., Cho, H.J., Ham, H.S., Yoo, Y.B., Ko, Y.C., Jun, W.T. and Park, H.J. (2002) Possible role of ginsenoside Rb1 on regulation of rat liver triglycerides. *Biol. Pharm. Bull.* **25**(4), 457–460.

Peng, S.H. and Zhou, T.H. (1996) Investigation on *in vivo* metabolism of *n*-butyl phthalide. *Acta Pharm. Sin.* **31**(10), 780–784.

Qiu, F., Chen, Y.J., Kano, Y.H. and Yao, X.S. (1999) Metabolism of orally administered icariin in rats. *Acta Pharm. Sin.* **34**(3), 22–26.

Raucy, J.L. (2003) Regulation of CYP3A4 expression in human hepatocytes by pharmaceuticals and natural products. *Drug Metab. Dispos.* **31**(5), 533–539.

Saruwatari, J., Nakagawa, K., Shindo, J., Nachi, S., Echizen, H. and Ishizaki, T. (2003) The *in vivo* effects of sho-saiko-to, a traditional Chinese herbal medicine, on two cytochrome P450 enzymes (1A2 and 3A) and xanthine oxidase in man. *J. Pharm. Pharmacol.* **55**(11), 1553–1559.

Song, Z.Y. and He, C.F. (1964) The physiological disposition of β-dichroine, an alkaloid of *Dichroa febrifuga* Lour. *Acta Pharm. Sin.* **11**, 437–443.

Sparreboom, A., Cox, M.C., Acharya, M.R. and Figg, W.D. (2004) Herbal remedies in the United States: potential adverse interactions with anticancer agents. *J. Clin. Oncol.* **22**(12), 2489–2503.

Xue, M., Cui, Y., Wang, H.Q., Luo, Y.J., Zhang, B. and Zhou, Z.T. (1999) Pharmacokinetics of cryptotanshinone and its metabolite in pigs. *Acta Pharm. Sin.* **34**(2), 81–84.

Xue, T.M. (1993) The metabolic activation of sennoside C in mice. *Plant Med. Foreign Med. Sci.* **8**(2), 84.

Yang, C.M., Hou, S.X., Zhang, Z.R., Wang, B.N. and Wang, X.C. (2001) Recent advances in metabolic chemistry of traditional Chinese medicine. *Asian J. Drug Metab. Pharmacokinet.* **1**(1), 57–62.

Yao, Q.Q. and Wang, M.Z. (1998) Metabolic transformation of (–)-clausenamide in rat liver microsomes. *Acta Pharm. Sin.* **33**(4), 296–299.

Ye, Y.P., Wang, S.Z. and Jiang, J. (1996) Studies on the metabolites of tetramethylpyrazine in human urine. *Acta Acad. Med. Sin.* **18**(4), 288–291.

Ye, Z.G. (1990) Pharmacological properties of galenical preparation. VII Components of Chinese traditional prescription "Kanzobusito" in rat portal blood after oral administration. *Tradit. Chin. Med. Foreign Med. Sci.* **12**(4), 44.

You, J.H., Tan, T.Z., Kuang, A.R., Zhong, Y.G. and He, S. (1994) Biodistribution of ^{3}H-gastrodigenin and ^{3}H-gastrodin in mice. *J. West China Univ. Med. Sci.* **25**(3), 325–328.

Yu, C.T., Chen, J., Teng, X.W., Tong, V. and Chang, T.K. (2004) Lack of evidence for induction of CYP2B1, CYP3A23, and CYP1A2 gene expression by *Panax ginseng* and *Panax quinquefolius* extracts in adult rats and primary cultures of rat hepatocytes. *Drug Metab. Dispos.* [Epub ahead of print].

Zhang, J. and Yang, K.W. (1996) Metabolites of puerarin in urine and bile of rats. *Tradit. Chin. Med. Foreign Med. Sci.* **18**(3), 46.

Zhang, W.J. and Zhou, T.H. (1998) Studies on urinary metabolites of HH07A, derivative of hainanensine, in rats. *Acta Pharm. Sin.* **33**(3), 212–216.

Zhang, W.J., Zhou, T.H. and Cui, Y.Y. (1997) The *in vitro* metabolism of hainanensine derivative HH07A by rat liver microsomes. *Acta Pharm. Sin.* **32**(2), 116–120.

Zhu, C.J., Zhang, J.T. and Qu, Z.W. (2000) Determination of plasma concentration of (−)-clausenamide and 6-hydroxyl-clausenamide in rats by HPLC and their pharmacokinetics. *Acta Pharm. Sin.* **35**(7), 500–504.

Chapter 11

Intestinal Metabolism of Traditional Chinese Medicine and Its Pharmacological and Toxicological Significance

Guozhu Han

Abstract

The intestine has a great ability to metabolise active constituents of traditional Chinese medicine (TCM). Since the majority of TCM are orally administered, the biological importance of such an ability of the gut must not be underrated. In the gut, TCM undergoes extensive metabolism by intestinal flora (IF) and enterocytes before and during absorption.

The metabolic reactions affected by IF tend to be reductive or deconjugative rather than oxidative or conjugative, and therefore appear to be antagonistic and complementary to those of liver, and as a result, lead to decreased molecular size, enhanced lipophilicity and increased biological activity. By now, a large amount of active constituents of TCM, especially glucosides such as glycyrrhizin, baicalin, sennoside, gerberinside, gensenosides, barbaloin, paeoniflorin, geniposide, etc., have been widely recognised as natural prodrugs, which are activated by IF and therefore produce their pharmacological effects. The toxicity of some active constituents has been attributed to IF-mediated hydrolysis or other forms of conversion. The metabolic reactions carried out by enterocytes are both degradative and synthetic, but mostly synthetic, frequently with detoxicative character, similar to that of the liver. Epithelium cells of intestinal mucosa have many important drug metabolising enzymes, leading to a significant first-pass metabolism and low bioavailability.

Great progress in the study on intestinal metabolism of TCM have been witnessed in recent years. A large amount of active constituents isolated from TCM have been studied extensively. New theories and ideas have been increasingly proposed. Today, a growing number of advanced micro-analytic techniques, methodologies and experiment models are used, which greatly promote the study on intestinal metabolism of TCM. However, much more work still needs to be urgently done to clarify the rules, mechanisms as well as biological significance of intestinal metabolism of TCM, particularly of compound prescriptions.

Keywords: Intestinal Flora; Metabolism; Traditional Chinese Medicine.

The intestine is not only a digestive but also a drug-metabolising organ, and has great ability to metabolise active constituents of traditional Chinese medicine (TCM). Such an ability has considerable impact on the fate of the body and therefore the biological activities of TCM. Since the majority of TCM are orally administered, the pharmacological/toxicological importance of intestinal metabolism of TCM must not be underrated. While one of the major metabolic sites of TCM is the liver, interest in intestinal metabolism having the highest extra-hepatic metabolic activity has increased markedly in recent years. Investigation and grasp of rules and mechanisms of intestinal metabolism of TCM have very important significance for the rational clinical uses and new drug development of TCM.

There are two ways for gut to metabolise active constituents of TCM: the metabolism could be mediated by intestinal flora (IF) within the gut lumen before absorption, or the metabolism could be carried out by intestinal mucosa during absorption.

11.1 Intestinal Metabolic Modes for Active Constituents of TCM and Their Characteristics

11.1.1 *Metabolic conversion mediated by IF*

The early studies on drug metabolism were focused on the hepatic metabolism. However, with the intensification of extra-hepatic metabolism research and rapid development of germ-free and gnotobiotic animal models, the metabolic effects of IF on drugs, especially active constituents of TCM have recently attracted much attention. IF have been shown to be capable of performing a large number of different metabolic reactions. Indeed, it has been estimated that the IF has an organ potential for the

Table 11.1. IF-mediated metabolic reactions for important active constituents of TCM.

Reactions	Structure of substrate	Product	Example
Hydrolysis			
Glucuronides	Drug-Gluceronic acid (GA)	Drug + GA	Glycyrrhizin, Baicalin
Glucosides	Aglycone-O-Sugar	Aglycone	Rutin, Amygdalin, Cycasin
Esters	RCOOR′	RCOOH + HOR′	Chlorogenic acid Acetyldigoxin, Cinobufagin
Amides	R–CO–NH–R′	RCOOH + H_2NR	4-Acetamidobenzoic acid
Reductions			
Double bonds	RCH=CHR′	R–CH_2CH_2R′	Cinnamic acid Caffeic acid
N-oxides	Ar–N. O		Oxymatrine Aristolochic acid Strychnine *N*-oxide Brucine *N*-oxide
Removal of functional groups			
Dealkylation	R–OCH_3	R–OH	3, 4-dimethoxycinnamic acid
Deamination	R–NH_2	R–H	Tryptophan
Decarboxylation	RCOOH	R–H	Phenolic acids, amino acids
Dehydroxylation	Ar–OH	Ar–H	Protocatechuic acid
C–C fission	C-glucosides	Aglycones	Aloin, Homoorientin Mangiferin, Bergenin, Aloesin
Other reactions			
Alkylation	Ar–COOH	Ar–COOMe	Gallate
Aromatisation	Cyclohexane derivatives	Ar	Quinic acid
Condensation	Various	Condensed compounds	Gerberinside
Polymerisation	Various	Polymer	Shikonin
Esterification	Various	Ester	Aconitine
Isomerisation	Various	Isomer	Glycyrrhetic acid Magnolol
Ring fission	Flavonoides	Phenolic acids	Quercetin, Rutin, Apigenin

metabolism of xenobiotics equivalent to or even greater than the liver (Testa and Jenner, 1976).

The IF-catalysed metabolic reactions often oppose the phase I and II reactions of mammalian tissues. The IF is highly anaerobic and thus tends to employ xenobiotic compound as electron acceptors. As a result, the IF-mediated phase I reactions are reductive rather than oxidative. Another contrast is that IF hydrolyses the conjugates formed in phase II mammalian reactions. As the metabolic reactions by IF tend to be degradative, this leads to decreased molecular size, enhanced lipophilicity, increased biological activity of drugs and thus tends to be antagonistic or complementary to those of liver (Rydstrom *et al.*, 1983; Sun *et al.*, 2001). The active constituents, especially glucosides, of TCM are more pre-disposed to the IF-mediated metabolic conversion, because glucoside compounds are IF important carbon sources under anaerobic conditions. The glucose molecules released by IF-mediated deglycosylation reaction will be utilised by IF bacteria as their nutrients. IF-catalysed hydrolysis of glycosidic bond becomes a major feature of IF-mediated drug metabolism (Liu *et al.*, 2000).

The metabolic reactions mediated by IF are many, but fall basically into the following four groups:

(1) Hydrolytic reactions, which serve as the main metabolic reactions occurring in the gut lumen and are catalysed by IF β-glucosidase, β-glucuronidase or β-rhamnosidase.
(2) Reductive reactions.
(3) Removal of chemical groups.
(4) Other reactions such as aromatisation, N-acetylation, ring-fission, isomerism, etc. (Han, 1999; George, 1982). See Table 11.1.

11.2 Metabolic Conversion Carried Out by Intestinal Mucosa

Intestinal mucosa has considerable metabolic capacity towards xenobiotics, involving both phase I (e.g. oxidation, C-hydroxylation, dealkylation, decarboxylation, reduction and hydrolysis) and phase II reactions (e.g. glucuronidation, sulfation, N-acetylation, O-methylation, glycine conjugation, glutathione conjugation, etc.). There are two reactions, hydrolysis and glucuronidation, that are very important for the metabolism of TCM during absorption.

The presence of glycosidases and esterase activity in the small intestine has been demonstrated (Day *et al.*, 1998). In general, monoglucosides are rapidly deglycosylated by the human small intestine, the hydrolytic mechanism being attributed to a broad specificity glucosidase, which catalyses the hydrolysis of the β-glucoside bond. The small intestine may be more active in this hydrolysis than the liver. It has been found that the biological activity of flavonoids depends on the presence or absence of the glycoside residue. Aglycone is likely to have a greater biological effects than the glycosides, so deglycosylation via β-glucosidase activity would be an important step in the metabolism of TCM (Day *et al.*, 1998). It has been shown that deglycosylation of monoglucosides is usually followed by conjugation reactions such as glucuronidation and methylation of catechol-containing structures.

The available data show that the enzyme activity in small intestine is less than that detected in the liver but that the ratio of hepatic to small intestine activity is highly variable. The literature contains several examples that show that the oxidative metabolic capacity of the intestinal mucosa is less than that of liver on a weight basis. However, when conjugation reactions are considered, the activity of the gut wall is close to that of the liver, and may in some cases exceed liver (Table 11.2) (Han, 1999; George, 1982). Intestinal mucosa contains high glucuronyl-transferase activity. It has been found that flavone and flavonol glucosides

Table 11.2. Oxidative and conjugative drug metabolism in the gut and liver of rabbit.

Metabolic reaction	Activity ratio (liver/intestine)
Oxidation	
Ethylmorphine N-demethylation	5.26
Biphenyl 4-hydroxylation	7.14
Glucuronic acid conjugation	
o-Aminophenol	0.24
Salicylic acid	0.09

and their corresponding aglycones can be glucuronidated during transfer across the small intestine. This glucuronidation can occur without the presence of IF (Spencer *et al.*, 1999).

Flavonoids after oral administration are usually present in blood circulation as glucuronides of their aglycones. In order to do so, the flavonoids must first be deglycosylated via glycosidase activity, then glucuronidated via UDP-glucuronyl-transferase activity (Rice–Evans *et al.*, 2000).

11.3 Pharmacological Significance of IF-Mediated Intestinal Metabolism of Active Constituents of TCM

11.3.1 *Metabolic activation by IF*

Currently, it has been widely accepted that "glucosides are natural prodrugs", which was first proposed by Dr. K. Kobashi, a famous pioneer of intestinal metabolic conversion research on TCM, at Toyama Medical and Pharmaceutical University, Japan (Han, 1999; Akao *et al.*, 1992; Kobashi, 1998). The great majority of the main active constituents of TCM are glycosides such as β-D-glucuronides, β-D-glycosides and C-glycosides that are poorly absorbed from the intestine, and reach lower bowels, which are abundant in IF, where they are activated by IF. They are first hydrolysed to release the respective lipophilic and absorbable aglycones by hydrolases of IF such as β-D-glucuronidase, β-D-glucosidase and C-glucosidase. Some aglycones are sequentially reduced by oxido-reductases of IF or subjected to other forms of metabolic conversions. In this way, these natural prodrugs are activated and therefore give rise to pharmacological activity and therapeutic effects. A great deal of active constituents of TCM, including glycyrrhizin, baicalin, sennoside, gerberrinside, gensenosides, barbaloin, paeoniflorin, geniposide, salicin, escin, saikosaponin, etc., have been demonstrated to be natural prodrugs.

11.3.1.1 Glycyrrhizin

Glycyrrhizin (GL), a triterpenoid glycoside with two glucuronic acids in the molecule, is a main effective principle from well-known TCM Radix Glycyrrhizae (*Gan Cao* in Chinese). It is a typical prodrug. The parent

GL is inactive because GL by itself is not absorbed from GI. After oral administration, it reaches large intestine and is hydrolysed by IF to glycyrrhentic acid (aglycone, GA) which is absorbed due to the high lipid solubility. It has been recognised that the pharmacological effects of GL is mediated by GA. IF play a key role in this metabolic conversion, as evidenced by the following facts (Han, 1999 and 2003; Kobashi, 1998):

(1) After oral administration of GL, GA was not detected in the faeces and caecal content of germ-free rats but was detected in the conventional and gnotobiotic rats.
(2) GL, given to above three rat models, was undetectable in the plasma using EIA, RIA and HPLC methods.
(3) Many experiments showed that after oral administration of GL to humans and rats, higher concentrations of GA but not GL in plasma was detected.
(4) GA was undetectable in intra-portal administration of GL to rats.
(5) A study on the hepatoprotective effects of GL against CCL_4-induced experimental liver injury in rats showed that oral administration of GL for three days resulted in significant (> 50%) inhibitory effects against serum AST and ALT activities in conventional and gnotobiotic rats but did not in germ-free rats.
(6) It has been found that a strain of predominant specific anaerobic bacterium designated as *Eubacterum sp.* GLH is responsible for the conversion of GL to GA in human gut. This bacterium has been found to have two kinds of β-glucuronidase, only one of them has hydrolytic activity against GL. Because of high substrate specificity for GL and inducibility by GL, this enzyme is designated as GL-β-glucuronidase.

These findings indicate that GL is a prodrug.

11.3.1.2 Sennosides

Sennoside A and B, the laxative constituents of Rhizoma Rhei (*Dahuang* in Chinese) and Folium Sennae (*Fanxieye* in Chinese), are dianthrono-diglucoside compounds. Their carthartic action has been found to be entirely dependent on the metabolic activation by IF (Han, 1999 and 2003; Akao *et al.*, 1992; Kobashi, 1998). Sennosides are inactive as themselves, but transformed via IF-mediated sequential deglucosylation and reduction reactions to rheinanthrone, which directly stimulates intestinal mucosa and hence promote defaecation. Sennosides A and B are hydrolysed in large intestine by β-glucosidase of IF to its aglycone sennidin, followed by reductive cleavage of at C–C bond linking the double anthraquinones by reductase of the IF to form rheinanthrone. This anthroglycoside is also able to be metabolised to rheinanthrone in the reverse order, namely, cleavage followed by hydrolysis.

The conclusion that sennosides act as a natural prodrug is supported by the following facts:

(1) No diarrhoea occurs after pro-administration of sennosides to germ-free rats and *IV* administration to conventional rats.
(2) Diarrhoea occurs after direct pro-administration of the metabolite rheinanthrone to animals.
(3) Cathartic effect of sennosides falls following pro-administration of chloramphenicol, while produced rheinanthrone decreases.
(4) Rheinanthroneis are detectable in the intestinal site where sennosides exert cathartic effect.
(5) *Clostridium sphenoides* and bifidobacterium adolecentis isolated from human gut have proved to be liable to convert sennosides to rheinanthrone.

Rheinanthrone as a purgative genuine component can only be formed in lower bowel with anaerobic condition and is found to be unstable in aerobic conditions where rheinanthrone is oxidised to inactive rhein. Due to its unstability, rheinanthrone cannot be administered directly as a therapeutic drug. Because of high lipophilicity, aglycone sennidin following oral administration is easily absorbed from small intestine and thus has difficulty exerts its laxative efficacy.

The above findings indicate that sennosides actually serve a carrier and thereby deliver the active constituent to large intestine where it exerts a laxative effect. This natural design confers on sennosides a targeting character. This special property is closely related to IF-mediated metabolic conversion.

11.3.1.3 Baicalin

Baicalin (5,6,7-trihydroxyflavone-7-β-D-glucuronide) is the main active constituent contained in *Scutellarieae Radix* (*Huang Qin* in Chinese), which is a most commonly used herbal medicine in complex TCM and oriented (kampo) medicine.

Early studies assumed that baicalin was absorbed directly as parent drug based on the findings that baicalin but not baicalein (aglycone) was detected in plasma of rats receiving oral administration of baicalin. However, when germ-free rat model, *in situ* jejunal loop method and *in vivo* intestinal absorption experiment were used, it was found out that baicalin was absorbed poorly from GI tract due to its high polarity, but absorbed as the aglycone baicalein resulting from IF-mediated hydrolysis of baicalin, and restored to its original form (baicalein-7-glucuronide) via glucuronic acid conjugation reaction occurring in gut mucosa (Han, 1999; Kobashi, 1998; Akao *et al.*, 2000; Lai *et al.*, 2003). So Baicalin is regarded as a restoration-type prodrug, as shown in Fig. 11.1.

A study showed that baicalin and baicalein administered orally to rats exclusively presented in the plasma as baicalein glucuronides (baicalin) and very small amount of baicalein sulfate, whereas baicalin and baicalein by thcmselves are negligibly absorbed. Therefore, the conjugated metabolites of baicalein are in fact responsible for the *in vivo* effects of baicalin and baicalein (Lai *et al.*, 2003).

In adition, *in vitro* experiments showed that small intestine microsomes of rats contained high activity of baicalein glucuronyltransferase (GT) with specific activity of 26.5 μmol/mg protein/min and k_m of

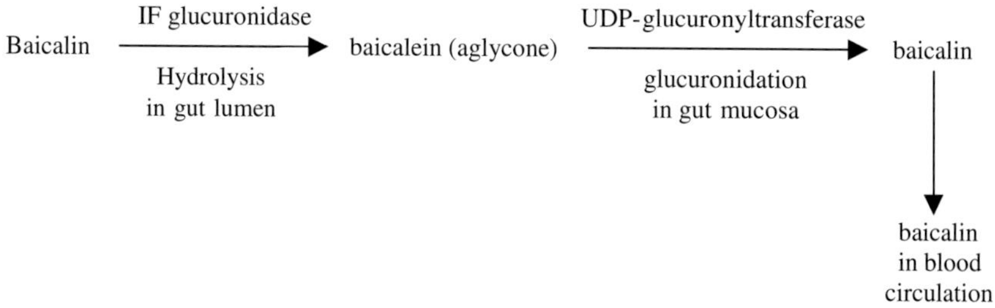

Fig. 11.1. Metabolic activation of baicalin in the gut.

16.7 μmol/L, opposed to low baicalein GT activity in the liver. The small intestine GT was also shown to be an highly specific distinct enzyme for baicalin. This enzyme exhibited much lower activity for *p*-nitrophenol (pNP) and glycyrrhentic acid (GA) and can be strongly inhibited by GA but not pNP.

11.3.1.4 Gerberinside

Gerberinside (4-hydroxy, 5-methyl-coumarin glycoside) is isolated from *Gerbera anandria* (L) (*Da dingcao* in Chinese) and exhibits no anti-bacterial activity *in vitro* but is active *in vivo*, especially against *Pseudomonas aeruginosa*. Two metabolites are isolated when the glycoside is incubated anaerobically with human IF: one is aglycone and the other is gerberindicoumarin (a condensed compound of the double aglycones via $-CH_2-$group). The aglycone and its condensive metabolite, but not its glycoside, exhibit bacteriostatic activity. The conclusion that the anti-bacterial activity of gerberinside is dependent on the IF-mediated metabolic transformation can thus be drawn, as presented in Fig. 11.2 (Han, 1999; Gu, *et al.*, 1988).

11.3.2 *Metabolic inactivation by IF*

In some cases, IF-mediated metabolic transformation results in formation of inactive or activity-diminished metabolic products. This metabolic inactivation by IF is rarely seen, as compared with metabolic activation. A study by Yang Suewei showed that the metabolic products deacetylcinobufagin and deacetulcinobufotalin by IF of cinbufagin and cinobufotalin

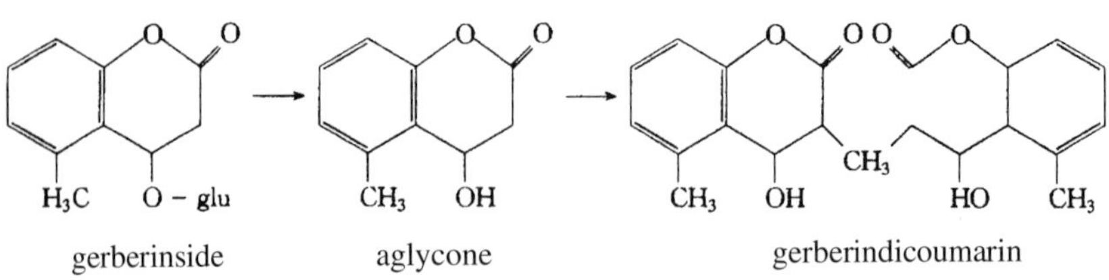

Fig. 11.2. Metabolic transformation of gerberinside by IF.

almost lose the anti-tumour activity, as indicated by IC_{50} data in activity screening experiments with human cancer cell strains (Yang and Hao, 2003a).

11.3.3 *Enterohepatic circulation by IF*

A large number of active constituents of TCM undergo conjugation, especially glucuronidation and sulfation, in the body and are excreted via bile. Frequently, however, re-absorption of unconjugated metabolites follows setting up the process known as enterohepatic circulation (EHC). IF-mediated hydrolysis of conjugates is a key step in the complex chain of events leading to EHC, resulting in delayed excretion of drugs from body and longer $t_{1/2}$. Indeed, the prolonged cardiac effects of digitalis appears to depend on the EHC (Han, 1988). Thus, IF-mediated metabolism and EHC can be regarded as a third phase in the transformation of drugs (phase III reaction) (Rydstrom *et al.*, 1983).

In recent years more and more active constituents of TCM have been reported to have EHC and consequently so-called double- or even multi-peak phenomenon of blood drug concentration (C)–time (T) curve, typified by GL and baicalin as shown in Fig. 11.3 (Han, 1999; Zhang *et al.*, 2005).

11.3.4 *Pre-systemic metabolism by enterocytes*

During absorption, the active constituents of TCM will be subjected to enterocyte-mediated metabolic transformation. Among the catalysed metabolic reactions by enterocytes, conjugative reactions by far predominate in comparison with degradative reactions, frequently resulting in formation of glucuronides and sulphate esters. Enterocyte-mediated metabolisms commonly give rise to a decrease in the amount of drugs entering systemic circulation, i.e. the so-called pre-systemic elimination or the first-pass metabolism, and therefore cause reduction in bioavailability and are often associated with a detoxication in nature (Han, 1999; George, 1982).

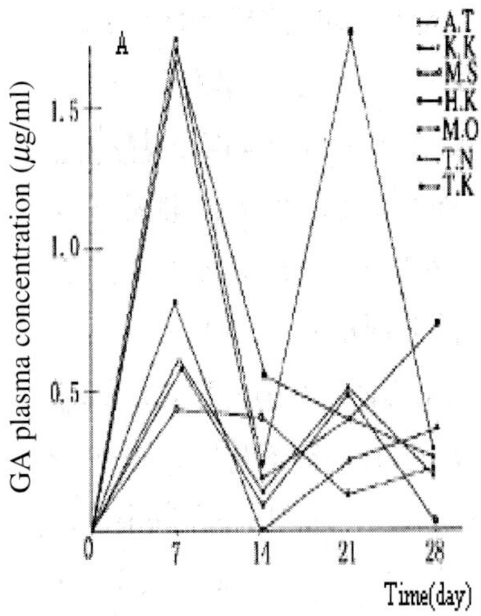

(A)

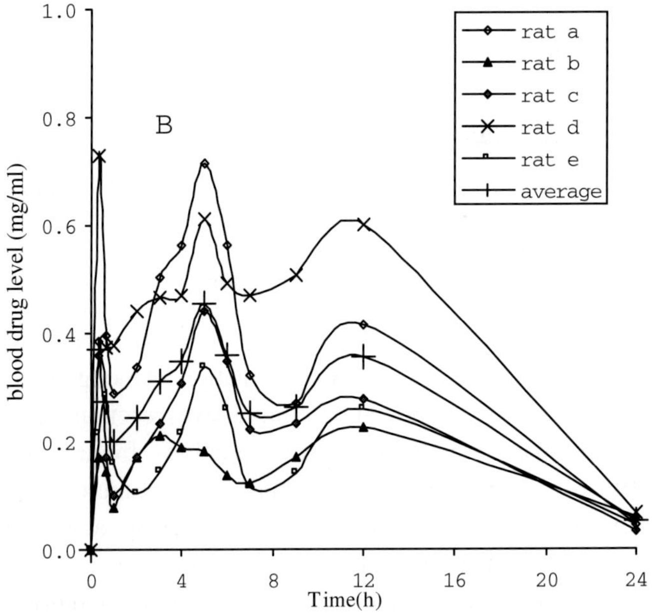

(B)

Fig. 11.3. The typical double- and multi-peak phenomenon of C-T curve of TCM. (A) GL given orally to seven healthy subjects. (B) Baicalin contained in the prescription Fever-Relieving Mixture given orally to five rats.

11.3.4.1 Morphine

Morphine provides a typical example (Han, 1999; George, 1982). Rat experiments showed that oral dose of ^{3}H-morphine resulted in a low bioavailability of only 18% on a parent drug basis but high bioavailability of 83% on a total radioactivity basis. Also, after intra-portal dose, the bioavailability calculated based on parent drug was elevated to 40%. This difference was attributed to the enzyme-catalysed metabolism of morphine in gut wall during absorption. This notion was also supported by rat isolated *in situ* intestine loop experiment, in which the effluent from gut loop at 30 minutes following injection of morphine 10 μmol/L in gut lumen contained 6.9% as free morphine and 6.1% as conjugated morphine of dose, respectively. This conjugation exhibited saturable property. Based on AUC data, extraction ratio of intestinal wall and liver was 55% and 60%, respectively. The further calculation yielded that 62% of the first-pass metabolism of morphine can be accounted for by intestinal mucosa. This, at least in part, explains why morphine is clinically given by parenteral instead of oral routes.

11.3.4.2 Ginsenoside Rg3

More recently, the intestinal uptake and metabolism of ginsenoside Rg3 (Rg3), a main active constituent of well-known TCM Panax Ginseng C.A. Meyer (Ren Sheng in Chinese), has been studied using the Caco-2 cell model (Xie *et al.*, 2004). The results showed that absorption process of Rg3 belongs to an M–M type active process. Its uptake is time- and concentration-dependent and is markedly reduced by metabolic inhibitors (sodium azide and 2,4-dinitrophenol). During uptake, Rg3 (a diglucoside) is deglucosylated to its secondary glycoside Rh2 (a monoglucoside), evidenced by a gradually increasing concentration of Rh2 in incubation solution. It is thought that Rg3 intestinal metabolism can partly contribute to its low oral bioavailability. Another study by the same authors on Rg3 metabolism in beagle dogs showed that after ig administration, the Rg3 and Rh2 were all detected using the HPLC-MS technique. It was assumed that Rg3 was absorbed from GI partly in a form of secondary saponin and thus exerted its therapeutic effects.

11.4 Toxicological Significance of IF-Mediated Intestinal Metabolism of Active Constituents of TCM

The IF-mediated degradative metabolic reactions often produce the more lipophilic, easily absorbable metabolites with stronger toxicity, thereby leading to drug toxic reactions. It is noteworthy that the IF is implicated in the carcinogenesis of certain compounds. The following are the good examples.

11.4.1 *Amygdalin*

A great deal of studies have shown that the IF is responsible for the toxicity of amygdalin, a cyanogenic glycoside, administered orally to humans and animals (Rydstrom *et al.*, 1983; Han, 1999; Li *et al.*, 1986). The conversion of amygdalin to cyanide involves initial enzymatic hydrolysis by a β-glucosidase to yield mandelonitrile and final chemical decomposition to form cyanide. Usually, drugs administered by an oral route produce toxicity lower than that by injection, but the contrary is the case with amygdalin. Oral administration of amygdalin results in significant toxicity.

The role of the IF in toxicity of amygdalin is supported by the following facts:

(1) Following oral dosing (500 mg/kg), 80% of mice died as compared with entire survival after *IV* dosing at the same dose and no overt toxicity after *IP* injection of up to 2500 mg kg^{-1} per day for 15 days.
(2) The oral administration of amygdalin (5000 mg kg^{-1}) produced high blood cyanide levels and toxicity in conventional rats but not in germ-free animals.
(3) The *IP* administration of large dose to mice gave blood cyanide levels similar to or marginally above control values.
(4) When a low, non-toxic dose (50 mg kg^{-1}) was given orally, the recovery of unchanged amygdalin in the urine was higher in germ-free than in conventional rats, whilst the unhydrolysed glycoside was detected in the faeces of germ-free rats only.
(5) The contents of the caecum of conventional but not germ-free rats metabolised amygdalin to benzaldehyde *in vitro*.

(6) The toxicity of orally administered amygdalin in mice was reduced by prior administration of lactose (a β-glucoside) but not maltose (an β-glucoside), and by suppression of the gut flora by kanamycin plus starvation.
(7) Oral but not *IV* dose to patients with cancer shows considerable toxicity. Furthermore, in the urine of patients with cancer who receive *IV* injection of amygdalin, the unchanged amygdalin is recovered at the amount close to the administered dose.

11.4.2 *Cycasin*

Cycasin (methylazoxymethanol-β-D-glucoside), a component of the seed of a subtropical plant *Cycas revolute* Thunb, also provides the classical and most convincing example of the role of the IF in toxicity and chemical carcinogenesis (Rydstrom *et al.*, 1983; Han, 1999), as evidenced by the following experiments:

(1) Oral administration of cycasin to conventional rats is hepatoxic and produces tumours in the liver, kidney and intestine; however, parenteral dose to conventional rats and oral dose to germ-free rats shows complete lack of hepatoxicity and carcinogenesis.
(2) Cycasin aglycone is toxic to both conventional and germ-free rats.
(3) The recovery in urine after oral administration of aglycone to conventional rats is less than 35%, but is almost complete in germ-free rats.
(4) Rats associated only with *Streptococcus faecalis*, a bacterium with strong glucosidase activity, developed typical cycasin lesions. The lesions did not develop, however, when associated with bacteria lacking glucosidase.

11.4.3 *Aristolochic acid (AA) and aristolochic acid I (AA I)*

AA and AA I are closely similar in chemical structure, differing only in that the AA I has an 8-methoxyl group whereas the AA does not. These two compounds are the special alkaloids contained in TCM *Fructus Aristolochiae* (*Madoling* in Chinese). After oral administration of herbal preparations containing AA/AA I, human IF can convert AA/AA I to aristololactam/aristololactam I, respectively. These two lactam-type metabolic products have high toxicity and can induce liver carcinoma and nephropathy.

In faeces and urine of animals administered AA I orally, the presence of aristololactam I has been detected. This metabolite can be further activated by hepatic cytochrome P-450 and hyperoxidase, and further forms adducts with DNA. The hyperoxidase-mediated two main adducts of AA I have been identified as 7-(deoxyguanosin-N_2-yl)-aristolactam I and 7-(deoxyadenosine-N_6-yl) aristolactam I. The fact that the adduct has been found in the human kidney and ureter supports the notion that the production of metabolite aristololactam and formation of the adducts are important causes of the so-called Chinese herbs nephropathy (Yang and Hao, 2003b).

11.5 Summary and Outlook

In the present paper, the IF- and enterocyte-mediated metabolic conversion of active constituents of TCM and its pharmacological/toxicological significance have been reviewed. In the former metabolism, degradative reactions predominate, tending to form the metabolic products with strengthened lipid solubility and enhanced biological activity. Its functions are quite different from that of the liver. In the latter, there are both degradative and synthetic reactions, but mostly synthetic reactions, tending to be detoxicative in nature. Its functions are often similar to that of the liver. We must be aware that intestinal metabolism of TCM play a key role in the pharmacological/toxicological and therefore therapeutic effects of TCM.

The study of intestinal metabolism of TCM has very important significance not only on clinical rational application but also on new drug development of TCM. Currently, discovery of genuine active constituents through study of intestinal metabolism/biological conversion *in vitro* mimicking the human intestinal environment has been considered to be a better model for the search of new drugs. This model complies with the theoretic system of Chinese traditional medicine (Yang *et al.*, 2004).

Great progress in the study of intestinal metabolism of TCM has been witnessed in recent years. A large amount of active constituents isolated from TCM have been extensively studied. Much data on chemical structure dependence on intestinal metabolism of TCM have been accumulated, especially flavonoid compounds as active constituents (Rice–Evans *et al.*, 2000; Zhang and Ma, 2004; Hong and Deng, 1998). New theories and ideas have been increasingly proposed. For example, "glucosides are natural prodrugs", "serum pharmacology" and "prescription of TCM-natural combinatorial chemical library and multi-target action mechanism", etc. (Kobashi, 1998; Han, 2003; Zhou, 1998). Today, growing use is made of advanced micro-analytic techniques, methodologies and experimental models such as LC/MS, NMR, Caco-2 cell line, "ADME/Tox experimental system", germ-free and gnotobiotic animal models (Zhang *et al.*, 2005; Wang, 2004). These greatly promote the study of intestinal metabolism of TCM, and undoubtedly accelerate the modernisation of TCM (Feng, 2003). However, there is still an urgent need for much more work on clarifying the metabolic rules, mechanisms as well as biological significance of TCM, particularly of compound prescriptions.

References

Akao, T., Hattori, M., Namba, T. and Kobashi, K. (1992) Metabolic activation of crude components by intestinal bacterial enzymes. *J. Med. Pharm. Soc. Wakan-Yaku* **9**, 1–13.

Akao, T., Kawabata, K., Yanagisawa, E., Ishihara, K. and Kobashi, K. (2000) Baicalin, the predominant flavone glucuronide of Scutellariae Radix, is absorbed from the rat gastrointestinal tract as the aglycone and restored to its original form. *J. Pharm. Pharmacol.* **52**, 1563–1568.

Day, A.J., Dupont, M.S., Ridley, S., Rhodes, M., Rhodes, M.J.C., Morgan, M.R.A. and Williamson, G. (1998) Deglycosylation of flavonoid and isoflavonoid glycosides by human small intestine and liver β-glucosidase activity. *FEBS Lett.* **436**, 71–75.

Feng, N. (2003) Drug metabolism and modernisation of traditional Chinese medicine. *World Sci. Technol./Modern. Tradit. Chin. Med. Mater. Med.* **5**(3), 5–7.

George, C.F. (1982) *Presystemic Drug Elimination.* Butterworth Scientific, London, pp. 3–68.

Gu, L.H., Li, X., Chen, Y.J. and Zhu, T.R. (1988) Studies on antibacterial constituents of Gerbera Anandria(L) Sch-Bip.: The metabolite of gerberinside and related compounds by human intestinal becteria *in vitro*. *Acta Pharm. Sin.* **23**(7), 511–515.

Han, G. (1988) Pharmacological metabolism by normal microbial flora. In: *Microecology* (ed.) Kang, B. Dalian Publishing House, Dalian, pp. 95–104.

Han, G. (1999) *Pharmacokinetics of Chinese Traditional and Herbal Drugs.* China Medico-Pharmaceutical Press, Beijing, pp. 139–165.

Han, G. (2003) Pharmacokinetics of traditional Chinese medicine. In: *Practice Pharmacokinetics* (ed.) Liu, C.X. China Medico-Pharmaceutical Press, Beijing, pp. 266–334.

Hong, Z. and Deng, H. (1998) Recent status of studies on pharmacokinetics of flavonoids. *Tradit. Chin. Med. Pharmacol. Clin.* **14**(6), 46–49.

Kobashi, K. (1998) Glucosides as natural pro-drugs — demonstration by germ-free rat model and human intestinal bacteria-infected rat model. *J. Kampo Med. Pharm. Sci.* **15**(1), 1–13. He, Y. (1999) (translation): *Foreign Med. (Sect. Chin. Tradit. Med.)* **21**(3), 14–18.

Lai, M., Hsiu, S., Tsai, S., Hou, Y. and Chao, P. (2003) Comparison of metabolic pharmacokinetics of baicalin and baicalein in rats. *J. Pharm. Pharmacol.* **55**, 205–209.

Li, X., Lu, W., Qin, Z., Jin, B. and Wu, F. (1986) Pharmacokinetics of amygdalin and its preliminary toxicological study. *New Remedy Clin.* **5**(3), 141–143.

Liu, T., Wang, Y. and Wang, B. (2000) Studies on the metabolism of icariin by intestinal bacteria. *Chin. Tradit. Herb. Drugs* **31**(11), 834–837.

Rice-Evans, C., Spencer, J.P.E., Schroeter, H. and Rechner, A.R. (2000) Bioavailability of flavonoids and potential bioactive forms *in vivo*. *Drug Metab. Drug Interact.* **17**(1–4), 291–310.

Rydstrom, J., Montelius, I. and Bengtsson, M. (1983) *Extrahepatic Drug Metabolism and Chemical Carcinogenesis.* Elsevier Scientific Publishers, New York, pp. 283–293.

Spencer, J.P.E., Chowrimootoo, G., Choudhury, R., Debnam, E.S., Srai, S.K. and Rice-Evans, C. (1999) The small intestine can both absorb and glucuronidate luminal flavonoids. *FEBS Lett.* **458**, 224–230.

Sun, Y., Li, X.-T. and Yin, S.-L. (2001) Effect of intestional microecological environment on internal metabolism of traditional Chinese herbs. *Chin. Tradit. Herb. Drugs* **32**(4), 375–377.

Testa, B. and Jenner, P. (1976) *Drug Metabolism: Chemical and Biochemical Aspects.* Marcel Dekker, Inc., New York, pp. 447–451.

Wang, K. (2004) *Modern Research Methodology of TCM.* Chemical Industry Press, Beijing, pp. 84–111.

Xie, H., Wang, G., Zhao, X. and Sun, J. (2004) Study on uptake and metabolism of ginsenoside Rg3. *Chin. J. Clin. Pharmacol. Ther.* **9**(3), 257–260.

Yang, S. and Hao, M. (2003a) *Metabolite Analysis for Chemical Constituents of Traditional Chinese Medicine.* China Medico-Pharmaceutical Press, Beijing, pp. 504–512.

Yang, S. and Hao, M. (2003b) *Metabolite Analysis for Chemical Constituents of Traditional Chinese Medicine.* China Medico-Pharmaceutical Press, Beijing, pp. 686–690.

Yang, S., Zhao, J., Cui, J. and Guo, W. (2004) Studies on the biotransformation of escin Ia by human intestinal bacteria and the antitimor activities of desacylescin I. *J. Peking Univ. (Health Sci.)* **36**(1), 31–35.

Zhang, G. and Ma, C. (2004) Advances in studies on pharmacokinetics of flavonoids. *Chin. Tradit. Herb. Drugs* **35**(5), 582–585.

Zhang, Y., Zhao, L. and Han, G. (2005) The pharmacokinetic study of baicalin in Qingre mixture in rats. *West. Chin. J. Pharm. Sci.* **20**(3), 232–234.

Zhou, J. (1998) Prescription of TCM — natural combinatorial chemical library and multi-target action mechanism. *Chin. J. Integr. Tradit. Chin. West. Med.* **18**(2), 67.

Chapter 12

Observation on the Effect of a Herbal Formula in Anti-metastasis of Post-operation Colorectal Cancer

Han-Chen Shen, Xian-Ru Zhu & Shen-Biao Luo

Abstract

Purpose: To investigate the effect of anti-metastasis of a herbal formula in operated colorectal cancer.

Methods: One hundred and one post-operation patients are randomly divided into two groups: patients in group 1 take a herbal formula capsule after operation and patients in group 2 performed operation without the herbal formula. Survival, metastasis and death rate were observed.

Results: Three-year survival rate of Dukes C period of group 1 is 70.83%, and that of group 2 is 41.66% ($p < 0.05$). Three-year metastasis and death rate of group 1 is 29.16%, and that of group 2 is 66.66%, $p < 0.01$. The results indicated that the herbal formula could improve the survival rate of colorectal cancer patients, particularly in Dukes C period.

Conclusion: Development of the herbal formula as an adjuvant medicine for post-operation colorectal cancer is feasible.

Keywords: Herbal Formula; Traditional Chinese Medicine; Colorectal Cancer; Metastasis.

Radical operation of colorectal cancer in the progressive stage usually results in metastasis and death within one to three years; therefore, prevention of post-operation metastasis is of significance in raising therapeutic efficiency. The study herbal formula is a drug developed on the basis of previous clinical practice and researches. From January 1997 to June 1998, we studied 101 post-operation colorectal cancer patients, who were divided into the post-operation long term taking the herbal formula group and the simple operation group without the herbal formula and we discovered that the herbal formula could improve the prognosis of Dukes C period colorectal cancer patients. It is summarised as follows:

12.1 Clinical Data

12.1.1 *General data*

A total of 101 studied patients were hospitalised. Among them, 61 cases male, 40 cases female — proportion of male to female 1.5:1. In the herbal formula treatment group (herbal formula + radical operation) there were a total of 51 cases: male cases 29, female cases 22 — male to female proportion 1.3:1. Contrast group (simple radical operation) had a total of 50 cases: male cases 32, female cases 18 — male to female proportion 1.8:1.

Herbal formula treatment group average age was 52.6 years and contrast group average age 54.20 years. The site of tumour was chiefly at rectum, in treatment group 74.5% located at rectum, contrast group 78.0%. All cases underwent pre-operative biopsy and diagnosed colorectal cancer; in the two groups most were adenocarcinoma with intermediate differentiation.

The clinical pathological stage of colorectal cancer is classified according to the Dukes classification. The patients of the two groups were of the Dukes B or C periods. In the treatment group, 27 cases were of the Dukes B period and 24 cases of the Dukes C period. In the contrast group, 26 cases belonged to the Dukes B period and 24 cases of the Dukes C period.

Scores of clinical symptoms before therapy: Before therapy 39 cases of the treatment group underwent score recording; in the contrast group 38 cases had score recording. Clinical symptoms were chiefly of the deficiency of *Qi* and *Yin*.

Immune function evaluation: Before therapy, 44 cases of the treatment group had examination of NK, CD_3, CD_4, CD_8, CD_4/CD_8 immune criteria and 41 cases of contrast group underwent the same examination.

Type of operation: All patients in the two groups had radical operations. For the patients with colonic cancer, the operation was colonectomy with anastomosis; for rectal cancer, artificial anus operation (Miles operation, Hartmann operation) and anus reservation operation (Dixon recto-anus anastomosis operation, draw out operation) were performed. In the two groups, the most frequently used operation was the Miles operation.

The baseline characteristics of sex, age, pathology, stage, clinical symptoms, immune function, type of operation before therapy in the two groups were no significant difference ($p > 0.05$).

12.1.2 *Selection of cases*

Inclusion criteria: Patient that had undergone pathological confirmation and colorectal cancer radical operation, the pathological stage being Dukes B or C and also those compatible with TCM forms deficiency of *Qi* and *Yin* or deficiency of *Qi* and stasis of blood.

Exclusion criteria: Patients to be excluded: (1) Pathological stage A or D colorectal cancer post-operation patients; (2) patients with severed cardiac, hepatic or renal disease or with psychotic disease; (3) aged below 18 years or over 70 years old or hypersensitive to herbal drug used; and (4) those who did not meet the inclusion criteria, not taking study medicine according to the study protocol, failed to assess the effectiveness, or clinical data incomplete.

12.2 Method

Total 101 patients who were hospitalised were randomly divided into two groups:

Treatment group (51 cases): Radical operation + herbal formula

Contrast group (50 cases): Radical operation only.

For patients in the treatment group, radical colonic operation (colonectomy with anastomosis, artificial anus operation, anus reservation operation) was conducted and herbal formula treatment was provided after operation, with a dose of four capsules each time, three times a day, continuously for three months as a treatment course. For control group, radical colonic operation (colonectomy with anastomosis, artificial anus operation, anus reservation operation) was conducted without herbal formula treatment after the operation.

The safety assessment is based on acute and sub-acute toxic effect manifestation and degree standard issued by the World Health Organization (WHO). Adverse effect episodes were recorded. The main observation parameters were the three-year survival rate and the three-year metastasis and death rate (which is defined as metastasis and death combined rate within three years).

All cases were followed-up by letter information; some cases were followed-up by telephone. In the treatment group, the follow-up rate was 78.43%, the control group was 80%. Those failed in follow-up were all considered metastasis and death cases. Follow-up rate of urban cases were significantly higher than rural. In the cases that failed to be followed-up, only two lived in the urban district.

Statistical analysis was conducted with t- and X^2-test.

Table 12.1. Three-year survival rate and metastasis and death rate comparison.

Period	Group	No. of cases	Survival cases	Survival rate	No. of metastasis and death	Metastasis and death rate
Dukes B	Herbal group	27	20	74.07	8	29.62
	Control group	26	20	76.92	7	26.92
Dukes C	Herbal group	24	17	70.83*	7	29.16**
	Control group	24	10	41.66	16	66.66
Total	Herbal group	51	37	72.54	15	29.41
	Control group	50	30	60.00	23	46

Note: $^{*}p < 0.05$, $^{**}p < 0.01$ compared with the control group.
No clinical adverse effects and abnormalities concerning blood, urine, faeces, heart, liver and renal functions were observed during the study period.

12.3 Result

12.3.1 *Post-operative survival and metastasis and death*

For the treatment group classified as Dukes C period the three-year survival rate was 70.83% and the control group was 41.66%. There was significant difference between the two groups ($p < 0.05$). For the treatment group in Dukes C period, the metastasis and death rate was 29.16%, while the control group (including two cases metastasis but still survived) was 66.66%. The difference was statistically significant ($p < 0.01$) (Table 12.1).

12.4 Discussion

12.4.1 *TCM theory basis in improving the prognosis of colorectal cancer post-operation patients by the herbal formula*

To improve the prognosis of colorectal cancer post-operation patients, it is necessary to aim at the chief factors that affect the prognosis of colorectal cancer — metastasis, relapse and to perform the respective therapy. The recognition of tumour metastasis in TCM may be traced to the time of "*Nei Jing*". In the book "*Ling Shu — The Origin of Diseases*" it was written: "When people are attacked by pathogenic factors taking advantage of lowered resistance ... the pathogenic factors are retained and they join the channels ... reside and transmit through the deep-sited past of the Chong channel ... reside and locate in the stomach and intestines ... reside and locate outside the stomach and intestines or between the Front-Mu and source points. When they reside in the channels, they will accumulate more and more. They may invade tiny branches of the channels, or the channels themselves, or the collateral branches of the large channels, or the Shu channel, or the deep-seated part of the Chong channel, or reside in the paravertebral musculature and tendons, or at the Front-Mu and source points of the intestines and stomach, connecting upwards with the moderate pulse so that the pathogens become abundant and over-flowing. These conditions are not easy to be described completely". Modern medicine considers tumour metastasis to be an extremely complex process that is caused by the interaction of multiple factors, numerous progressive steps and multiple genes involved. It is a manifestation of pathological imbalance resulted from the positive and negative regulatory factors between the tumour and the tissues of the host. If the *Yin Yang* theory is used to elucidate the process of tumour metastasis, the recognition is that the cancer patient who is undergoing operation, chemotherapy and radiotherapy, has his body material basis greatly consumed, so that clinically most of the patients show *Yin* deficiency and at this time, the cancer cells, detaching from the primary site, pass through four stages (*Yang*) to form the metastatic focus and this process indicates abundance of *Yang*. It is therefore necessary to establish the therapeutic principle of "regulation of *Yin* and *Yang*" and to correct the pathologic process of deficiency of *Yin* and abundance of *Yang* with "expulsion of the overload and supplement of the deficiency". When metastatic focus has not appeared treatment should be done according to the principle of "deficiency" and "not to mind about the amount of evil, but should aim at the correction of deficiency". Supplement of *Yin* should be used to suppress *Yang* for the regulation of *Yin* and *Yang* in the post-operation cancer patient and through the bidirectional regulation of TCM drugs, deficiency is supplemented and abundance is pared off to prevent metastasis. There are at least four stages in tumour metastasis: invasion, spread through circulation, distant clone, and angiogenesis; therefore, promotion of *Qi* and activation of blood is applied to treat tumours in the process of metastasis.

When cancer is diagnosed, usually sub-clinical metastasis is present, and the latter is the target of immunotherapy; therefore, the principle of strengthening body resistance and eliminating pathogenic factors should be applied to treat sub-clinical metastasis. If cancer is confirmed, the patient is in a state of exhaustion of *Qi* and injury of blood and if operation, radiotherapy or chemotherapy is administered, the body energy would be further lowered. In clinical practice, most of the patients with post-operation metastasis have deficiency of *Qi* and *Yin* and stasis of blood, and deficiency of both *Qi* and *Yin* is usually seen and therefore treatment should be instituted under the principle of supplement *Qi* and nourish *Yin*. In the syndrome differentiation of post-operation cancer patients, we intermixed the knowledge of modern medicine in cancer metastasis with TCM syndrome differentiation and also with the recognition of disease pathology, and finally we established the principle of strengthening the body resistance and eliminating the pathogenic factor and the therapeutic rule of supplementing *Qi* and nourishing *Yin*, promoting *Qi* and activating blood. On this basis, we investigated and developed a herbal formula capsule. The herbal formula consists of astragalus root, tortoise-plastron, chuanxiong rhizome, fresh-water turtle shell, bighead astractylodes rhizome, motherwort and hawthorn fruit, in which the prepared astragalus root supplements *Qi* and resists evil, tortoise-plastron nourishes *Yin* and suppresses *Yang*, softens hardness and abolishes stasis. These two are the monarch drugs which enter the lung and kidney and supplement the insufficiency of *Qi* and *Yin*. Bighead astrartylodes rhizome resists many evils and strengthens the six Fu organs; if the spleen is weak, it can do the supplement and if the stomach is weak and the food intake decreases, this drug is helpful. Fresh-water turtle shell softens hardness and abolishes nodules; it joins the liver channel, searches for evils, resists coldness, nourishes *Yin* but does not injure *Qi* so that these two drugs serve as minister. The coordination of monarch and minister can supplement deficiency and eliminate evil. Chuanxiong rhizome is helpful in the promotion of *Qi* circulation and activation of blood, in elimination of stasis and growth of new tissues. Motherwort activates blood circulation, eliminates stasis and promotes diuresis; hawthorn fruit promotes digestion and eliminates stasis and stagnation. All drugs of the formula act coordinatively to attain the supplement of *Qi* and nourishment of *Yin*, circulation of *Qi* and activation of blood and strengthening of body resistance, elimination of evil and finally to reach the perspective of anti-metastasis and lengthening of survival period.

12.4.2 *Significance of clinical and laboratory investigation results of the herbal formula*

Before clinical research, we performed some laboratory investigations with the herbal formula and found that it could inhibit intestinal cancer cell growth and promote death of the tumour cells, inducing retardation of intestinal cancer cell $G_2 + M$ stage and apoptosis of these cells (Qian *et al.*, 1999). For S180, the tumour inhibition rate was 37%; for Lewis lung cancer, the lung inhibition rate was 26%; for Lewis lung cancer with blood metastasis, the inhibition rate was 12%; for B16 melanoma with lung metastasis, the inhibition rate was 13.26% (Sheng *et al.*, 1999a). For mouse CA795 lung adenocarcinoma, spontaneous metastasis inhibition rate was 29.34%; used synergetically with cisplatinum for mice implanted with human ovarian cancer, the metastasis inhibition rate was 57.2% (Sheng *et al.*, 1999b). At the same time, through immune function examination, it was found that the immune function was increased and through molecular biological study, it was shown that the cancer inhibition gave P^{53}, the cancer metastasis inhibition gene nm^{23} was elevated, the cancer metastasis gene mdm^2 and metastasis-related gene CD_{44} were lowered. The above laboratory investigation provided basis for clinical research. The present clinical study, as a comparison, demonstrates that in the herbal formula treatment group, the three-year survival rate for Dukes C period was 70.83%, while in the control group it was only 41.66% ($p < 0.05$); in treatment group three-year metastasis and death rate was 29.16%, while in the control group it was 58.33% ($p < 0.05$). It suggests that the herbal formula can improve the prognosis, increase survival rate and decrease metastasis and death rate of colorectal cancer post-operation Dukes C period patients.

12.5 Summary

From the result of this clinical study, it is shown that the herbal formula can improve the prognosis of post-operation colorectal cancer patients, its effect on increasing colorectal cancer survival rate and decreasing the metastasis and death rate are chiefly manifested in the Dukes C period patients, its action is related to the improvement of internal environment of the body and anti-metastasis ability by the herbal formula. It is anticipated that the development of the herbal formula as an adjuvant drug for post-operation colorectal cancer is feasible.

References

Qian, L.-J., Mu, H.-Z. and Xu, S.-H. (1999) The mechanism of Chinese medication Chang Bi An on tumour cells of large intestine. *Zhejiang J. Med. Pharm. Tech.* **1**, 38.

Sheng, H.-C., Yang, F. and Shen, X. (1999a) Experimental study of Chang Bi An capsules on anti-cancer and metastasis through blood verrales. *Zhejiang J. Tradit. Chin. Med.* **34**(2), 81.

Sheng, H.-C., Yang, F. and Shen, X. (1999b) Experimental study of Chinese medicine Chang Bi An capsule on immune function of tumour-borned mice. *Zhejiang J. Tradit. Chin. Med.* **39**(3), 124.

Chapter 13

Evaluation of Research on Diabetes with Combined TCM and WM

Lan Ling & Qing Ni

Abstract

The research on the protection and treatment of diabetes and its complications has received significant achievement with the principle of mainly using Chinese medicine (CM) combined with Western medicine (WM). Research of combined CM and WM on diabetes has already become the main part in medical research areas in China. The theory of combined CM and WM is advanced with inheritance and new ideas. The basis of combined CM and WM is established by the permeation of theory of aetiology and pathogenesis. The prevention and treatment of diabetes with combined CM and WM are improved by the new ideas, which depend on the basis of inheritance. The method of differential types, which are standardised scientifically, is the new model for studying diabetes with combined CM and WM. Researchers should pay attention not only to diabetes treatment, but also to the prevention and treatment of its complications. The advantage of combined CM and WM should be developed; we should look for the combined point between CM and WM and absorb the modern pharmacological results from past research. Much achievement is obtained through the research on clinical trials and experimental studies of diabetes and its complications, and through the rational selection of Chinese herbs and WM. Some new, effective and easily ingested herb products are developed and widely used in the clinics.

Keywords: Diabetes; Combined Chinese and Western Medicine; Standardised Differential Types; Prevention and Treatment of Complications; Experimental Research.

Along with the changes of living patterns, increase in the proportion of the elderly in society and enhancement of self-consciousness of health protection, the incidence of diabetes has increased dramatically worldwide. The incidence of diabetes in China in the eighties of the past century was 0.6–1.0% and since then, it has risen to 3.6–5.0%, in which those above 60 years of age have an incidence of 6% and the number of patients has increased from six million to 24 million. The incidence in Western countries is 2.5–5.0% and the number of patients worldwide has increased from 30 million in the period of the eighties to 120 million, and it is estimated that in 2025 it will increase to 299 million (Jiang, 1992). In the recent years, countries in America, Europe and South-eastern Asia, have begun to appreciate physiotherapy, so that TCM now receives increasing favour. The advantages of traditional Chinese medicine and pharmaceutics are given full play in our country and the principle instituted is the combination of TCM and WM with TCM as the main core, and because of this, the research on prevention and treatment of diabetes and its complications have achieved significant results (Ling, 1999). These have become an important part of the medical researches of our country. The following comments are based on data collected from the literature.

13.1 Coordination Permeation of TCM and WM Theories, Inheritance and New Ideas

Coordination permeation of aetiological and pathogenetic theories provide the basis for combined TCM and WM therapy.

Diabetes is a disease of complex aetiology; its cause is heterogenetic, to which its clinical polymorphism is ascribed. In studies of diabetic aetiology, investigators in the field of combined TCM and WM usually use systemic methods in a comprehensive manner and allow the two medical systems to permeate each other coordinatively, pushing forward development of the academic research. Attention is paid on congenital deficiency and weakness of five viscera as chief aetiology and internal cause of diabetes. "Those with weak five viscera are susceptible to diabetes" — as written in the "*Nei Jing*" — similar to the saying of WM about the genetic and body building factors (Chi, 1986). The external factor must act through the presence of the internal factor. Congenital deficiency and weakness of five viscera produce weakness of kidney, dryness of lung, heat of stomach and weakness and dryness-heat of *yin*, all of which form the chief pathogenetic bases. The invasion of six climatic factors, the injury of *yin* by heat and the simultaneous attack of external and internal factors eventually lead to the formation of diabetes. The concept that damage to *yin* by injury of lung exists through attack of six climatic factors is basically similar to the recognisation of WM that virus infection affects the auto-immune system, leading to the damage of pancreatic cells and finally to the development of diabetes. Emotional instability, if prolonged, may turn into fire; flaring upwards, it may hurt the lung fluid, towards the middle, it may impair gastric secretion, and downwards to the lower past, it causes exhaustion of kidney water and eventually diabetes is formed. This is similar to the theory of WM that emotional stress may lead to dysfunction of the endocrine-immune network and also anxiety, which causes decrease of insulin secretion and induced diabetes. Irregular diet intake and body fluid hurt by heat can cause abundance of gastric fire, which, flashing upwards, consumes lung fluid, running downwards, hurts kidney *yin* and consequently diabetes is formed. This is one of the external factors in the causation of the disease. WM also gives much attention to obesity caused by loss of diet control; it causes insulin resistance and induces diabetes. Disorder in the regulation of relaxation and work and too frequent sexual intercourse can hurt the kidney, rendering further consumption of body tissues; this causes increase of adrenaline and adrenocorticosteroids, which counteract insulin, promote glyconeogenesis, raise blood glucose and produce diabetes. Hence, we can see that the causes of diabetes are complicated; they may be congenital deficiency, improper food intake, lack of rest, sexual intercourse, the six climatic factors and emotional instability. These factors may consume and hurt the *yin* of lung, stomach, spleen and kidney. Weakness of viscera like lung, spleen and kidney, disorder of fluid metabolism, stagnation of liver *qi* and unsmooth excretion or discharge all may produce stagnation of *qi*, stasis of blood and coagulation of sputum, leading to prolongation of the course of disease and appearance of various complications. Researchers in WM also demonstrate that hyperlipaemia, abnormal haemokinetics, slow blood flow, and tissue hypoxia are not the only factors causing diabetes, but are also the results of the disease pathology, and are important causes leading to complications and aggravation of the disease (Zhang, 1989).

From the point of pathogenesis, diabetes is chiefly related to abnormal metabolism of glucose, fat and protein and also to insufficient insulin secretion. Glucose, fat and protein are the basic material formed during the metabolic procreates in the body viscera and they belong to the category of "genuine energy" in TCM. Under physiologic conditions, the "wondering and overflowing genuine energy" of stomach, the "scattered essence" of spleen, the "smooth communication of water pathways", and the "differentiation of the clear and turbid" by the small intestines are all put into work through vaporisation of kidney. Congenital deficiency and weakness due to consumption of kidney *qi* after birth or weakness of kidney *qi* due to injury may cause pathologic changes of the lung, spleen and kidney, presenting with kidney weakness as the chief pathology, from which a series of pathologic changes may ensue. No matter what is the cause, the result will be consumption of kidney *yin*, internal production of fire of the deficiency type, consumptive drying of body fluid and eventual formation of diabetes. Hyperglycaemia is due to the permeation of pathologic products like wetness, sputum and coagulants into the blood and they become components of blood glucose. It is a concrete presentation resulting from obstruction of *qi* following lack of fluid, stasis of blood following consumption of fluid, abundance of sputum following overloading wetness and intermingling obstruction following blood stasis. *Qi* weakness of spleen and kidney and loss of function in raising the clear and lowering the turbid are the criteria of pathogenesis, but the lung, stomach and liver also play an important role. The pathogenesis of diabetes should be considered as a whole; congenital deficiency and weakness of five viscera are the basis of illness; weakness of *qi* and *yin* is the chief pathogenesis; the site of disease is mainly located at the spleen, kidney, lung, and stomach. Moreover, the liver and small intestines also have close relationships. Weakness of *yin* pierces through the entire course of illness. In the early stage, diabetes usually presents symptoms of *yin* weakness and dryness heat, but it may rapidly turn to the stage of deficiency of *qi* and *yin*. Deficiency of *qi* and *yin* changes from deficiency of *qi* in spleen and kidney, from deficiency of *yin* in liver or kidney, or from deficiency of *yin* and dryness heat when the course of disease is prolonged and when the deficiency of *qi* affects *yin* or when the deficiency of *yin* affects *qi*. The above condition constitutes a rather prolonged pathologic interval. When chronic complications occur in diabetes, the terminal stage of the disease may present deficiencies of *yin* and *yang*. Metabolic dysfunction of visceral organs and circulatory disorders of *qi*, blood and fluid can give rise to wetness, blood stasis and wetness-heat, which may mingle with one another and retain in the body during the entire course of diabetes (Zhong, 1989).

13.2 Inventiveness on the Basis of Inheritance Raises the Combined TCM and WM Therapeutic Level of Diabetes

According to the TCM theory of weakness of spleen, it is proposed that the pancreas is an important component of the fire of gate of life. Some scholars consider that, in discussion, the function of pancreas belongs to the field of "spleen" in TCM. From the point of view of the physiologic function of pancreas in modern medicine, the pancreas is affiliated to the "spleen" in TCM. In food, the nutritious materials like glucose, fat, protein and various micro-elements must be acted upon by pancreatic amylase, pancreatolipase and trypsinase secretion by the pancreatic exocrine cells for digestion and absorption. If there is insufficient secretion of these digestive enzymes or abnormality of their functions, difficulties in absorption occur and the body is unable to obtain enough nutrition so that the presence of insufficient activation of *qi* and blood from weakness of spleen exists and this is disorder of the "pituitary-hypothalamus-pancreas axis" and the "intestine-pancreas axis". Insulin is the primacy impetus of body energy and is also the first step in the chain of disintegration and composition of glycogen. If insulin is deficient, glucose cannot be utilised and disintegration of fat and protein is increased so that there is accumulation of lactic acid and production of ketone bodies. Manifestations of heat would appear, the ingested food cannot nourish the skin and muscles and the body becomes thinner day by day. Therefore, pancreas is an important component of the fire of gate of life and the material basis of body fluid. If this part of the fire of gate of life is not sufficient, not only will the symptoms of *yang* deficiency such as retardation of development, thinness, mental fatigue and weakness of skeleton occur, but also fire heat manifestations like thirst, heat restlessness and internal heat-toxin, causing increase of blood glucose. Clinically, supplement of spleen *qi* can enhance the utilisation of various nutrients by the body as well as increase the secretion of insulin. When the nutritious materials cannot be utilised by the body and when they become hear evil, then the stomach heat should be classified, the *yin* protected and the fluid increased so as to facilitate the utilisation and metabolism of various nutritious materials.

According to the theory of spleen dominating transportation, it is suggested that the transportation property of spleen includes the endocrine and exocrine functions of the pancreas. According to TCM theory, some scholars consider the dominant transport function of spleen to include the endocrine and exocrine function of the pancreas. The spleen digests and absorbs the micro-ingredients of food and water and raises the classified parts; this is similar to the exocrine function of pancreas, where the various digestive enzymes are the material bases for the fulfillment of this function. The micro-ingredients of food and water are transported by spleen to various parts of the body, internally to the five *zang*-organs and six *fu*-organs, externally to the limbs, skeleton, skin, hairs and tendons, for the nourishment of the organs and tissues of the whole body and insulin is the material basis for the fulfillment of this function. In diabetes, there is hypofunction of the pancreatic β cells and insulin is insufficient in absolute or selective amounts, therefore transportation of nutritious micro-ingredients by spleen is insufficient. The spleen transports liquid for the stomach and when the material basis of this function is insufficient, diabetic symptoms with weakness of spleen as the chief manifestation are produced. Treatment with formulas and drugs to replenish *qi* and invigorate the spleen in experimental condition proves that these kind of formulas can increase the number of pancreatic β cells and recover their function, and therefore this fact demonstrates from another viewpoint that weakness of spleen is the chief pathologic aspect of diabetes. Deficiency of insulin receptors and post-receptors is usually found in more or less obese patients, presenting clinical symptoms of weakness of spleen *qi* and internal retention of sputum-wetness. Treatment with supplement of *qi* and clearance of sputum method often gives good results.

According to the TCM principle of balance of *yin* and *yang*, the theory of glucose autostability and autoregulation is suggested. This theory proposes that the regulation of glucose, fat and protein depends on hormones that raise and lower the glucose level separately. The hormone that lowers glucose is insulin and those that increase glucose are glucagons, growth hormone, adrenaline and noradrenalin. The two are similar to the *yin* and *yang* in TCM, existing in a balance state normally, but under stress and emotional injury, glucose autostability is impaired and the glucose level may be high or low, and factors causing increase of blood glucose belong to *yang*, and those causing decrease of blood glucose belong to *yin*. Insulin renders lowering of blood glucose and gives rise to a picture of deficiency of *qi* and deficiency of *yang*. The hormones causing rise of blood glucose contribute to the picture of *yang* heat and abundance of fire. This heat fire usually comes from enclosure of *qi*, which turns into fire, or the fire may be caused by enclosure of wetness or by enclosure of blood. What we want is to balance *yin* and *yang*; the energy and blood should be made to relax and guided to attain a state of peace. If the cause is of the emotional type, treatment should aim at soothing the lover and regulating *qi*; if there is change of fire from enclosed *qi*, treatment is to soothe the lover and relieve the stasis. For the internal retention of sputum wetness, treatment is to dry the wetness and eliminate the sputum; for heat produced from retention of sputum, treatment is to eliminate the heat and clear away the sputum. Those with stasis of blood should be treated by activation of blood and clearing away clots; if stasis of blood produces heat, treatment should be clearance of stasis and elimination of heat. If *yin* is injured, one should take the case of *yin* and those having heat should be treated by elimination of heat. Treatment by syndrome treated by differentiation should be carried out flexibly so as to obtain a higher clinical effect (Ling, 1992).

13.3 Scientific Standardisation of TCM Syndrome Differentiation Becomes a New Combined TCM and WM Research Model in Diabetes

According to the coordinative relation between individuality and generality and between gross differentiation and microcosmic differentiation, 900 cases of diabetes were differentiated into three forms, namely, deficiency of *yin* and abundance of heat form, deficiency of both *qi* and *yin* forms, and deficiency of both *yin* and *yang* forms. These three forms represent separately the early, middle and late stages of diabetes. Deficiency of *yin* is the common character of these three forms, summing through the whole course of the disease and is the internal factor in the formation and development of diabetes. The fundamental of the deficiency of *yin* and abundance of heat form is deficiency of *yin* with abundance of heat as the incidental, its formation and development are related to congenital deficiency of *yin* and invasion of evil, or to irregular intake of food and internal retention of wetness-heat, or to injury from seven emotions and consumption of lung *yin*, or related to exopathy from six climatic conditions which turn into heat and hurt the body fluid leading to deficiency of *yin* in lung and stomach associated with abundance of heat and symptoms of weakness of the fundamental and excess of the incidental. In this condition, the course of disease is short, the age of patient younger, the complications less and milder and the disease usually belongs to the simple type. The deficiency of both *qi* and *yin* form shows a prolonged course and develops on the basis of deficiency of *yin* and blood and insufficiency of kidney water. It is the most common clinical form, showing a longer course of disease, an older age group, with the association of some chronic complications such as early stage nephrosis and early stage retinal disease. This is a critical form showing that the disease is undergoing an important change. The deficiency of both *yin* and *yang* type indicates that diabetes has been a long-term condition and insufficiency of kidney water further causes weakness of kidney *yang*. These patients are older in age, with more severe chronic complications and presenting symptoms of nocturia premature ejaculation, impotence, coldness of limbs, and these are usually seen in diabetes complicated with nephrosis or coronary disease. Investigations on the relation between syndrome forms and objective criteria show that deficiency of *yin* and abundance of heat form, on account of prolonged disease course, has a milder hyperglycaemia and also disturbance of lipid metabolism and, therefore, its vascular pathologic changes are less and milder. For the deficiency of both *yin* and *yang* forms, there is significant increase of cases with hyperlipaemia, but cases with high density lipoprotein are less in number, therefore, the course of this form is prolonged and usually accompanied by various vascular pathologic changes. The deficiency of *qi* and *yin* forms is a transient stage between the above two forms. The above three forms all present abnormalities of haemokinetics. The deficiency of *yin* and abundance of heat form has lower hyperviscosity, hypercoagulability and hyperaggregation as compared with the deficiency of both *yin* and *yang* forms, and the deficiency of *qi* and *yin* forms lies between the above two forms. As to clinical albuminuria, the positive rate in the deficiency of both *yin* and *yang* forms is significantly higher than the deficiency of *yin* and abundance of heat form. The deficiency of both *qi* and *yin* forms is located between the above two forms. These three forms of syndrome differentiation of diabetes are adopted as the standard TCM forms of diabetes in the current "Guidelines of clinical trial for new traditional Chinese medicine in treatment of diabetes mellitus", issued by the Ministry of Health.

There is an enormous amount of research reports about the three forms of diabetes and their related microcosmic criteria and these research increase the field of clinical application of these three forms, using them as the chief differentiating basis for diabetes and its complications in our country. This not only demonstrates the scientific aspect, its objectiveness and practicability, but also renders the form differentiation of diabetes and its complications towards unity, and also increases the comparability of research data as well as the current level of combined TCM and WM research in diabetes in China. Combined TCM and WM research in diabetes usually adopt this standard from differentiation and these three forms have become the model forms of diabetes investigated with combined TCM and WM method and this has directive significance in combined TCM and WM research on diabetes (Ling, 1999).

13.4 Efforts have been put on the Research of Diabetes, yet More Attention should be Paid on Treatment and Prevention of Its Complications

Research effort in diabetes is chiefly put on the control of blood glucose. Research on TCM and pharmaceutics by modern medical means can absorb the essences of TCM and WM and gain better results. According to former results on syndrome classification of diabetes, in China, we were the first to adopt the therapeutic measures with supplement *qi* and nourish *yin* method as the main method in treating diabetes, and we formulated a Chinese proprietary drug mainly to supplement *qi* and nourish *yin*. Investigation results revealed that this proprietary drug can promote insulin secretion, lower hyperglycaemia, increase the number of insulin receptors and improve glucose tolerance. Its chief action is lowering blood glucose and its regulation on insulin is bidirectional. It acts through supplementing *qi* and nourishing *yin*, regulating visceral *yin* and *yang*, especially through improvement of the deficiencies of *qi* and blood *yin* of the three *zang* organs, lung, spleen and kidney and thus, it further promotes the secretion of insulin by pancreatic β cells, improves the function of pancreatic α cells, lowers high blood glucose level and at the same time, it increases the number of insulin receptors with the result of lowering blood glucose and improvement of clinical symptoms, reaching the state of "regulation of *yin* and *yang* to attain a balanced condition".

Large amounts of research work proved that simple use of Chinese drugs to lower blood glucose did not show significant effects, but a few Chinese drugs combined with WM hypoglycaemic agents showed a synergetic effect, and it appeared that the combined use of two was superior to simple use of one. According to the reports from five hospitals — PUMC hospital, Hua Shan hospital, Rui Gin hospital, Hua Xi, Medical University, Zhong Shan Medical University — the addition of certain Chinese drugs to glyburide yields better results than simple use of the latter and simple use of certain Chinese drugs has no significant effect.

Chronic vascular changes are the chief causes of death or disability in diabetes. It was reported that 74.2% of diabetic patients died of cardiovascular changes and in developed countries, its mortality is comparable to malignant tumours and coronary diseases, occupying the third place. How to control the chronic vascular complications and reduce mortality is a medical research problem that has not been ideally solved because of the lack of effective drugs. The use of a comprehensive preventive and therapeutic combined TCM and WM method can not only relieve symptoms of the patient but also can raise his living quality, alleviate as well as delay the process of the chronic complications (Cai, 2001).

According to TCM theory, blood stasis is related to hyperviscosity and hypercoagulability of blood and to the formation and development of diabetic vascular and capillary complications. Activation of blood and elimination of stasis is an important therapeutic principle in the prevention and treatment of diabetic complications. In China, investigations applied the activation of blood and elimination of stasis method combined with modern medical research achievements and obtained prominent therapeutic effects in prevention and treatment of diabetic complications. The Guang An Men Hospital of Traditional Chinese Medicine Research Institute of China, since the seventh decade of the last century, used the Chinese drug "*Qiang Tang Tong Mai Ning* capsule" that could supplement *qi*, nourish *yin*, activate blood and eliminate stasis. It is used to treat various vascular complications of diabetes and reported good results. This drug can correct the abnormalities of haemokinetics, lower blood viscosity as well as haematocrit, sedimentation rate, platelet aggregation, fibrinogen and its degradation products; it can also improve lipid metabolism, correct the function of pancreatic islets, lower blood glucose and relieve clinical symptoms. Clinical observations also showed that this capsule could nourish heart *yin* and supplement heart *qi*, improve myocardial hypoxia, correct abnormal EKG and improve cardiac function, indicating good effects on treatment of diabetic cardiovascular diseases. Cephalic CT demonstrated that this drug can activate blood and eliminate stasis, counteract coagulation and haemolyze thrombin, improve cephalic haemokinetics and possesses some effect on treatment of cephalic thrombus formation. Ultrasound of limbs showed that this drug could dilate the diameter of the arterial lumen of lower limbs and promote its blood circulation, and it contributed greatly to the prevention and treatment of vascular diseases of lower limbs. Using the fluorescent funduscopy and ophthalmoscopy for examination, it was demonstrated that this drug had a good effect on early diabetic retinal changes and at the same time, it could improve the related biochemical parameters as well as the clinical symptoms of diabetic nephrosis. Basic laboratory investigations showed that the drugs action on activation of blood and elimination of stasis was reflected on its improvement of microcirculation, relief of vascular spasm, lowering of vascular permeability, on anti-coagulation, disconglomeration of red cells, dissolution of thrombus, promotion of vascular neogenesis and establishment of collateral circulation, enhancement of blood circulation and absorption of blood clots and also regulation of immune function. In animal experimental diabetes, it can significantly lower blood glucose, cholesterol triglyceride and vascular tension, and it can retain vascular elasticity, increase red cell deformability, inhibit platelet aggregation, lower blood lipid, blood viscosity and decrease vascular wall injury. It has significant effects on the prevention and treatment of diabetic nephrosis, diabetic cardiovascular disease, diabetic neuropathy, diabetic cardiovascular disease, diabetic retinal disease and diabetic lower limb vascular disease.

It is now clear that the complications of diabetes are mainly related to the resistance of insulin, reductase activity of aldose and protein non-enzyme glycosylation. Investigators did a lot of research work and gained many gratifying results. Some used the insulin-resistant large mouse model and found that the Chinese drugs, astragalus root, liquorice, red sage root, gentian root, as well as the drugs *quercetin sylibin*, *baicalin*, *puerarin* and *naringenin* could significantly inhibit the reductase activity of aldose, its effect approaching the aldose reductase inhibitor of Western medicine. Aminoguanidine is an internationally accepted classical anti-protein non-enzyme glycosylation and oxygenation agent. Research has demonstrated that the Chinese drugs *quercetin*, *sylibin*, *baicalin*, *baicalein*, *rutin* and *hydroxyethylrutin* had a aminoguanidine-like effect; it could interrupt protein non-enzyme glycosylation and oxygenation, decrease the terminal products of glycosylation of protein in aortic collagen, renal cortex and crystals, decrease urine albumin and total protein excretion and interrupt oxygenation.

13.5 Take Advantage of the Combination of TCM and WM; Rational Selection of TCM and WM Drugs

Both TCM and WM have their advantages and disadvantages in the treatment of diabetes. Simple use of WM treatment, although liable to develop drug resistance (i.e. secondary loss of effect, epigastric discomfort, eruptions and other adverse effects) has the efficient ability to decrease blood glucose and is easily accepted by patients. Simple use of TCM drugs in treatment would not result in adverse effects and is better for the control of clinical symptoms and complications in amplitude. Only when TCM is combined with WM in treatment that the clinical symptoms can be improved, complications prevented and the adverse reactions and secondary loss of effect can be avoided (Ling, 1999). At present, the advantages of combined TCM and WM in treatment of diabetes are chiefly manifested in the following aspects.

Search for point of TCM and WM combination

Practical experience demonstrates that TCM treatment by syndrome differentiation combined with WM small doses of agents for lowering glucose level is a feasible method of treatment. It is noticed that although the associated application of WM small doses of agents for lowering glucose level is used, it is still necessary to have a dialectical materialist point of view, to cleverly combine the syndrome differentiation of TCM with the disease diagnosis of WM and to consider comprehensively the patient's age, height, body weight, working and the fluctuation of his blood glucose to select respectively the appropriate WM drug to lower blood glucose.

According to TCM syndrome differentiation principle, absorb previous pharmacological research achievements

Large amounts of research confirm that the TCM drugs that have the effect of lowering blood glucose are those that have supplementing property, such as ginseng, astralagus root, Siberian solomonseal rhizome, Chinese yam, wolfberry fruit, rehmaunia root, Tuckahoe, *herba epimedii*, dogwood fruit, Chinese angelica, those having cleansing activity and detoxification power, and regulation of *qi* and activation of blood action such as atractylodes rhizome, corn stigmz, litchi reed, gallnut, root of red rooted salvia, white mulberry leaf, root-bark of white mulherry, rhizome of wind-weed, sauna leaf; those that can decrease glucosuria are Chinese yam, dogwood fruit, Cherokee rose-hip, mantis egg-case, Gordon euryale seed, these drugs can also supplement kidney and reserve sperms. The above drugs also include large-herded atractylodes, atractylodes rhizome, chicken's gizzard-skin, astralagus root; they can supplement *qi* and invigorate the spleen. According to our experience, in hyperlipaemia, we can select drugs among chicken's gizzard-skin, *alisma orientalis*, sophora flower-bud, rhubarb; for abnormalities of haemokinetics or disturbances of microcirculation one may use drugs like Chinese angelica, root of red rooted salvia, peach kernel, safflower, *chuanxiong* rhizome, red peony root, leech, 土元, motherwort, *alisma orientalis*, notoginseng, dragon's blood. Rational selection of drugs on the basis of syndrome differentiation can certainly increase effectiveness, but one must do the proper syndrome differentiation, otherwise effectiveness would not be obtained, for example, for a patient with deficiency of *yang*, it is not appropriate to give drugs like rhizome of wind-seed and phellodendron bark.

For metabolic disorders of glucose and lipids, select detoxifying drugs and formulas

Research demonstrate that accumulation of glucose in blood can lead to "chronic toxication of glucose" and accumulation of lipid to "hyperlipaemia" "obesity" and "fatty liver". Hyperglycaemia and hyperlipaemia belong to "sputum wetness" and "sputum turbidity" of TCM. If there are harmful substances that are retained in the body for a long period, they would interfere with the activity of spleen and stomach, of *qi* and blood and of the distribution of body fluid; therefore, in clinical practice, we should eliminate sputum and drive away turbidity to abolish toxin, activate and cool down blood, to excrete toxins and thus allow the harmful substances in the body be metabolised and excreted. In routine treatments, it is feasible to add drugs such as honeysuckle flower, forsythia fruit, *alisma orientalis*, Moutan bark, lithosperm root, red peony root, dried rehmannia root, scrophilaria root, coptis root, wolf's milk, houttuynia, rhubarb, Oriental wormwood, plantain seed and shell of areca nut so as to obtain better effectiveness (Zhu, 2000).

According to pathologic changes of islets of pancreas, select respective drugs and formulas

Quite a few scholars have noted that type I diabetes patients usually have history of upper respiratory tract infection, at the onset of which inflammation occurs in the pancreas where the pancreatic islets are gradually destroyed leading to absolute insufficiency or lack of insulin. Therefore, in early type I diabetes, having chiefly heat symptoms of upper respiratory tract infection drugs for treatment should be used for clearing of heat with detoxification and nourishment of *yin* as subsidiary. For elimination of pancreatic local inflammation and protection of pancreas, drugs like plaster stone, rhizome of wind-seed, ophiopogon root, dried rehmaunia root, honeysuckle flower, forsythia fruit and dandelion herb should be used. In the middle stage of the disease, the chief manifestation is deficiency of *yin*, and thus treatment should aim at nourishment of *yin* with drugs for activation of blood as subsidiary. The drugs for selection are pseudostellaria root, ophiopogon root, rehmaunia root, resophularia root, fragrant solomonseal rhizome, pollen and Siberian solomonseal rhizome. If there is an association of abundant heat, it is appropriate to give heat clearance drugs; if there is an association of stasis of blood, to give blood activation drugs. In the late stage, when there is absolute insufficiency of insulin and appearance of deficiency of both *qi* and *yin* or deficiency of both *yin* and *yang*, it is appropriate to follow in treatment the principle of supplement *qi* and nourish *yin*, supplement and nourish *qi* and blood or supplement both *yin* and *yang* to improve the weak condition of the body and increase insulin secretion. The following drugs may be used: Astragalus root, pilose asiabell root, ophiopogon root, Chinese yam, schisandra fruit and siberian solomonseal rhizome. For those having masked deficiency of kidney *yang*, add drugs like pilose antler, desertiving cistanche, dodder seed and morinda root; for those having significant deficiency of kidney *yin*, add prepared rehmaunia root, dogwood fruit, glossy privet fruit, wolfberry fruit and glue of tortoise shell. As for type II diabetes, besides using drugs according to syndrome differentiation, it is also rational to select pilose asiabell root, or astragalus root to promote insulin secretion of β cells of the pancreatic islets. The drugs, Chinese angelica, root of red rooted salvia, red peony root, notoginseng and peach kernel can improve microcirculation; the drugs fritillary bulb, moutan bask, oyster shell, prunella spike can improve pancreatic filrosis or starch deposition and the drugs coptis root, rhubarb, smilax glabra rhizome can improve insulin resistance and increase sensitivity of peripheral tissues to insulin.

Development of special drugs and formulas according to pathogenesis of disease

It is important to aim at the particular stage or a certain form of diabetes and its complications for the determination of the principle of treatment and for development of special drugs and formulas. This is the aspect that the current literature is most concerned about; it involves the prevention and treatment of diabetes and its complications and the advantages in development of special drugs and formulas. For example, based on the pathogenesis of deficiency of both *qi* and *yin* in diabetes, we developed the "*Qiang Tong A* tablet" and the "*He Fok Ning* capsule", which have the properties of supplementing *qi* and nourishing *yin*; and based on the characteristic of deficiency of *qi* and *yin* associated with stasis of blood in diabetic pathogenesis, we developed the drug "*Qiang Tang Tong Mai Ning*", which is able to supplement *qi*, nourish *yin*, activate blood and eliminate stasis. These drugs had significant clinical effects and were given awards in China. They are currently sold in the market. We treat diabetic nephrosis with the new drug "*Tang Wei Kong*" and diabetic cardiac disease with "*Tang Sin Ping*". Pharmacological studies show that they can significantly lower blood glucose and lipids. We have done some work in providing effective drugs for prevention and treatment of diabetes and its complications.

13.6 Brief Summary and Prospects

In the past 20 years, the combined TCM and WM research on prevention and treatment of diabetes has made comparatively great advances. Problems encountered in the research and the solutions are briefly listed in the following.

Intensify education and nursing; concentrate research efforts on prevention and treatment

Treatment of diabetes is a long term and painstaking work, and for the patient, it requires meticulous education and persuasion, and comprehensive nursing care is crucial in raising the living quality of the patient in addition to the prevention and treatment of the disease. The contents of education, besides a guide to drug administration and diet control, include also avoidance of affection by adverse living environment, habits and working conditions. Supplementing with kinesitherapy may help in raising the patient's living quality and in controlling complications.

Standardise research systems and encourage new ideas

At present, for intensification of diabetes TCM research, it is necessary first to standardise the research work. For example, the various complications of diabetes do not yet have a unified TCM diagnosis, forms of syndrome differentiation and also a standard effect evaluation, thus there is great difference between data and comparison is impossible. As to effective screening of drugs and prospective research of large number of cases, there exists a great disadvantage. In the literature, most of the clinical studies are based on small groups of patients and there is a lack of massive retrospective research, so that the methods of therapy and quality level are difficult to estimate. Therefore, it is imperative to establish a national standard on TCM diagnosis, differential diagnosis, syndrome differentiation and curative effect of diabetes and its complications. Clinical studies should choose research items strictly, design the research based on the principle of "randomised, compare, blind method" so that the investigation is objective and standardised. People in ancient times as well as modern have accumulated profound experiences in the treatment of diabetes. Many drugs and formulas can be found throughout the literature, spanning many centuries, and the drugs that may lower blood glucose found in current TCM pharmacological studies are also mentioned in various scientific works. To systematically collect these findings and summarise the rules in drug usage of the old and modern times remain important tasks in TCM research of diabetes.

Improve the animal models and develop laboratory research

At present, reports in the literature concerning TCM and combined TCM and WM research in diabetes mostly belong to clinical studies, and basic experimental researches that have a high level and acceptable to Western medical scholars are comparatively few. This raises some difficulty in further investigations on combined TCM and WM research on diabetes as well as in making their research achievements suitable for international study. The animal models used in combined TCM and WM studies of diabetes are derived from the methods used in WM so it is worthwhile for us to consider the establishment of an animal model suitable for combined TCM and WM research. The authors think that from now on, we should make use of modern technology, bravely develop new ideas and proceed with deeper investigations on TCM pathogenesis to fully comprehend the diabetic aetiology, its multiple factor character and the complexity of disease onset. We should do synchronous research on the disease and its syndrome manifestation, and should have a steady and reliable combined TCM and WM animal model for the study of disease pathogenesis and also for practical needs of clinical work. If these are fulfilled, we can evaluate objectively the results of TCM drugs, and can, from multiple aspects, reveal the pathogenesis of diabetes and its complications and the principles involved in its prevention and treatment by TCM drugs.

References

Cai, Y. (2001) *Modern Chinese Medicine and Western Medicine — Clinical Endocrinology.* China Press of Traditional Chinese Medicine (in Chinese).

Chi, Z. (1986) *Diabetes.* People's Medical Publishing Press (in Chinese).

Jiang, G. (1992) *Practical Diabetes.* People's Medical Publishing House (in Chinese).

Ling, L. (1992) *Treatment on Diabetes with Combined Chinese Medicine and Western Medicine.* Beijing Science and Technology Press (in Chinese).

Ling, L. (1999) *Diabetes Study with Combined Chinese Medicine and Western Medicine.* China Medical Science and Technology Press (in Chinese).

Zhang, J. (1989) *Endocrinology Manual.* People's Medical Publishing Press (in Chinese).

Zhong, X. (1989) *Clinical Diabetes.* Shanghai Scientific and Technical Publishers (in Chinese).

Zhu, X. (2000) *Modern Diabetes.* Press of Shanghai Medical University (in Chinese).

Chapter 14

Research on Depth and Angle of Dangerous Acupoints

Zhengguo Yan, Jue Bai, Baishui Shao & Jianhua Zhang

Abstract

In this article, we describe the theory of acupuncture manipulation of dangerous acupoints in ancient classic works; introduce the methods of stratified anatomy and layer anatomy; and sum up the safe needling depths, dangerous needling depths and needling angles for dangerous acupoints on the cervical part, chest, abdomen and back. This paper serves as a reference for clinical acupuncturists seeking to improve therapeutic effects and prevent accidents.

Keywords: Acupoints; Acupuncture Contraindication; Dangerous Acupoints; Needling Angle.

14.1 Introduction

Dangerous acupoints are those which cause accidents when needlings hurt brain, spinal cord, main blood vessel and important organs such as the heart, lung, liver and kidney. Ancient Chinese doctors are very careful with the dangerous acupoints. As mentioned in *Plain Questions*, "there are important organs in the body and a doctor has to know them — it is safe to obey the needling principles, otherwise it is dangerous". There are many descriptions on acupuncture contraindication of dangerous acupoints in classic works. Usually, the dangerous acupoints are exactly those that have good therapeutic effects in the acupuncture clinic. But there are different descriptions about needling depths and angles among these works. For example, the most shallow depth permitted for inserting Yamen and Renying is 0.3 cun (China Academy of TCM, 1978) and 0.2 cun (Acupuncture and Moxibustion Department of the First Affiliated Hospital of Tianjing College of TCM, 1981), respectively, while the deepest ones are both 2 cun (Yang, 1984; Wang, 1996). The locations of dangerous acupoints have special and complex anatomic structures. It is risky when the reasonable needling depth and angle cannot be decided. So we use fresh adult cadavers to study the safe needling depth, dangerous needling depth and anatomic structures of important dangerous acupoints on the cervical part, chest and abdomen (Yan *et al.*, 1996; Zhang *et al.*, 1998a; 2001a). In this article, we will be introducing the above research and some related researches.

14.2 Historic Origin for the Dangerous Acupoints Researches

Ancient Chinese doctors have acknowledged the existence of dangerous acupoints during the course of their clinical experience, and have thoroughly described the locations that cannot be needled, needling depths and needling manipulation. The descriptions on acupuncture contraindication are extensive in classical works, such as *The Yellow Emperor's Internal Classic*, *A-B Classic of Acupuncture and Moxibustion* and *Prescriptions Worth a Thousand Gold*. These provide basis for the posterior researches.

14.2.1 *Important organs cannot be hurt*

The heart, liver, spleen, lung and kidney, which lie on the chest and abdomen, are very important organs of the human body. "Vital essence and energy need to be held and not to be purged". Acupuncture must not touch or hurt these organs otherwise accidents may occur.

Plain Questions — the "Zhen Yao Jing Lun" chapter: "When needling the chest and abdomen, the five organs must be avoided to touch. If the heart is hurt, the patient will die at once; if the spleen or lung are hurt, the person will die in five days; if the kidney is hurt, the person will die in seven days; if the diaphragm is hurt, the person will die within one year although his/her disease is healed. If a doctor knows to avoid hurting the five organs, he must understand the proper place his needles should arrive. The place is between the diaphragm and spleen, kidney. Accidents may happen if a doctor does not know the place".

Plain Questions — the "Si Shi Ci Ni Cong" chapter: "When needling the five organs, if the heart is hurt, the person will die in one day with the symptom hiccup; if the liver is hurt, the person will die in five days with the symptom speak; if the lung is hurt, the person will die in three days with the symptom cough; if the kidney is hurt, the person will die in six days with the symptom sneeze; if the spleen is hurt, the person will die in ten days with the symptom swallow. A person will die if all his five organs are hurt and the day of death depends on his symptom according to the hurt organ".

Plain Questions — the "Ci Jin" chapter: "If the heart is hurt, the person will die in one day with the symptom hiccup; if the liver is hurt, the person will die in five days with the symptom speak; if the kidney is hurt, the person will die in six days with the symptom sneeze; if the lung is hurt, the person will die in three days with the symptom cough; if the spleen is hurt, the person will die in ten days with the symptom swallow; if the gallbladder is hurt, the person will die in one and a half days with the symptom vomit".

Plain Questions — the "Ci Jin" chapter: "If the depth is deeper than it should be when needling Quepen, the Qi will leak and so make the patient cough and develop asthma. If the lung is hurt when needling Yingzhong, then symptoms such as cough, asthma and sigh will occur. If the depth is deeper than it should be when needling the intercostals place, the patient will develop cough and asthma. If the needle touches and hurts the bladder, the urine will leak and the patient will feel full in his lower abdomen".

Miraculous Pivot — the "Jiu Zhen Shi Er Yuan" chapter: "If the needle touches the important organ and does not pull up immediacy, the vital essence will leak; if the needle inserts and pull out immediately, the Qi will be put together; if the vital essence leaks, then the disease will be worse; if the Qi is put together, ulcer will occur".

The five organs are very important to the human body. If the needling depth is superficial, the injury is light. But if the depth is deep, it can be fatal. Thus, clinical doctors must be extremely cautious with needling depth.

14.2.2 *The brain and blood vessels cannot be hurt*

The points on the cervical part are of equal importance in ancient acupuncture contraindication. "The brain is the reservoir of the marrow".

There are many important blood vessels and nerves on the neck leading to the brain, so it is the most dangerous region for acupuncture. Governor Vessel lies on the spine, and the spinal cord will be hurt if needling is too deep in this region. If the blood vessels are hurt, the patient will bleed and may die since the vessels are passages for Qi and blood. The organs will be affected if the blood vessels around them are hurt.

Plain Questions — the "Ci Jin" chapter: "The patient will die at once if the needle inserts into the brain when needling the Naohu. Rickets will occur if the spinal cord is inserted and hurt; if the needle hurts the Taiying Meridian on the arm or the thigh and the bleeding cannot be stopped, the patient will die; if the needle hurts the blood vessel on the dorsum of the foot and the bleeding cannot be stopped, the patient will also die".

Plain Questions — the "Ci Jing" chapter: "If the vessel of Shaoyin Meridian of foot is hurt by needling, the patient will be very fatigue because of loss of large amounts of blood and experience inability to speak; if the vessel is hurt when needling the cleft between bones, the patient will become pale, faint and syncope; if the main vessel is hurt when needling Qijie and do not bleed, the local skin will swell and syncope".

Miraculous Pivot — the "Ben Shu" chapter: "The ulnar artery of Yin lies on Wuli, which is not permitted to be at the Five-shu location".

Plain Questions — the "Jin Ci" chapter: "Inserting and hurting the related vessel when needling the supraorbital depression bone, symptoms such as leaking and blinding may occur; inserting and hurting the related vessel when needling the face, blinding may occur; inserting and hurting the related vessel when needling the place under the tongue, alalia may occur if bleeding cannot be stopped; inserting and hurting the related vessel when needling Kezuren, leaking and loss of hearing may result".

Prescriptions Worth a Thousand Gold — Chapter 29: "For bleeding, avoid hurting the central vessel when needling the two sides of the big vessels under the tongue, otherwise the patient will die if the bleeding cannot be stopped".

About the acupoint Renying, *A-B Classic of Acupuncture and Moxibustion* said "Moxibustion is not permitted. The depth of needling can only be 4 Fen, otherwise the patient will die".

So, deep depth, improper angle and excessive manipulation can cause serious dangerous results.

14.2.3 *Needling after learning the deep structure of acupoints*

A doctor should select treatment according to differential diagnoses in clinical experience. Also, a doctor should learn the anatomical location and deep structure of acupoints before he/she decides the needling depth.

Plain Questions — the "Ci Yao" chapter: "A disease has a deep and shallow nature and the needling depth is deep and superficial accordingly. A doctor would not make a mistake when he/she knows this principle".

Miraculous Pivot — the "Xiao Zhen Jie" chapter: "If needling is too deep, the evil-qi will enter the deep tissue. It is named "Fancheng", i.e. the diseases with superficial nature cannot be given deep needling, otherwise the evil-qi will enter the deep tissue. Skin, tendon and meridian have their own place, i.e. meridians are owned respectively".

Miraculous Pivot — the "Guan Zhen" chapter: "If the disease is superficial and a doctor punctures deeply, the healthy muscle may be hurt and carbuncle may occur; if the disease is deep and is needled superficially, the evil-qi cannot be expelled and pus is caused".

Plain Questions — the "Ci Yao" chapter: "Diseases are located on fine hairs and seat pores, skins, muscles, vessels, tendons, bones or marrows. Do not hurt skins when needling fine hairs and seat pores, otherwise the lung will be injured. Do not hurt muscles when needling skins, otherwise the spleen will be injured. Do not hurt vessels when needling muscles, otherwise the heart will be injured. Do not hurt tendons when needling vessels, otherwise the liver will be injured. Do not hurt bones when needling tendons, otherwise the kidney will be injured. Do not hurt marrows when needling bones, otherwise the bone will ache and be destroyed, and the patient might die".

Plain Questions — the "Ci Qi" chapter: "Do not hurt tendons when needling bones. The tip of the needle withdraws when it is inserted into the tendons and does not touch the bones; do not hurt muscles when needling tendons. The tip of the needle withdraws when it is inserted into the muscles and does not touch tendons; do not hurt vessels when needling muscles. The tip of the needle withdraws when it is inserted into the muscles and does not touch vessels; do not hurt vessels when needling skins. The tip of the needle withdraws when it is inserted into the vessels and does not touch skins. Do not hurt muscles when needling skins, as it is believed that when a disease occurs on skins, one just has to puncture the skin without hurting the muscles. Similarly, do not hurt tendons when puncturing muscles and do not hurt bones when puncturing tendons. It is called contrary if needling is too deep and the tendons or bones are hurt accordingly".

Miraculous Pivot — the "Jiu Zhen Shi Er Yuan" chapter: "The most dangerous adverse results caused by improper acupuncture, such as inducing to lose large amounts of Yin or Yang, are death or mania accordingly".

Mastering the needling depth correctly depends on learning the mechanism of relation between Zang and Fu, meridian passages and anatomical structures (Han, 2003).

14.3 Anatomical Methods for Dangerous Acupoints Research

The development of modern medicine provides basis for researches on meridian morphology. The stratified and layer anatomical methods are used to study the dangerous acupoints. The stratified anatomical method of acupoints is first used to locate an acupoint correctly on the cadavers, then the acupoint is stratified after freezing the body at 20–30°C below zero, so as to show the laminar anatomical structures at different angles, depths and ranges involved in the needling procedure. There are three kinds of stratified anatomy: coronary laminar for cutting a sample into anterior and posterior parts; sagittal plane for cutting a sample into left and right parts, and level laminar for cutting a sample into up and down parts. Layer anatomy is first used to locate an acupoint correctly on the cadavers, and then every layer is anatomised after inserting or dyeing with a steel needle, so as to express the anatomical structure on the acupoint region.

14.3.1 *Materials*

Fifty-seven fresh adult cadavers (24 males and 33 females) were randomly chosen from our Shanghai University of Traditional Chinese Medicine

(TCM) (Zhang *et al.*, 2000). In total, ten adult cadavers for anatomical teaching use (eight males and two females) were chosen from the Anhui College of TCM (Shen *et al.*, 1999). Twenty adult cadavers (17 males and three females) and five cadavers from the Wenzhou Medical College (Cui *et al.*, 2002) and the Nanjing University of TCM (Zhang *et al.*, 1998b) were used, respectively.

14.3.2 *Stratified anatomical method*

Acupoints underline and location

The skin point located by an acupoint is called the superficial point. The location of the superficial point complies with the *Standards of Acupoints Location*. Briefly, the acupoint was located and a tangential underline was made on the skin with a colour pencil, then the superficial point and tangential underline were dyed with red or blue paint. The tangential line of Conception and Governer Vessels lies on the anterior or posterior median line accordingly. The tangential line of acupoints on abdomen lies on the superior or inferior directions. The direction of the tangential line of left acupoints depends on the needling direction.

Freezing bodies with low temperature

Then all cadavers were put into refrigerators at −30°C for four days.

Incision cadavers

The cadavers were incised into coronary, sagittal and level laminas with an incision machine through tangential lines at the skin of superficial points. The cross-sections of acupoints were those locations where needles have passed. There was an angle of 90° between the serrated ruler of the incision machine and the acupoint skins.

Observation and measurement

The structures passing through by needles were observed after the cross-sections thawed and the distance between superficial points and deep points was measured using an electronic ruler. The deep points were the nearest points to the superficial points before the needles reached and hurt important organs.

Data analysis

All data were analysed using a special statistic software. The unit of measure was millimetre.

14.3.3 *Layer anatomical method*

Location, dye and fixture

The method of location was the same as that used in stratified anatomy. We dyed every layer of deep tissues by rough needles with gentian violet so as to decide the location of acupoints in every layer (Zhang *et al.*, 2001b). Steel needles of 60 mm in length and 0.8 mm in diameter were used in the Anhui College of TCM (Shen *et al.*, 1999). Needles were left in the local region after they were inserted in the Wenzhong Medical College (Cui *et al.*, 2002).

Layer anatomy

Each layer was dissected and the anatomical structures of dyed area were observed using surgical lancets and forceps. The structures within 0.5 mm diameter region around needles was also observed and the needling depth between inserting points and every layer of deep tissues was measured (Zhang *et al.*, 2002).

14.4 Safe Depth, Dangerous Depth and Angle of Dangerous Acupoints

The dangerous acupoints mainly lie on the cervical part, chest and abdomen and the primary affected organs are the brain, spinal cord, heart, liver, gallbladder, kidney, spleen, stomach and bladder, when needles are inserted too deeply or at improper angles. With the methods of anatomy, the dangerous depths of 75 acupoints located on the cervical part, chest and abdomen were studied, and a formula for safe needling depths of these acupoints was summed up as: safe needling depth = dangerous needling depth × 70% (Zhang *et al.*, 2000).

14.4.1 *Research of dangerous acupoints on cervical part*

Acupoints on cervical part are usually chosen when treating optical, cerebrobascular and cardiovascular diseases. The cervical part regions are the most dangerous because of the complication of local anatomical structures and the importance of deep organs. Our research is aimed at providing reference for clinical acupuncturists.

The safe and dangerous needling depths

At the cross-sections, the above formula was used to calculate the safe needling depth of these acupoints, and the related vulnerable organs and the dangerous needling depths were pointed out accordingly. Results of the ten dangerous acupoints on cervical part are shown as follows (Table 14.1):

Table 14.1. Safe and dangerous needling depths and vulnerable organs of dangerous acupoints on cervical part.

Acupoint	Safe needling depth (mm)	Dangerous needling depth (mm)	Vulnerable organs
Jingming	29.97	42.81	Anterior optical canal
Chengqi	27.30	39.00	Optic nerve or ophthalmic artery
Renying	21.70	31.00	Common carotid artery, vagus nerve or sympathetic trunk
Fengfu	35.07	50.10	Brain stem or spinal cord
Yamen	33.33	47.62	Brain stem or spinal cord
Fengchi	34.80	49.71	Brain stem or vertebral artery
Jianjin	39.17	55.96	Lung
Tianliao	42.19	60.27	Lung
Jianzhongshu	40.08	57.25	Lung
Jianwaishu	38.79	55.42	Lung

Source: Yan *et al.* (1996).

Needling directions and related local anatomical structures

Jingmin and Chengqi are located inside the orbita. Bleeding, ocular proptosis and even loss of sight can easily result when these points are needled too deeply or at improper angles. When needling Jingmin, the needles should be perpendicular or slightly oblique to the posterior and external direction depending on the correct location. If slightly oblique to the superior direction, the anterior ethmoidal artery may be hurt when the needling depths are deeper than 18 mm (Li *et al.*, 1997). For Chengqi, acupuncturists should puncture along the infraorbital ridge. If the infraorbital ridge is touched too tightly, the infraorbital vessels may be hurt when the needling depths are deeper than 12 mm. If needles are inserted towards the superior and external directions, the ciliary artery may be hurt and bleeding may result when the needling depths are more than 25 mm (Lui and Huang, 1997).

When needling Fengfu, Yamin and Fengchi, the patient should lower his head and use a flexion position on a table since all the acupoints are located on the nape. The needle should be inserted towards the mandible projection when needling Fengfu. The medulla oblongata and spinal cord will be affected or the subarachnoid space will bleed if the needling direction is towards the tip of the nose when needling Fengfu and Yamen. The needle should be inserted towards the inner canthus of the opposite side when needling Fengchi. The medulla oblongata or vertebral artery will be hurt accordingly if the needling depth is too deep when needling towards the outer canthus of the opposite side or the inner one of the homolateral side (Yan, 1996).

Renying is located on the anterior region of the neck, and there are important structures such as common carotid artery, internal jugular vein, vagus nerve and sympathetic trunk in the deep tissues. When needling this point, keep away from the common carotid artery, put it towards the outer side and insert the needle along the anterior margin of the m. sternocleidomastoideus or slightly towards the inner side perpendicularly. Otherwise, the bifurcating place of the common carotid artery and cervical arterial bulbus will be hurt and blood pressure will be changed abnormally when the needling depth reaches 0.5 cun. The vagus nerve or sympathetic trunk will be affected when the needling depth reaches 0.6–0.8 cun or over 1.0 cun accordingly. And a fatal outcome will result from the above conditions. The hypoglossal nerve and superior thyroid artery may be hurt if the needle inserts towards the outer side (Tai, 2002).

Jianjing lies on the shoulder near the apex and superior lobe of the lung. Pneumatothorax may happen if this point is needled improperly. On this acupoint, the needle should be inserted perpendicularly or obliquely towards the posterior and inferior directions and the needling angle between the needle body and local skin should be smaller than 67.5 ± 10.0°. It is prohibited to insert towards the anterior and inferior directions or towards the inner and inferior directions deeply to avoid stabbing the pleura and hurting the lung (Cui *et al.*, 2002).

14.4.2 *Research of dangerous acupoints on chest and abdomen*

The dangererous acupoints on the chest and abdomen lie mainly on Conception Vessel, Kidney Meridian of Zu-shaoyang, Stomach Meridian of Zu-yangmin and Spleen Meridian of Zu-taiying. These acupoints are widely used in clinic and have been proven to have good therapeutic effects. Namely, heart and lung in the thoracic cavity, liver, gallbladder, stomach, intestine, kidney, spleen and bladder in the abdominal cavity. These organs are vulnerable to hurt if inserted too deeply when needling dangerous acupoints on chest and abdomen. Deep insertion and strong manipulation may cause serious damage to the above organs and result in adverse effects.

The safe and dangerous needling depths

Twenty-three dangerous acupoints on the chest and 17 on the abdomen were studied systemically. The dangerous needling depths of all these acupoints were measured and their safe needling depths were calculated. The results are shown in Table 14.2.

Needling directions and related local anatomical structures

Tiantu is located on the depression superior of the suprasternal notch. The direction of needling this acupoint is based on superficial or deep needling. Superficial needling is to puncture perpendicularly within 0.5 cun depth, while deep needling is to first puncture perpendicularly 0.3 cun, then insert the needle tip downward along the posterior aspect of

Table 14.2. Safe and dangerous needling depths and vulnerable organs of dangerous acupoints on chest and abdomen.

Acupoint	Safe needling depth (mm)	Dangerous needling depth (mm)	Vulnerable organs
Shufu	18.72	26.31	Lung
Yuzhong	9.51	13.59	Lung
Shencang	8.31	11.87	Lung
Lingxu	9.15	13.08	Lung or heart
Shenfeng	10.09	14.41	Lung or heart
Bulang	11.25	16.09	Lung or heart
Quepen	26.83	38.34	Lung
Qihu	21.43	30.62	Lung
Kufang	13.65	18.66	Lung
Wuyi	10.79	15.42	Lung
Yingchuang	10.32	14.74	Lung
Rugeng	8.55	12.21	Lung
Qimen	8.97	12.81	Lung
Riyue	10.63	15.19	Liver
Tianchi	10.50	15.00	Lung
Yuanye	13.61	19.44	Lung
Dabao	12.74	18.19	Lung
Zhejing	11.55	16.50	Lung
Zhongrong	17.29	24.70	Lung
Xiongxiang	13.84	19.77	Lung
Tianxi	12.08	17.26	Lung
Shitou	10.62	15.17	Lung
Tiantu	13.41	22.91	Trachea or lung
Burong	10.87	15.53	Liver
Chengman	9.56	13.63	Liver
Liangmen	9.14	13.06	Liver or stomach
Guanmen	9.19	13.13	Liver or stomach
Youmen	9.32	13.31	Liver
Futonggu	8.13	11.62	Liver
Yingdu	7.99	11.11	Liver
Changqu	8.23	11.75	Stomach
Henggu	17.60	25.14	Bladder or small intestine
Fuai	8.88	12.69	Liver, gallbladder or transverse colon
Zhangmen	10.90	15.57	Liver, colon or spleen
Jingmen	11.75	16.79	Inferior margin of Liver or kidney

Table 14.2. (*Continued*)

Acupoint	Safe needling depth (mm)	Dangerous needling depth (mm)	Vulnerable organs
Jiuwei	10.29	14.70	Liver
Juque	8.06	11.52	Liver
Shangwan	8.22	11.74	Liver
Zhongwan	8.51	12.16	Stomach or transverse colon
Qugu	16.58	23.68	Bladder or small intestine

Source: Zhang *et al.* (1998a) and Zhang *et al.* (2001a).

the sternum. The tracheal rings or ligaments between neighbouring rings will be hurt if it is perpendicularly punctured at more than 0.5 cun. When needling deeply, the aortic arch, left common carotid artery or brachiocephalic trunk will be hurt accordingly if the needles are oblique to the posterior direction, left or right sides. The lung will be inserted if the needling depth is more than 1.5 cun. The anterior margin of the lung will be hurt if the tip of the needle is oblique to the two sides or the patient has pulmonary emphysema (Li *et al.*, 2001).

Quepan is located on the midpoint of the supraclavicular fossa and the vulnerable organ is the lung if puncturing is done improperly. The safe needling method of this acupoint is to puncture perpendicularly towards the posterior direction or puncture towards the inferior and lateral direction at an angle greater than 45° (Zhang *et al.*, 2001b).

Jiuwei lies on the anterior median line of the upper abdomen at the thoracoepigastric combination. There are left lobe of liver in the deep tissues and heart in the left superior direction. The direction of needling this acupoint is based on superficial or deep needling. Superficial needling is to puncture obliquely towards the superior or inferior direction and the needling depth is within 0.6 cun at an angle within 25°. Deep needling is to puncture perpendicularly at 0.3 cun, then obliquely insert close to skin towards the superior or inferior directions. The subcutaneous tissue and tendon are weak on the location of this acupoint and xiphoid process is inserted when puncturing perpendicularly. If the needle is inserted more than 1.2 cun the depth of the xiphoid process, the tip of the needle will reach peritoneal cavity and hurt the liver. If the needling direction is left and superior and the depth is more than 25°, the needle will reach pleural cavity and hurt the heart. If the needling direction is obliquely to the left or right sides, the needle will hurt the internal and inferior angles of two sides of the lung (Yan, 2001).

Zhongwan lies on the anterior median line of the upper abdomen and the needling direction is at perpendicular insertion or oblique insertion around. The needle will touch the gastric wall with perpendicular insertion when the stomach is full. The transverse colon will be inserted with perpendicular insertion over 0.5 cun when the patient is hungry. If inserted deeper, the transverse colon, central and upper part of the pancreas will be penetrated. If the needling depth reaches above 70 mm with a Mang-needle, the rate of organs inserted will be: stomach 56%, transverse colon 48%, small intestine 44%, pancreas 36%, left renal vein 16%, left lobe of liver 16%, splenic vein 12% and duodenum 4% (Chuai and Wang, 2002). Although the body of the Mang-needle is very slim, repeated and intense manipulations should be avoided to prevent against organ damage (Song, 1999; Peng, 2000).

14.4.3 *Research of dangerous acupoints on lumbar and back*

The lumbar and back are parts to the compound pleural cavity and peritoneal cavity which house important organs, such as the heart, lung, liver and kidney. Since the kidney locates tightly with the abdominal wall on two sides of the spine, it is easily hurt when needling dangerous acupoints on the lumbar, such as Huangmen and Zhishi, with deep insertion. The chest wall is also weak, just like the ancients' description: "The lumbar is as thin as a piece of paper". The Bei-(Shu) points, located on the back of the Bladder Meridian of Zu Tai-yang, are close to important organs, thus the heart, liver and lung will be affected and death may result if these points are needled too deeply or improperly (Lun and Rong, 1997).

The safe and dangerous needling depths

We studied 24 dangerous acupoints on the lumbar and back systemically, measured the dangerous needling depths of all these acupoints and calculated their safe needling depths. The results are shown in Table 14.3.

Table 14.3. Safe, dangerous needling depths and vulnerable organs of dangerous acupoints on lumbar and back.

Acupoint	Safe needling depth (mm)	Dangerous needling depth (mm)	Vulnerable organs
Dazhu	43.77	62.54	Lung
Fengmen	41.17	58.82	Lung
Feishu	35.42	50.60	Lung
Yueyingshu	29.58	42.25	Lung
Xinshu	25.56	36.52	Lung
Dushu	22.96	32.80	Lung
Geshu	21.13	30.18	Lung
Weiwanxiashu	21.54	30.77	Lung
Ganshu	22.45	32.07	Lung
Danshu	25.01	35.73	Lung
Qishu	26.68	38.11	Lung or liver
Weishu	29.86	42.65	Liver
Fufen	36.98	52.83	Lung
Pohu	31.09	44.42	Lung
Gaohuang	25.34	36.20	Lung
Shentang	20.50	29.28	Lung
Yixi	16.55	23.65	Lung
Geguan	14.43	20.61	Lung
Huenmen	13.78	19.68	Lung
Yanggang	14.34	20.49	Lung
Yishe	15.90	22.71	Lung or liver
Wenchang	19.73	28.19	Liver
Huangmen	22.53	32.18	Kidney
Zhishi	23.32	33.32	Kidney

Source: Zhang *et al.* (2000).

Needling directions and related local anatomical structures

Bei-(Shu) points, Feishu, Xinshu, Ganshu and Weishu, lie on the back with 1.5 cun lateral to the lower border of the spinous process. When needling these acupoints, the needling direction should be towards the spinous process, that is inward oblique insertion, with the needling angle at 65°. Do not puncture more than 0.8 cun if inserting perpendicularly. It is very dangerous to obliquely puncture outward since in this situation the lung may be hurt, and pneumatothorax and hematopneumothorax can result (Lui, 1998).

Geguan, Hunmen and Yanggang are located on the back at 3.0 cun lateral to the lower border of the spinous process. The values of their dangerous needling depths are extremely small since they are so close to the important organs and are highly likely to cause accidents. When needling these acupoints, the needles should be inserted perpendicularly or obliquely towards the superior and inferior directions. The lung will be punctured and so pneumatothorax may happen if needled too deeply.

Huangmen and Zhishi located on the lumbar and kidney lies under their deep location. There are spinal muscles and quadratus lumborum there but it is usually safe if the needling direction and depth are proper. Needles should be inserted perpendicularly or obliquely towards the anterior and inferior directions. The kidney will be hurt if inserted too deeply.

Most dangerous acupoints are those used widely in clinic with good therapeutic effects. But the anatomical structures of places where these acupoints are located are complicated and there are important organs in their deep location. As the descriptions of needling depths and angles in various ancient works are different, it is necessary to study the dangerous acupoints using the stratified anatomical and layer anatomical method. The results serve as a reference of safe needling depth for clinical acupuncturists, thus avoiding fatal accidents.

References

Acupuncture and Moxibustion Department of the First Affiliated Hospital of Tianjing College of Traditional Chinese Medicine (1981) *Applied Acupuncture and Moxibustion*. Tianjing Science and Technology Press, p. 138.

China Academy of Traditional Chinese Medicine (1978) *Concise Compilation of Acupuncture and Moxibustion*. People's Medical Publishing House, Beijing, p. 73.

Chuai, Z. and Wang, Z. (2002) Study on safe factors of deep needling at Zhongwan point with elongated needle. *Chin. Acupunct. Mox.* **22**(8), 535–536.

Cui, H., Lou, X., Jiang, S., *et al.* (2002) Local anatomic research on needling location of Jianjing. *J. Clin. Acupunct. Mox.* **18**(9), 3–4.

Han, H. (2003) Research of natural opinion and humanistic opinion on theory of acupuncture contraindication in *Internal Classic*. *J. Clin. Acupunct. Mox.* **19**(5), 1–2.

Li, W., Kong, L. and Fang, Z. (1997) Anatomic structures and safe needling methods of Jingmin and Chengqi. *J. Anhui Tradit. Chin. Med. Coll.* **16**(1), 44–45.

Li, W., Yin, L. and Yang, H. (2001) Research on needling ancient prohibited acupoints of the conception vessel. *J. Clin. Acupunct. Mox.* **17**(12), 1–2.

Lui, Y. (1998) *Rescue and Prevention for Acupuncture Accidents*. Chinese Medical Ancient Books Publishing House, Beijing, pp. 66–68.

Lui, W. and Huang, J. (1997) Research on relationship between bleeding of Jingmin and acupuncture manipulation. *Chin. Med. Res.* **13**(6), 45–46.

Lun, X. and Rong, L. *Analysis on Acupuncture Accidental Cases*. People's Medical Publishing House, Beijing, pp. 198–205.

Peng, L. (2000) Clinical application of deep insertion with Mang-needle. *Chin. Acupunct. Mox. Suppl.* 50–51.

Shen, G., Wang, L. and Yan, G. (1999) Research on safe needling depth of Renying. *J. Anhui Tradit. Chin. Med. Coll.* **18**(5), 57–58.

Song, H. (1999) Clinical application on puncturing Zhongwan deeply by Mang-needle. *Liaoning J. Tradit. Chin. Med.* **26**(2), 81–82.

Tai, H. (2002) Research on acupuncture contraindication and morphosis on cervical part. *J. Chengdu Univ. Tradit. Chin. Med.* **25**(1), 3–7.

Wang, Y. (1996) Review on researches of Renying. *Shanghai J. Acupunct. Mox.* **2**, 36–37.

Yan, Z. (1996) *Anatomic Basis for Usually Used Acupoints*. Press of Shanghai University of Traditional Chinese Medicine, Shanghai, pp. 160–163.

Yan, Z. (2001) *Applied Acupoints Anatomy*. Press of Shanghai University of Traditional Chinese Medicine, Shanghai, pp. 98–104.

Yan, Z., Zhang, J., Gu, H., *et al.* (1996) Research of dangerous acupoints on cervical part. *Shanghai J. Acupunct. Mox.* **15**(3), 37–38.

Yang, J. (1984) *Acupoints*. Shanghai Science and Technology Press, Shanghai, p. 44.

Yang, Z. (1987) *Acupuncture Accidents Prevention*. Shanxi Science and Education Press, Shanxi, pp. 153–258.

Zhang, J., Yan, Z., Gu, H., *et al.* (1998a) Research of dangerous acupoints on chest. *Shanghai J. Acupunct. Mox.* **17**(6), 24–25.

Zhang, J., Yan, Z., Yu, A., *et al.* (2000) The safe needling depth in the accidental acupoints. *Acupunct. Res.* **25**(3), 233–235.

Zhang, J., Yan, Z., Yu, A., *et al.* (2001a) Research of dangerous acupoints on abdomen. *Chin. Acupunct. Mox.* **21**(2), 83–84.

Zhang, J., Yu, A., Zhao, Y., *et al.* (2001b) Anatomic structure and needling depth of Quepen point. *Chin. Acupunct.* **21**(8), 493–494.

Zhang, J., Yu, A., Zhao, Y., *et al.* (2002) Study on the anatomic structure and safe needling depth of Jianjing (GB 21) point. *Acupunct. Res.* **27**(2), 152–154.

Zhang, S., Xu, H. and Wang, Y. (1998b) Analysis on local anatomic sign and therapeutic functions of Renxing. *J. Zhengjiang Med. Coll.* **8**(4), 448–449.

Chapter 15

Acupuncture in Cancer Patient Care

Gary Deng, Andrew Vickers, K. Simon Yeung & Barrie R. Cassileth

Abstract

Background: Acupuncture has been evaluated in clinical studies for its effect in reducing some of the common symptoms experienced by cancer patients.

Methods: Clinical studies of acupuncture in cancer-related symptoms, published in the English language, are reviewed. The data are summarised. Implications in cancer care are discussed.

Results: There is good evidence supporting acupuncture's effects in the reduction of cancer-related pain and chemotherapy-induced acute nausea and vomiting. There are preliminary data suggesting that acupuncture may help reduce post-chemotherapy fatigue, hot flashes resulting from hormonal treatment and xerostomia caused by radiation. Acupuncture has a good safety record when performed by qualified practitioners.

Conclusion: Acupuncture is a useful complementary therapy in cancer care. Integration of acupuncture into regular oncology practice can improve supportive care of cancer patients.

Keywords: Cancer; Integrative Oncology; Acupuncture; Complementary Therapies.

15.1 Introduction

Acupuncture is an integral part of traditional Chinese medicine (TCM). It originated in China more than 2000 years ago, spread to other East Asia countries in the sixth century and later to Europe and North America in the 17th and 19th centuries.

Historically, acupuncture was used as a modality to prevent and treat many ailments, but its efficacy has been evaluated with rigorous scientific research methodology only in the last few decades. During that time frame, research on acupuncture's physiological effects, possible mechanisms of action and its clinical efficacy for specific indications has produced a large body of cumulative data. It is perhaps the most accepted TCM modality in Western countries, in a large part due to these studies. Acupuncture can induce objective, measurable neurophysiologic changes in animals and humans. It has been shown to be efficacious in randomised controlled clinical trials for pain, nausea and vomiting, and other symptoms. There are excellent review articles of acupuncture in general (Kaptchuk, 2002; Han, 2004; NIH, 1998).

Given the cumulative evidence, acupuncture has been increasingly incorporated into mainstream Western health care as a complementary therapy. There is no evidence that acupuncture has direct effects against cancer. However, there is evidence showing acupuncture can help reduce some of the common symptoms experienced by cancer patients, hence improving their quality of life. Here we review data from clinical studies on acupuncture relevant to cancer patient care.

Although there are numerous publications on acupuncture in the Chinese, Japanese and Korean scientific literature, this review focuses on studies that are published in English and accessible via international biomedical bibliography indexes such as Medline. We will also discuss briefly how acupuncture can be integrated into the health care system in the United States as a complementary therapy for cancer patients.

15.2 Methods

Medline was searched using "acupuncture" and the specific symptoms as keywords, with limits to the English language and Clinical Trials. Resultant publications were evaluated for their relevance to cancer medicine. We summarised and provide commentary on data from key publications. This is not a systemic review.

15.3 Results and Discussion

15.3.1 *Pain*

Almost every cancer patient experiences pain at one time or another. Pain is the indication for which acupuncture has been studied the most, producing a large body of data. Cancer patients with difficult-to-control pain are a heterogeneous group, most often suffering from chronic pain caused directly by tumour invasion or treatment, such as chemotherapy-induced mucositis. They also may experience acute pain, such as that following surgery or procedures. Mastectomy and other pain syndromes are unique to cancer, and pain in terminal stages of disease has its own characteristics and special issues. Clinical research broadly supports acupuncture for the relief of pain.

Most pain research addresses non-cancer acute or chronic pain. Pain after dental surgery provides a good model of acupuncture analgesia due to its limited and predictable course and good control of co-interventions. Patients undergoing third molar extraction were randomised to acupuncture or guide tube placebo on a double-blind basis. Mean duration of the pain-free interval following surgery was 181 minutes in acupuncture patients versus 71 minutes in controls, a statistically significant difference (Lao *et al.*, 1995). A systematic review of 16 such studies concluded that acupuncture was effective for pain after dental surgery (Ernst and Pittler, 1998).

There is also evidence for acupuncture against chronic pain. In one report, 52 athletes suffering from rotator cuff tendonitis were randomised to eight treatments of true or placebo acupuncture. Outcome was assessed with a combined pain and function score at four weeks by an orthopaedist blinded to treatment allocation. Differences between groups at the end of treatment were statistically and clinically significant, with improvement among patients receiving true acupuncture more than twice that of controls. These improvements were maintained at six-month follow-up (Kleinhenz *et al.*, 1999). A systematic review of acupuncture for chronic headache pain found that most placebo-controlled trials favoured acupuncture. A meta-analysis of ten such studies estimated the chance of a response to be approximately 50% greater after treatment with acupuncture than placebo (Melchart *et al.*, 1999).

A large trial of 401 patients with chronic headache, predominantly migraine, showed that acupuncture led to persisting, clinically relevant benefits (Vickers *et al.*, 2004a). Patients were randomised to receive up to 12 acupuncture treatments over three months or to a usual care control intervention. Headache score at 12 months fell by 34% from baseline in the acupuncture group, but only by 16% in controls. Patients in the acupuncture group experienced fewer days of headache per year, used less medication, made fewer visits to primary doctors, and took fewer days of sick leave (Vickers *et al.*, 2004a). A recent randomised controlled trial of 570 patients with osteoarthritis of the knee found that a 26-week course of acupuncture significantly improved pain and dysfunction when compared to sham-acupuncture control. In this study all patients received other usual care for osteoarthritis. At week 8, improvement in function but not in pain was observed, indicating that long term treatment may be required to achieve full effects (Berman *et al.*, 2004). A companion paper reported the results of a randomised controlled trial of acupuncture for chronic neck pain. A statistically significant but not clinically significant (12%) reduction of pain was reported (White *et al.*, 2004). This study was criticised for using only one acupuncturist to deliver the intervention (Ernst, 2005).

There has been only limited research on acupuncture for chronic pain in cancer patients. Most reports are restricted to case series. An early study reported that approximately half of a series of over 300 cancer patients obtained clinically relevant, persisting pain relief from acupuncture (Filshie and Redman, 1985) and a further 20% had pain relief lasting at least a few days. A similar level of activity was reported in a subsequent study of 47 hospice patients, 40 of whom had cancer: 62% reported pain relief as "excellent" or "good" on a five-point scale; visual analog scores (VAS) improved from 64 to 32 mm (Leng, 1999). A second study in the hospice setting included 28 patients, 22 of whom had advanced cancer. Treatment was by insertion of semi-permanent needles at acupuncture points on the auricle. Despite only minor changes in analgesic intake, pain scores fell immediately following acupuncture and continued to fall over the course of the four-week follow-up. At two weeks, pain fell on average by slightly less than 3 points on a 0–10 numerical rating scale, with all but two patients reporting at least moderate pain relief (Dillon and Lucas, 1999). In another paper, 20 cancer patients with continuing severe pain after one month of stable treatment with WHO level 2 or 3 analgesics received treatment with semi-permanent needles on the auricle. Mean baseline VAS pain of 76 mm was reduced by an average of 33 mm at 60-day follow-up (Alimi *et al.*, 2000).

Recently, a randomised placebo-controlled trial tested auricular acupuncture for patients with pain despite stable medication. This is by far the most rigorous study reported. A total of 90 patients were randomised to have needles placed at correct acupuncture points (treatment group), versus acupuncture or pressure at non-acupuncture points. Pain intensity decreased by 36% at two months from baseline in the treatment group, a statistically significant difference compared with the two control groups, for whom little pain reduction was seen (Alimi *et al.*, 2003). Skin penetration alone showed no significant analgesic effect. These results are especially important because most of the patients had neuropathic pain, which is often refractory to conventional treatment.

Brain imaging technology is now used to examine the specific nervous pathways involved in acupuncture. In functional MRI studies, true acupuncture induces brain activation in the hypothalamus and nucleus accumbens, and deactivates areas of the anterior cingulate cortex, amygdala, and hippocampus. Such changes are not observed in control stimulations, which affect only sensory cortex change. De-activation of the amygdala and hippocampus is observed with electroacupuncture. These data suggest that acupuncture modulates the affective-cognitive aspect of pain perception (Wu *et al.*, 1999). Correlations between signal intensities and analgesic effects also are reported (Zhang *et al.*, 2003). In another study, positron emission tomography (PET) was carried out in 14 osteoarthritis patients to image cerebral functional changes associated with real acupuncture, placebo acupuncture and skin-prick, using a single-blind, randomised crossover design. The insula ipsilateral to the site of needling was activated to a greater extent during real acupuncture than during the placebo intervention. Both real acupuncture and placebo caused greater activation than skin prick in the right dorsolateral prefrontal cortex, anterior cingulate cortex, and midbrain. The results suggest that real acupuncture has a specific physiological effect and that patients' expectation and belief regarding a potentially beneficial treatment modulate activity in component areas of the reward system (Pariente *et al.*, 2005).

15.4 Nausea and Vomiting

Acupuncture helps lessen chemotherapy-induced nausea and vomiting (Lee and Done, 2004). In one study, 104 breast cancer patients receiving highly emetogenic chemotherapy were randomised to receive electro-acupuncture at the PC6 and ST36 acupuncture points, minimal needling at non-acupuncture points, or pharmacotherapy alone. Electroacupuncture significantly reduced the number of episodes of total emesis from a median of 15 to five when compared with pharmacotherapy only, or with minimal needling as sham acupuncture control. Most patients did not know the group to which they had been assigned (Shen *et al.*, 2000). The effects of acupuncture do not appear entirely due to attention, clinician-patient interaction, or placebo.

The combination of acupuncture and serotonin receptor antagonists, the newest generation of antiemetics, has shown mixed results. In a trial of patients with rheumatic disease, the combination decreased the severity of nausea and the number of vomiting episodes more than ondansetron alone in patients on methotrexate (an agent also used in chemotherapy) (Josefson and Kreuter, 2003). However, a study of cancer patients receiving high dose chemotherapy and autologous stem cell transplantation reported no significant benefit for ondansetron plus acupuncture versus ondansetron plus placebo acupuncture (Streitberger *et al.*, 2003). Acupuncture also suppresses nausea and vomiting caused by pregnancy (Rosen *et al.*, 2003), surgery (Streitberger *et al.*, 2004) and motion sickness (Bertolucci and DiDario *et al.*, 1995; Ming *et al.*, 2002).

Acupressure wrist bands that render continuous stimulation of the PC6 point also have been tested for chemotherapy-related nausea and vomiting. In a randomised, controlled trial of 739 patients, nausea on the day of chemotherapy was reduced significantly in patients wearing wrist bands compared with no-band controls. No significant differences were found for delayed nausea or vomiting (Roscoe *et al.*, 2003). Unlike acupressure wrist bands, electrostimulation wristbands do not significantly reduce nausea or antiemetic use. The stimulus generated by the electrostimulation band may act as a conditioned stimulus (akin to a reminder) of the nausea that patients are trying to control, and thereby actually accentuate nausea in some individuals (Roscoe *et al.*, 2003).

A meta-analysis of 11 randomised trials confirms the above findings. Overall, acupuncture reduced the proportion of acute vomiting, but not the mean number of acute emetic episodes or acute or delayed nausea severity compared with controls. Electroacupuncture reduced the proportion of acute vomiting, but manual acupuncture did not. Acupuncture's effect on delayed nausea/vomiting were not reported. Acupressure reduced mean acute nausea severity and most severe acute nausea, but not acute vomiting or delayed symptoms. Non-invasive electrostimulation (transcutaneous stimulation) showed no benefit for any outcome (Ezzo *et al.*, 2005).

15.5 Fatigue

Fatigue is prevalent in cancer patients, particularly among those undergoing chemotherapy or radiation therapy. Its most readily identifiable cause is anaemia. Treatment with erythropoietin improved anaemia and reduced fatigue in a randomised trial (Littlewood *et al.*, 2001). Other causes of fatigue in cancer patients include depression, sleep disorder, deconditioning, infection, thyroid disorders, side-effects of medications such as opiates or anti-histamines, nutritional factors, cytokine induction during therapy and electrolyte imbalance. However, many patients with cancer-related fatigue have none of these aetiologies (Lesage and Portenoy, 2002).

Conventional approaches to symptomatic treatment of fatigue without identified correctable conditions include administration of psychostimulants, treatment of co-morbidities and behavioural techniques. Acupuncture was tested as a treatment for fatigue in a single-arm trial (Vickers *et al.*, 2004b). Patients who completed cytotoxic chemotherapy at least three weeks previously but still complaining of persisting fatigue were treated with acupuncture twice a week for four weeks or once weekly for six weeks. Of the 31 patients who completed the study, most of whom had experienced fatigue for many years, 12 patients (39%) improved by 40% or more and three experienced near total (> 75%) resolution of fatigue symptoms. The mean improvement of fatigue scores from baseline to follow-up was 31.1% (95% confidence interval 20.6–41.5%). Younger, less depressed, and more anxious patients showed a greater response. Although this was a single-arm study, the results compare favourably to other reports where cancer patients received usual care. In another report, fatigue scores were followed in four to six weeks of multidisciplinary treatment, including pharmacotherapy (Escalante *et al.*, 2001). Four of the 17 patients (24%) with severe fatigue at baseline (BFI 7 or above) had non-severe fatigue on follow-up. The corresponding figures from the acupuncture study are 11 of 14 patients (79%) severe at baseline and non-severe on follow-up ($p = 0.002$ for the comparison between trials). Such comparison suggests that acupuncture may be superior to usual care, although this needs to be tested in controlled trials.

15.6 Hot Flashes

Hot flashes is a common problem experience by breast and prostate cancer patients undergoing hormonal therapies. It is also experienced by other menopausal cancer patients. The standard oestrogen or progesterone/oestrogen treatment is not widely used for cancer patients, in particular breast cancer patients, because it might stimulate the growth of oestrogen receptor positive cancer cells. Alternatives such as anti-depressants (venlafaxine, paroxetine), clonidine, megastrol acetate, soy phytoestrogens or black cohosh showed limited efficacy or other limitations (Loprinzi *et al.*, 1998; Stearns *et al.*, 2000; Weitzner *et al.*, 2002; Goldberg *et al.*, 1994; Pandya *et al.*, 2000; Quella *et al.*, 2000; Van Patten *et al.*, 2002).

Several single-arm and randomised studies of acupuncture for hot flashes are available. The first trial involved 24 menopausal women who were randomised to receive ten treatments of either acupuncture with electrical stimulation (EA) or "superficial needle insertion" (SNI) acupuncture. Similar point locations were used in both arms (Wyon *et al.*, 1995). As such, this was a trial of high versus low intensity stimulation (or "dose"). During the ten-week treatment period, visual analog scale scores of symptom severity approximately halved in the EA group and were significantly reduced by a third in those receiving SNI. At six-month follow-up, scores remained low in EA patients but returned toward baseline in the SNI group. Large and statistically significant falls also were observed for both groups in calcitonin-gene related peptide (CGRP), a potent vasodilator. Higher levels of CGRP are found in menopausal women with hot flashes compared to those without symptoms (Wyon *et al.*, 1998); moreover, increased serum levels of CGRP can be detected during a hot flash (Wyon *et al.*, 2000). This trial not only suggests an effect of acupuncture on hot flashes and provides a biological mechanism, but also supports a dose-effect for strength of acupuncture stimulation.

Other trials studied hot flashes related to cancer treatment. Towlerton *et al.* (1999) detailed a case series of 12 women with tamoxifen-related hot flashes. Six remained symptomatic after pharmacological management and two discontinued tamoxifen because of symptoms. The women were treated with semi-permanent studs sited at acupuncture points. Patients were able to replace these themselves and were instructed to stimulate the studs in the prodromal period. The studs remained in place for an average of 13 months (range four to 36 months) and were well tolerated by all but two patients. Hot flashes were abolished or attenuated in eight of the 12 women. Porzio *et al.* (2002) report a case series of 15 breast cancer patients with tamoxifen-induced menopausal symptoms treated by weekly acupuncture for three months. Vasomotor symptoms improved by 55% from baseline to six-month follow-up.

A similar study was conducted in prostate cancer patients (Hammar *et al.*, 1999). Seven men with prostate cancer experiencing hot flashes during hormonal therapy received 14 sessions of electroacupuncture over a 12-week period. One patient dropped out after two weeks for an apparently unrelated medical problem. Average number of daily hot flashes for the remaining six patients fell from 7.9 at baseline to 2.5 after treatment, rising only slightly to 3.6 at a six-month follow-up. These reductions are very much greater than would be expected given control arm data from previous randomised studies.

A randomised trial of acupuncture for cancer-related hot flashes was published in abstract form (Hammar *et al.*, 1999). Thirty-eight breast cancer patients received either acupuncture or relaxation therapy. As relaxation therapy has previously been shown in a randomised trial to reduce hot flashes in menopausal women (Irvin *et al.*, 1996), this can be considered to be an active control trial. Mean number of daily hot flashes at baseline, three and six months were 8.5, 4.1 and 3.7 in patients receiving acupuncture and 8.0, 4.9 and 2.8 in the relaxation group. These falls were statistically significant for both treatment arms.

15.6.1 *Xerostomia*

Xerostomia, the subjective experience of dry mouth, is one of the most common complaints experienced by cancer patients treated with radiation therapy to the head and neck region (Guchelaar *et al.*, 1997). It is caused by salivary gland dysfunction as a result of damage in the field of radiation (Valdez, 1991). Xerostomia has a debilitating impact on health and overall quality of life in head and neck cancer survivors because decreased salivation can lead to dental caries, periodontal diseases, a shift of oral flora, poor tolerability to dental prosthesis and inflammation, atrophy and ulceration of mucosa. In addition, salivary gland dysfunction contributes to systemic problems including loss of appetite, chronic oesophagitis, gastroesophageal reflux, and sleep disruption due to the need for frequent mouth moistening and subsequent polyuria (Vissink *et al.*, 1988). Current treatment of radiation-induced xerostomia includes dietary and oral hygiene, saliva substitution or stimulation of salivation by moistening agents or medications such as pilocarpine (Nieuw-Amerongen and Veerman, 2003; Johnson *et al.*, 1993; LeVeque *et al.*, 1993; Rieke *et al.*, 1995). However, the temporary nature of the relief, the inconvenience, social embarrassment, and side effects limit their use in all patients (Atkinson and Fox, 1992; Levine *et al.*, 1987; Kusler and Rambur, 1992).

Studies show that acupuncture can influence salivary production. Its effect has been studied in healthy subjects (Dawidson *et al.*, 1997), patients with Sjögren's Syndrome (an autoimmune disorder that can result in salivary dysfunction) (List *et al.*, 1998; Blom and Lundeberg, 2000), and head and neck cancer patients treated with radiation (Wong *et al.*, 2003; Johnstone *et al.*, 2001, 2002a and b; Rydholm and Strang, 1999; Blom *et al.*, 1993; Andersen and Machin, 1997; Blom *et al.*, 1996). In a small study of eight healthy volunteers, unstimulated, chewing-stimulated, and citric acid-stimulated salivary flows were investigated in combination with manual and electrically stimulated acupuncture before, during, and after every acupuncture session (Dawidson *et al.*, 1997). The unstimulated salivary flow increased significantly both during and after manual acupuncture stimulation when compared to baseline. No effect on the unstimulated salivary flow with electroacupuncture was observed. The authors postulated that salivary secretion might be influenced by the release of neuropeptides caused by acupuncture. A significant increase in the salivary levels of calcitonin gene-related peptide (CGRP), neuropeptide Y (NPY) and vasoactive intestinal polypeptide (VIP) both during and after acupuncture stimulation was reported (Dawidson *et al.*, 1998a and b; 1999).

List *et al.* (1998) randomised 21 patients with Sjögren's syndrome to acupuncture or no treatment control. Although the trial was too small for meaningful statistical analysis, several interesting trends are apparent. Visual analog scores of subjective mouth dryness fell from a median of 7.2 at baseline to 5.5 after treatment in the acupuncture group, but increased from 6.3 to 6.8 in controls. Stimulated saliva secretion approximately doubled after acupuncture treatment, with no change in controls.

In a single-arm study of 20 palliative care patients (17 of them cancer patients), acupuncture reduced xerostomia, dysphagia, and articulation (Rydholm and Strang, 1999). The patients reported improvement after five treatments. Another study tested an acupuncture-like transcutaneous nerve stimulation device in 46 patients (Wong *et al.*, 2003). All patients had received more than 50 Gy of radiotherapy to bilateral head and neck fields, including the parotid glands, and all had residual salivary function. Two six-week courses of treatment, separated by a two-week break, were given. Xerostomia symptoms, unstimulated saliva production, and citric acid-primed saliva production all improved. The improvement persisted at the six-month follow-up. An investigator in the current proposal, Dr. Peter Johnstone, reported that even patients refractory to pilocarpine treatment may respond to acupuncture treatment (Johnstone *et al.*, 2001). In a study of 50 patients, Johnstone showed that 70% of patients improved 10% or more in xerostomia scores after a mean of six acupuncture treatments. Interestingly, the effects of acupuncture appear to persist for many months after initial treatment. Additional acupuncture therapy can maintain improved salivary flow for up to three years (Blom and Lundeberg, 2000).

A group from McMaster University published results of a phase I–II study with transcutaneous electrical stimulation using a proprietary device (CODETRON) (Wong *et al.*, 2003). Forty-six patients were randomised between three different groups of body acupoints. Points were stimulated for random ten-second intervals for 20-minute sessions twice weekly for six weeks, then for another six weeks after a two-week break. For 37 patients who completed therapy, statistically increased salivation using a visual analog scale was reported at both three- and six-month follow-up. Further, statistically increased basal and stimulated salivation was noted at both follow-up durations (Wong *et al.*, 2003).

Blom *et al.* (1996) published a small randomised controlled trial of acupuncture for radiotherapy-induced xerostomia. Forty-one patients were treated either with traditional acupuncture or by a placebo technique that involved shallow needling away from true acupuncture points. The endpoint was salivary flow rates, with patients experiencing an increase in salivary flow of 20% or more considered as having responded. The statistical approach of the paper is somewhat flawed, but fortunately, the authors present individual patient data allowing full re-analysis. Andersen and Machin (1997) published a re-analysis based on a survival approach, comparing the time between groups to achieve a 0.1 g/minute increase in salivary flow rates. They report a hazard ratio of 2.4 (95% C.I. 0.8, 6.8; $p = 0.11$), and conclude that the study suggests a benefit.

15.6.2 *Dyspnoea*

Shortness of breath, or dyspnoea, is a common symptom in cancer patients, particularly those with advanced cancer. In some situations, only symptomatic treatment can be offered due to absence of treatable aetiology or patient's inability to tolerate treatment. Symptomatic treatment of shortness of breath includes bronchodilators, steroids, opiates and oxygen. Acupuncture has also been evaluated for treatment of dyspnoea.

Randomised controlled trials have examined acupuncture for shortness of breath. Tashkin *et al.* (1977) used a laboratory-based model of methacholine-induced asthma. The laboratory setting allowed good experimental control and the study was double-blind, placebo-controlled and randomised. Significant differences in lung function emerged between needling true versus inactive ("sham") points. A similar randomised, double-blind, placebo-controlled study in a laboratory setting involved a standardised running test to induce bronchorestriction in asthmatics. Exercise-induced reductions in lung function were significantly lower in real compared to sham acupuncture (Fung *et al.*, 1986). A trial of acupressure for chronic obstructive pulmonary disorder (COPD) reported significant differences between groups for subjective breathlessness. Thirty-one patients were randomised to self-administer acupressure at true or sham acupuncture points on a double-blind, crossover basis. Acupressure led to approximately a one-third reduction of scores on a VAS of dyspnoea compared to about a 20% improvement in placebo controls (Maa *et al.*, 1997).

In an uncontrolled trial 30 cancer patients in palliative care experiencing dyspnoea received a single session of acupuncture. The mean visual analog score for breathlessness before treatment was 42; this fell to 24 immediately following ten minutes of needle insertion, an improvement that was maintained at six-hour follow-up. Breathlessness scores returned to baseline 24 hours later (Filshie *et al.*, 1996).

In a randomised controlled trial of 47 patients with lung or breast cancer presenting with dyspnoea, patients received a single session of true or placebo acupuncture in addition to their usual care for dyspnoea, followed by placement of miniscule acupuncture needles at certain points or placebo needles at non-acupuncture points. Patients were instructed to apply pressure to these studs twice a day to provide ongoing stimulation to acupuncture points. Dyspnoea scores were slightly higher for patients receiving true versus placebo acupuncture, for both the period immediately following acupuncture treatment and for the daily one week follow-up. The 95% confidence interval excludes the pre-specified minimum clinically significant difference of a 20% greater improvement in dyspnoea for patients receiving acupuncture. It was concluded that the acupuncture technique used in this trial is unlikely to have effects on dyspnoea significantly larger than placebo for patients with advanced cancer (Vickers *et al.*, 2005).

15.6.3 *Risks and adverse events*

Acupuncture is a generally safe treatment modality. A prospective survey of well-qualified Japanese acupuncture practitioners recorded only 94 minor adverse events, the most common being forgotten needles and faintness, but no serious adverse events across 65,000 treatments (Yamashita *et al.*, 1999). Similar findings were reported in a study from Norway (Norheim and Fonnebo, 1996).

A study of Swedish physiotherapists practicing acupuncture prospectively recorded side-effects during more than 9000 episodes of care. Although minor bleeding or haematoma was reported following nearly one in five treatments, fatigue, sweating and other minor adverse effects were rare and there were no serious complications (Odsberg *et al.*, 2001). More recently, a UK study involving 574 acupuncturists evaluated adverse events and treatment reactions associated with 34,407 treatments. No serious adverse events were reported although there were 43 minor adverse events, about a quarter of which were severe nausea and fainting (MacPherson *et al.*, 2001).

A recent prospective survey of 32,000 consultations with physicians and physiotherapist acupuncturists found no serious adverse events and 14 minor adverse events per 10,000 acupuncture consultations (White *et al.*, 2001). In the most recent study of over 760,000 treatments in 97,733 patients receiving acupuncture in Germany, only six cases of potentially serious adverse events were reported. They included exacerbation of depression, hypertensive crisis, vasovagal reaction, asthma attack, and pneumothorax. The most common non-serious adverse events included local bleeding and needling pain. Only six serious adverse events were reported (Melchart *et al.*, 2004).

15.6.4 *Integration of acupuncture into mainstream oncology care in the United States*

The availability of acupuncture therapy and the degree of integration into mainstream health care varies by geographic location, institution type and the demographics of the patient population. Laws regulating the practice of acupuncture vary across states. In most states, acupuncture falls within the scope of practice for conventionally trained physicians. Some states require additional training on acupuncture from 100 to 300 hours. Others do not require such training. Most states also grant licenses or certifications to individuals who are not graduates of conventional medical schools but have successfully completed training in a qualified educational programme focusing on the practice of acupuncture and traditional Oriental medicine, such as an acupuncture school in the U.S. or other countries. In some states, acupuncture can also be provided by chiropractors, dentists and podiatrists who may or may not receive additional acupuncture training (Leake and Broderick, 1999; Eisenberg *et al.*, 2002).

Despite substantial progress during the last decade, acupuncture is not routinely integrated into mainstream cancer care in the U.S. We believe this situation will change, and that acupuncture eventually will become as central to supportive care as are pain and palliative care services, physical therapy and rehabilitation, or speech therapy. This will depend on the amount and quality of rigorous scientific evidence produced. Equally important is the dissemination of such research data to practicing physicians and physicians-in-training, as complementary therapies are not part of the regular medical school curriculum. An international organisation, the Society of Integrative Oncology (*http://www.integrativeonc.org*), has been established to encourage appropriate scientific evaluation and clinical integration, as well as the dissemination of evidence-based information. Health care professionals interested in the use of acupuncture in the care of cancer patients should become actively involved in these activities to help create a critical mass of information and people for the advancement of the field.

References

Alimi, D., Rubino, C., Leandri, E.P. and Brule, S.F. (2000) Analgesic effects of auricular acupuncture for cancer pain. *J. Pain Symptom Manage.* **19**(2), 81–82.

Alimi, D., Rubino, C., Pichard-Leandri, E., Fermand-Brule, S., Dubreuil-Lemaire, M.L. and Hill, C. (2003) Analgesic effect of auricular acupuncture for cancer pain: a randomised, blinded, controlled trial. *J. Clin. Oncol.* **21**(22), 4120–4126.

Andersen, S.W. and Machin, D. (1997) Acupuncture treatment of patients with radiation-induced xerostomia. *Oral Oncol.* **33**(2), 146–147.

Atkinson, J.C. and Fox, P.C. (1992) Salivary gland dysfunction. *Clin. Geriatr. Med.* **8**(3), 499–511.

Berman, B.M., Lao, L., Langenberg, P., Lee, W.L., Gilpin, A.M. and Hochberg, M.C. (2004) Effectiveness of acupuncture as adjunctive therapy in osteoarthritis of the knee: a randomised, controlled trial. *Ann. Intern. Med.* **141**(12), 901–910.

Bertolucci, L.E. and DiDario, B. (1995) Efficacy of a portable acustimulation device in controlling seasickness. *Aviat. Space Environ. Med.* **66**(12), 1155–1158.

Blom, M., Dawidson, I. and Angmar-Mansson, B. (1993) Acupuncture treatment of xerostomia caused by irradiation of the head and neck region: case reports. *J. Oral Rehabil.* **20**(5), 491–494.

Blom, M., Dawidson, I., Fernberg, J.O., Johnson, G. and Angmar-Mansson, B. (1996) Acupuncture treatment of patients with radiation-induced xerostomia. *Eur. J. Cancer B Oral Oncol.* **32B**(3), 182–190.

Blom, M. and Lundeberg, T. (2000) Long-term follow-up of patients treated with acupuncture for xerostomia and the influence of additional treatment. *Oral Dis.* **6**(1), 15–24.

Dawidson, I., Angmar-Mansson, B., Blom, M., Theodorsson, E. and Lundeberg, T. (1998a) The influence of sensory stimulation (acupuncture) on the release of neuropeptides in the saliva of healthy subjects. *Life Sci.* **63**(8), 659–674.

Dawidson, I., Angmar-Mansson, B., Blom, M., Theodorsson, E. and Lundeberg, T. (1998b) Sensory stimulation (acupuncture) increases the release of vasoactive intestinal polypeptide in the saliva of xerostomia sufferers. *Neuropeptides* **32**(6), 543–548.

Dawidson, I., Angmar-Mansson, B., Blom, M., Theodorsson, E. and Lundeberg, T. (1999) Sensory stimulation (acupuncture) increases the release of calcitonin gene-related peptide in the saliva of xerostomia sufferers. *Neuropeptides* **33**(3), 244–250.

Dawidson, I., Blom, M., Lundeberg, T. and Angmar-Mansson, B. (1997) The influence of acupuncture on salivary flow rates in healthy subjects. *J. Oral Rehabil.* **24**(3), 204–208.

Dillon, M. and Lucas, C. (1999) Auricular stud acupuncture in palliative care patients. *Palliat. Med.* **13**(3), 253–254.

Eisenberg, D.M., Cohen, M.H., Hrbek, A., Grayzel, J., Van Rompay, M.I. and Cooper, R.A. (2003) Credentialing complementary and alternative medical providers. *Ann. Intern. Med.* **137**(12), 965–973.

Ernst E. (2005) Acupuncture for chronic mechanical neck pain. *Ann. Intern. Med.* **142**(10), 873; author reply 873–874.

Ernst, E. and Pittler, M.H. (1998) The effectiveness of acupuncture in treating acute dental pain: a systematic review. *Br. Dent. J.* **184**(9), 443–447.

Escalante, C.P., Grover, T., Johnson, B.A. *et al.* (2001) A fatigue clinic in a comprehensive cancer center: design and experiences. *Cancer* **92**(6 Suppl), 1708–1713.

Ezzo, J., Vickers, A., Richardson, M.A. *et al.* (2005) Acupuncture-point stimulation for chemotherapy-induced nausea and vomiting. *J. Clin. Oncol.* **23**(28), 7188–7198.

Filshie, J. and Redman, D. (1985) Acupuncture and malignant pain problems. *Eur. J. Surg. Oncol.* **11**(4), 389–394.

Filshie, J., Penn, K., Ashley, S. and Davis, C.L. (1996) Acupuncture for the relief of cancer-related breathlessness. *Palliat. Med.* **10**(2), 145–150.

Fung, K.P., Chow, O.K. and So, S.Y. (1986) Attenuation of exercise-induced asthma by acupuncture. *Lancet* **2**(8521–8522), 1419–1422.

Goldberg, R.M., Loprinzi, C.L., O'Fallon, J.R. *et al.* (1994) Transdermal clonidine for ameliorating tamoxifen-induced hot flashes. *J. Clin. Oncol.* **12**(1), 155–158.

Guchelaar, H.J., Vermes, A. and Meerwaldt, J.H. (1997) Radiation-induced xerostomia: pathophysiology, clinical course and supportive treatment. *Support Care Cancer* **5**(4), 281–288.

Hammar, M., Frisk, J., Grimas, O., Hook, M., Spetz, A.C. and Wyon, Y. (1999) Acupuncture treatment of vasomotor symptoms in men with prostatic carcinoma: a pilot study. *J. Urol.* **161**(3), 853–856.

Han, J.S. (2004) Acupuncture and endorphins. *Neurosci. Lett.* **361**(1–3), 258–261.

Irvin, J.H., Domar, A.D., Clark, C., Zuttermeister, P.C. and Friedman, R. (1996) The effects of relaxation response training on menopausal symptoms. *J. Psychosom. Obstet. Gynaecol.* **17**(4), 202–207.

Johnson, J.T., Ferretti, G.A., Nethery, W.J. *et al.* (1993) Oral pilocarpine for post-irradiation xerostomia in patients with head and neck cancer. *N. Engl. J. Med.* **329**(6), 390–395.

Johnstone, P.A., Niemtzow, R.C. and Riffenburgh, R.H. (2002a) Acupuncture for xerostomia: clinical update. *Cancer* **94**(4), 1151–1156.

Johnstone, P.A., Peng, Y.P., May, B.C., Inouye, W.S. and Niemtzow, R.C. (2001) Acupuncture for pilocarpine-resistant xerostomia following radiotherapy for head and neck malignancies. *Int. J. Radiat. Oncol. Biol. Phys.* **50**(2), 353–357.

Johnstone, P.A., Polston, G.R., Niemtzow, R.C. and Martin, P.J. (2002b) Integration of acupuncture into the oncology clinic. *Palliat. Med.* **16**(3), 235–239.

Josefson, A. and Kreuter, M. (2003) Acupuncture to reduce nausea during chemotherapy treatment of rheumatic diseases. *Rheumatology* **42**(10), 1149–1154.

Kaptchuk, T.J. (2002) Acupuncture: theory, efficacy, and practice. *Ann. Intern. Med.* **136**(5), 374–383.

Kleinhenz, J., Streitberger, K., Windeler, J., Gussbacher, A., Mavridis, G. and Martin, E. (1999) Randomised clinical trial comparing the effects of acupuncture and a newly designed placebo needle in rotator cuff tendinitis. *Pain* **83**(2), 235–241.

Kusler, D.L. and Rambur, B.A. (1992) Treatment for radiation-induced xerostomia. An innovative remedy. *Cancer Nurs.* **15**(3), 191–195.

Lao, L., Bergman, S., Langenberg, P., Wong, R.H. and Berman, B. (1995) Efficacy of Chinese acupuncture on postoperative oral surgery pain. *Oral Surg.* **79**(4), 423–428.

Leake, R. and Broderick, J.E. (1999) Current licensure for acupuncture in the United States. *Altern. Ther. Health. Med.* **5**(4), 94–96.

Lee, A. and Done, M.L. (2004) Stimulation of the wrist acupuncture point P6 for preventing postoperative nausea and vomiting. *Cochrane Database Syst. Rev.* 3:CD003281.

Leng, G. (1999) A year of acupuncture in palliative care. *Palliat. Med.* **13**(2), 163–164.

Lesage, P. and Portenoy, R.K. (2002) Management of fatigue in the cancer patient. *Oncology* **16**(3), 373–377.

LeVeque, F.G., Montgomery, M., Potter, D. *et al.* (1993) A multicenter, randomised, double-blind, placebo-controlled, dose-titration study of oral pilocarpine for treatment of radiation-induced xerostomia in head and neck cancer patients. *J. Clin. Oncol.* **11**(6), 1124–1131.

Levine, M.J., Aguirre, A., Hatton, M.N. and Tabak, L.A. (1987) Artificial salivas: present and future. *J. Dent. Res.* **66**, 693–698.

List, T., Lundeberg, T., Lundstrom, I., Lindstrom, F. and Ravald, N. (1998) The effect of acupuncture in the treatment of patients with primary Sjögren's syndrome. A controlled study. *Acta. Odontol. Scand.* **56**(2), 95–99.

Littlewood, T.J., Bajetta, E., Nortier, J.W.R., Vercammen, E. and Rapoport, B. (2001) Effects of epoetin alfa on hematologic parameters and quality of life in cancer patients receiving non-platinum chemotherapy: results of a randomised, double-blind, placebo-controlled trial. *J. Clin. Oncol.* **19**(11), 2865–2874.

Loprinzi, C.L., Pisansky, T.M., Fonseca, R. *et al.* (1998) Pilot evaluation of venlafaxine hydrochloride for the therapy of hot flashes in cancer survivors. *J. Clin. Oncol.* **16**(7), 2377–2381.

Maa, S.H., Gauthier, D. and Turner, M. (1997) Acupressure as an adjunct to a pulmonary rehabilitation program. *J. Cardiopulm. Rehabil.* **17**(4), 268–276.

MacPherson, H., Thomas, K., Walters, S. and Fitter, M. (2001) The York acupuncture safety study: prospective survey of 34,000 treatments by traditional acupuncturists. *Br. Med. J.* **323**(7311), 486–487.

Melchart, D., Linde, K., Fischer, P. *et al.* (1999) Acupuncture for recurrent headaches: a systematic review of randomised controlled trials. *Cephalalgia* **19**(9), 779–786; discussion 765.

Melchart, D., Weidenhammer, W., Streng, A. *et al.* (2004) Prospective investigation of adverse effects of acupuncture in 97,733 patients. *Arch. Intern. Med.* **164**(1), 104–105.

Ming, J.L., Kuo, B.I., Lin, J.G. and Lin, L.C. (2002) The efficacy of acupressure to prevent nausea and vomiting in post-operative patients. *J. Adv. Nurs.* **39**(4), 343–351.

Nieuw-Amerongen, A.V. and Veerman, E.C. (2003) Current therapies for xerostomia and salivary gland hypofunction associated with cancer therapies. *Support Care Cancer* **11**(4), 226–231.

NIH Consensus Conference (1998) Acupuncture. *J. Am. Med. Assoc.* **280**(17), 1518–1524.

Norheim, A.J. and Fonnebo, V. (1996) Acupuncture adverse effects are more than occasional case reports: results from questionnaires among 1135 randomly selected doctors, and 197 acupuncturists. *Complement. Ther. Med.* **4**, 8–13.

Odsberg, A., Schill, U. and Haker, E. (2001) Acupuncture treatment: side effects and complications reported by Swedish physiotherapists. *Complement. Ther. Med.* **9**(1), 17–20.

Pandya, K.J., Raubertas, R.F., Flynn, P.J. *et al.* (2000) Oral clonidine in postmenopausal patients with breast cancer experiencing tamoxifen-induced hot flashes: a University of Rochester Cancer Center Community Clinical Oncology Program study. *Ann. Intern. Med.* **132**(10), 788–793.

Pariente, J., White, P., Frackowiak, R.S. and Lewith, G. (2005) Expectancy and belief modulate the neuronal substrates of pain treated by acupuncture. *Neuroimage* **25**(4), 1161–1167.

Porzio, G., Trapasso, T., Martelli, S. *et al.* (2002) Acupuncture in the treatment of menopause-related symptoms in women taking tamoxifen. *Tumouri* **88**(2), 128–130.

Quella, S.K., Loprinzi, C.L., Barton, D.L. *et al.* (2000) Evaluation of soy phytoestrogens for the treatment of hot flashes in breast cancer survivors: A North Central Cancer Treatment Group Trial. *J. Clin. Oncol.* **18**(5), 1068–1074.

Rieke, J.W., Hafermann, M.D., Johnson, J.T. *et al.* (1995) Oral pilocarpine for radiation-induced xerostomia: integrated efficacy and safety results from two prospective randomised clinical trials. *Int. J. Radiat. Oncol. Biol. Phys.* **31**(3), 661–669.

Roscoe, J.A., Morrow, G.R., Hickok, J.T. *et al.* (2003) The efficacy of acupressure and acustimulation wrist bands for the relief of chemotherapy-induced nausea and vomiting. A University of Rochester Cancer Center Community Clinical Oncology Program multicenter study. *J. Pain Symptom Manage.* **26**(2), 731–742.

Rosen, T., de Veciana, M., Miller, H.S., Stewart, L., Rebarber, A. and Slotnick, R.N. (2003) A randomised controlled trial of nerve stimulation for relief of nausea and vomiting in pregnancy. *Obstet. Gynecol.* **102**(1), 129–135.

Rydholm, M. and Strang, P. (1999) Acupuncture for patients in hospital-based home care suffering from xerostomia. *J. Palliat. Care* **15**(4), 20–23.

Shen, J., Wenger N., Glaspy, J. *et al.* (2000) Electroacupuncture for control of myeloablative chemotherapy-induced emesis: a randomised controlled trial. *J. Am. Med. Assoc.* **284**(21), 2755–2761.

Stearns, V., Isaacs, C., Rowland, J. *et al.* (2000) A pilot trial assessing the efficacy of paroxetine hydrochloride (Paxil) in controlling hot flashes in breast cancer survivors. *Ann. Oncol.* **11**(1), 17–22.

Streitberger, K., Diefenbacher, M., Bauer, A. *et al.* (2004) Acupuncture compared to placebo-acupuncture for postoperative nausea and vomiting prophylaxis: a randomised placebo-controlled patient and observer blind trial. *Anaesthesia* **59**(2), 142–149.

Streitberger, K., Friedrich-Rust, M., Bardenheuer, H. *et al.* (2003) Effect of acupuncture compared with placebo acupuncture at P6 as additional antiemetic prophylaxis in high-dose chemotherapy and autologous peripheral blood stem cell transplantation: a randomised controlled single-blind trial. *Clin. Cancer Res.* **9**(7), 2538–2544.

Tashkin, D.P., Bresler, D.E., Kroening, R.J., Kerschner, H., Katz, R.L. and Coulson, A. (1977) Comparison of real and simulated acupuncture and isoproterenol in methacholine-induced asthma. *Ann. Allergy* **39**(6), 379–387.

Towlerton, G., Filshie, J., O'Brien, M. and Duncan, A. (1999) Acupuncture in the control of vasomotor symptoms caused by tamoxifen. *Palliat. Med.* **13**(5), 445.

Valdez, I.H. (1991) Radiation-induced salivary dysfunction: clinical course and significance. *Spec. Care Dent.* **11**(6), 252–255.

Van Patten, C.L., Olivotto, I.A., Chambers, G.K., *et al.* (2002) Effect of soy phytoestrogens on hot flashes in postmenopausal women with breast cancer: a randomised, controlled clinical trial. *J. Clin. Oncol.* **20**(6), 1449–1455.

Vickers, A.J., Feinstein, M.B., Deng, G.E. and Cassileth, B.R. (2005) Acupuncture for dyspnoea in advanced cancer: a randomised, placebo-controlled pilot trial [ISRCTN89462491]. *BMC Palliat. Care* **4**, 5.

Vickers, A.J., Rees, R.W., Zollman, C.E. *et al.* (2004a) Acupuncture for chronic headache in primary care: large, pragmatic, randomised trial. *Br. Med. J.* **328**(7442), 744.

Vickers, A.J., Straus, D.J., Fearon, B. and Cassileth, B.R. (2004b) Acupuncture for postchemotherapy fatigue: a phase II study. *J. Clin. Oncol.* **22**(9), 1731–1735.

Vissink, A., Panders, A.K., Gravenmade, E.J. and Vermey, A. (1988) The causes and consequences of hyposalivation. *Ear Nose Throat J.* **67**(3), 166–168, 173–176.

Weitzner, M.A., Moncello, J., Jacobsen, P.B. and Minton, S. (2002) A pilot trial of paroxetine for the treatment of hot flashes and associated symptoms in women with breast cancer. **23**(4), 337–345.

White, A., Hayhoe, S., Hart, A. and Ernst, E. (2001) Adverse events following acupuncture: prospective survey of 32,000 consultations with doctors and physiotherapists. *Br. Med. J.* **323**(7311), 485–486.

White, P., Lewith, G., Prescott, P. and Conway, J. (2004) Acupuncture versus placebo for the treatment of chronic mechanical neck pain: a randomised, controlled trial. *Ann. Intern. Med.* **141**(12), 911–919.

Wong, R.K., Jones, G.W., Sagar, S.M., Babjak, A.F. and Whelan, T. (2003) A Phase I–II study in the use of acupuncture-like transcutaneous nerve stimulation in the treatment of radiation-induced xerostomia in head-and-neck cancer patients treated with radical radiotherapy. *Int. J. Radiat. Oncol. Biol. Phys.* **57**(2), 472–480.

Wu, M.T., Hsieh, J.C., Xiong, J. *et al.* (1999) Central nervous pathway for acupuncture stimulation: localization of processing with functional MR imaging of the brain — preliminary experience. *Radiology* **212**(1), 133–141.

Wyon, Y., Hammar, M., Theodorsson, E. and Lundeberg, T. (1998) Effects of physical activity and acupuncture on calcitonin gene-related peptide immunoreactivity in different parts of the rat brain and in cerebrospinal fluid, serum and urine. *Acta. Physiol. Scand.* **162**(4), 517–522.

Wyon, Y., Lindgren, R., Lundeberg, T. and Hammar, M. (1995) Effects of acupuncture on climacteric vasomotor symptoms, quality of life and urinary excretion of neuropeptides among post-menopausal women. *Menopause* **3**(1), 3–12.

Wyon, Y.A., Spetz, A.C., Theodorsson, G.E. and Hammar, M.L. (2000) Concentrations of calcitonin gene-related peptide and neuropeptide Y in plasma increase during flushes in postmenopausal women. *Menopause* **7**(1), 25–30.

Yamashita, H., Tsukayama, H., Tanno, Y. and Nishijo, K. (1999) Adverse events in acupuncture and moxibustion treatment: a six-year survey at a national clinic in Japan. *J. Altern. Complement. Med.* **5**(3), 229–236.

Zhang, W.T., Jin, Z., Cui, G.H. *et al.* (2003) Relations between brain network activation and analgesic effect induced by low versus high frequency electrical acupoint stimulation in different subjects: a functional magnetic resonance imaging study. *Brain Res.* **982**(2), 168–178.

Index